BARBERSHOPS OF AMERICA THEN & NOW

ROB HAMMER

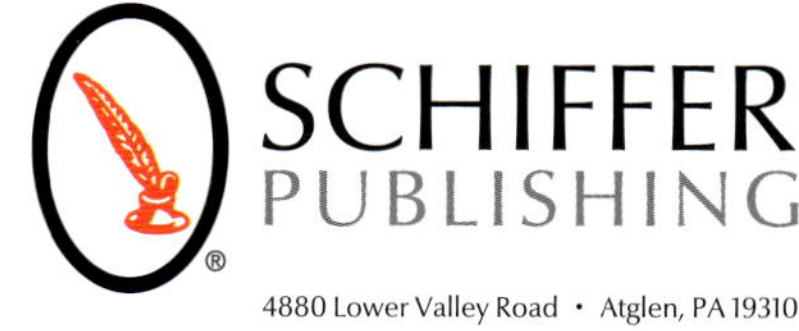

4880 Lower Valley Road • Atglen, PA 19310

Library of Congress Control Number: 2019947345

Edited by Ian Robertson
Designed by Justin Watkinson
Type set in Gotham Light/Univers LT Std

ISBN: 978-0-7643-5928-6
Printed in China

Published by Schiffer Publishing, Ltd.
4880 Lower Valley Road
Atglen, PA 19310
Phone: (610) 593-1777; Fax: (610) 593-2002
E-mail: Info@schifferbooks.com
Web: www.schifferbooks.com

For our complete selection of fine books on this and related subjects, please visit our website at www.schifferbooks.com. You may also write for a free catalog.

Schiffer Publishing's titles are available at special discounts for bulk purchases for sales promotions or premiums. Special editions, including personalized covers, corporate imprints, and excerpts, can be created in large quantities for special needs. For more information, contact the publisher.

We are always looking for people to write books on new and related subjects. If you have an idea for a book, please contact us at proposals@schifferbooks.com.

CONTENTS

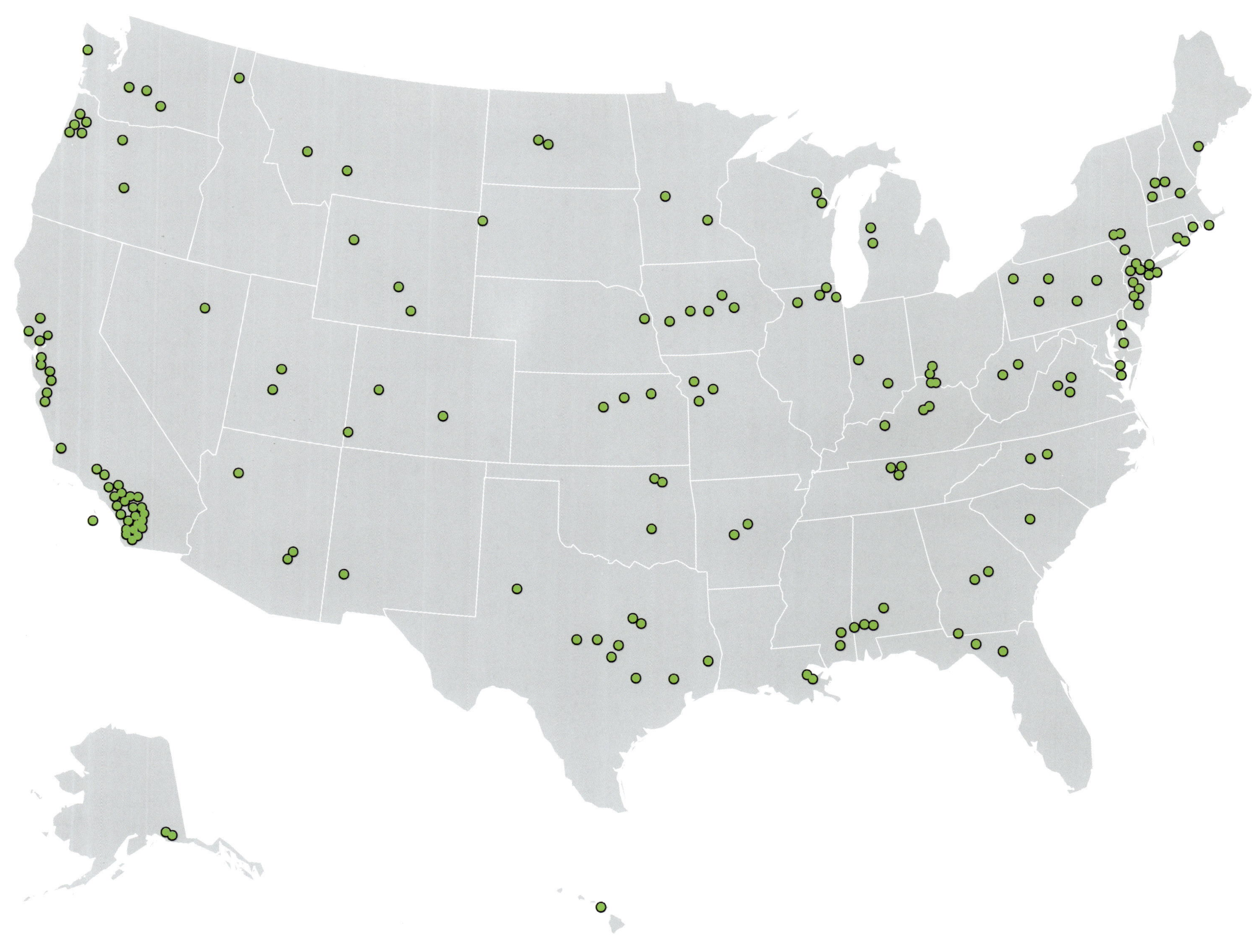

FOREWORD

I never really enjoyed getting a haircut when I was a kid. I'm sure I'm not the only guy who thought that getting a haircut as a kid was more of a chore than a luxury. Growing up in the islands of Samoa (a small chain of islands in the South Pacific), schools started their morning with a student assembly and inspection of all the students. Teachers checked to make sure that our school uniforms were clean, our fingernails were cut, and for us boys, that our hair never touched the back of our shirt collars. To get away with not getting called out for failing inspection, most of us boys would tilt our heads down, hoping that whatever was touching our collars would slightly distance itself, but there was no fooling the teachers as they came down the lines and rows of sitting kids. "Solofa! Get your haircut by tomorrow!" is something that I commonly heard throughout my elementary- and middle-school years.

As a young boy, haircuts for me weren't done at a barbershop. The poverty level in the islands meant that many families like my own couldn't afford the luxury of paying someone else for something that our mum could do for free. So my haircuts were done sitting outside in the hot and humid island heat, on an empty bucket turned upside down, having a towel wrapped around my shoulders, and having Mum use whatever pair of scissors we had lying around the house (usually the blunt ones from her sewing kit). She'd start grabbing and cutting hair wherever she saw or felt it needed trimming as I fought off the mosquitos that took full opportunity of my defenseless state. Now mind you, Mum wasn't giving me a haircut of style, but rather a haircut of purpose, and if given an option, I would have chosen style. But back then I didn't even know what that consisted of. Of course I'd show up the next morning to school, envious of the ones whose families could afford the barbershops and their nice haircuts, but the ends justified the means: my hair was shorter and worthy of passing the inspection.

My haircuts during my college years in Hawaii in the late '80s got much better. This was an era in American pop culture where MTV and VH1 ruled supreme, and music videos of every genre would be playing constantly throughout the day. I was now among kids from all over the world, who had flare and style unlike anything I'd ever seen before growing up in Samoa, where everyone wore school uniforms and there was no such thing as embracing individuality, no cable television, and no malls, and there definitely wasn't any exposure to the styles and expressiveness of fashion and pop culture happening in the good old US of A.

There was a guy on the basketball team named Deon, and he was the appointed barber to all of the basketball players living in the dorms. Deon was our small forward from Antigua, and his roommate was our point guard Eric from Los Angeles. I was immediately drawn to how Deon and Eric dressed and carried themselves, and particularly how clean and precise their haircuts always looked. One day I asked Deon who cut their hair, and he told me that he did it himself, and that for $8 he could do the same for me.

My first time getting a haircut by Deon was unlike any haircut experience I had ever had prior. His and Eric's room had all kinds of hip-hop posters on the walls, and the entire time he cut my hair he was playing the hits from Eric B & Rakim, Public Enemy, EPMD, and KRS-1. He had only one pair of clippers (which I remember getting hot to the touch during the haircut), a bunch of plastic attachments, one comb, and scissors so tiny that they got lost in his massive hands. I'd ask him questions on how to improve my hoop game, where he bought his clothes, and what it was like growing up back in his home of Antigua (which sounded not much different from growing up in Samoa). And whenever he was done with my haircut, I was amazed at both how great my hair looked and how much it made me feel good, as if maybe I might be on the same level of cool as he and Eric. Unbeknown to me, getting a haircut from Deon was my first small taste of what a barbershop experience was like, and it is something that still resonates with me more than thirty years after the fact.

I didn't actually go to a proper, traditional barbershop until I was in my mid-twenties, and I had left Hawaii and returned to American Samoa to help with the family business (my haircuts after graduating college typically ended up being by my own hand with a cheap pair of clippers). When I returned to Samoa, I went to one of the only barbershops in town, behind the main market place. It was literally a shack built out of old wood and corrugated iron, and had one chair in a room the size of a small kitchen. There was no decor, just an air-conditioning unit crudely installed into one of the walls. The only barber working there was the owner, named "Fale," and he looked like the Samoan version of James Brown: his hair was worn in a perfect pompadour, and he was always dressed in a long, red high school graduation gown as his smock. His tiny shop was always filled with older Samoan men—usually about eight of them—all crammed inside the small space, waiting their turn. Almost all of them got the same haircut from Fale: short, high, and tight haircuts or flat tops—never anything fancy or overly stylized, and always clean and precise clipper cuts. If I was lucky enough to get a space to sit inside and wait, I'd usually be the youngest one in the room filled with old men who often just laughed and talked about things that in any language would be considered "grown men's talk." Every time I left Fale's Barbershop, I always felt that same sense of confidence that came with getting one of his $10 haircuts, the same feeling that I got after walking out of Deon's dorm room with one of his $8 fades . . . there was an undeniable correlation between the two that, at the time, I couldn't put my finger on other than just getting a good haircut.

When I chose to become a barber more than ten years ago, I left behind a seventeen-year career in banking, insurance, and finance that never really brought me fulfillment, although it was a career that allowed me to get from one check to the next. I vividly remember being laid off from the mortgage bank I was working for when the financial market crashed in 2008, wondering what my next career choice would be, and as I sat at my desk, cycling through my options, I thought of Deon and Fale, and the simple joy they seemed to get out of cutting hair, as well as the simple joy I experienced getting my haircut, the confidence I felt after, and the sense of fellowship and community that came with sitting among like-minded men who had come together in one room to share advice, stories, and laughter.

I signed up for barber college within the week and haven't looked back since. I can't say that I fully knew eleven years ago how valuable a barbershop was to a community (a neighborhood, town, or city), or how much value it brought to building a community within its own walls with the men gathered there, but if hindsight is truly 20/20, then I can definitely speak to this truth today being both a barber and a barbershop owner.

Merriam-Webster Dictionary defines the word "community" as being "a unified body of individuals; such as the people with common interest living in a common area." Throughout the ages, there have been very few known places where common men could go and sit among other like-minded men and genuinely feel like they belonged. Sure, men have always had their social groups, from country clubs and car clubs to lodges and bars, and even boys have had the Boy Scouts and college men have had their fraternities. But the dilemma that each of these groups and places presented was that they came with an exclusivity that often required an application, an initiation, an approval, and a membership based on specific interests, causes, and economic classes. More often than not, many of these places weren't willingly open to all men regardless of their backgrounds, beliefs, likes, dislikes, color, creed, religion, or social standing. However, there has always been one place that throughout history has kept its doors open and welcomed men from every single walk of life, never discerning whether they were worthy of entering the room or not, and that special common-area place has been the barbershop.

Barbershops can be found in many a common area, in every city, town, and even in small neighborhoods, and now they come in as diverse a variety as the men and customers that they serve. My perception of a barbershop was definitely molded by my experiences as a kid with Mum, as a teenager with Deon, and as a young man with Fale, but after entering the trade eleven years ago, it quickly became more refined and heavily influenced by the traditional barbershops of the 1950s and 1960s. What do traditional barbershops look like to me? They are places where a bunch of old men cut hair long after they should have retired, because they still enjoy doing it. It's a place where men try to convince each other who the greatest boxer of all time is. It's a place where every man becomes a professional sports analyst, can break down an entire NFL draft, and believes that he would have made a different play call on fourth and goal with seconds left to win the game, even though he's never coached a football game in his entire life. It's a place where men enter as complete strangers and leave as friends. It's a place where grown men embrace and hug. It's a place where these said grown men will confide in their barber about things that they wouldn't share with their priest, rabbi, parents, wives, or best friends. It's a place where no man is better than another. It's a place that doesn't care what your job is, what your social class is, what your ethnic background is, or how much money you have, because everyone pays the same price and everyone gets the same treatment. It's a place where soon-to-be dads get advice about raising children that's not in any book, it's where soon-to-be husbands get advice from men who have been married many times over, and it's where boys get advice on manhood that their mothers would rather they didn't hear . . . ever! It's a place where opinions will differ, but opinions expressed with respect will be heard. It's a place filled with laughter, encouragement, support, and wisdom, and, on a good day, filled with legendary tall tales told by old men that all start with "Well, back in my day!" or "Back when I was your age!"

The photographs presented in this book offer a unique and intimate look inside the world of traditional barbershops throughout America, whose legacies, reputations, and histories are now synonymous with the red, white, and blue poles that can be found spinning inside their front windows or outside their front doors. Whether or not you've ever stepped foot into a barbershop, or recall hearing stories about them as a kid from your dad or grandpa, or perhaps you're even a barber yourself now, you are encouraged to study every photo in detail and imagine the scents of bay rums and colognes and aftershaves, imagine the sounds of scissors and clippers as they snip hair and straight razors as they shave stubble, but, most importantly, as you study and appreciate these photos, imagine the sounds of a crowded room of men from all walks of life laughing together. Imagine them debating together, encouraging and supporting each other, and imagine the great sight of these men seeing no division among themselves other than those who are sitting in the barber chairs getting a haircut, those standing behind the barber chairs giving the haircuts, and those sitting in the waiting chairs preparing to be called up next to get their hair cut. In a world that has always had so much division, this book will serve as a constant reminder that the men of today (and those of generations before us) will always have a place of community to call their own, and a special place to call their home away from home. As both a barber and a barbershop owner, I can attest that a barbershop *is* a place of community, and the most rewarding part of what I do is being part of a "unified body of individuals" each and every day in which I am blessed to work.

Mark-Jason Solofa

INTRODUCTION

There is nothing else in the world like a traditional barbershop, so to still be working on this project eight years later makes me feel very fortunate. After hundreds of thousands of miles on the road with my dog Mojo, it's connected me with some very real people, brought me to places I probably wouldn't otherwise see, and allowed me to explore a beautiful piece of American culture during a time in its history that won't ever be repeated. In 2012, when I first started shooting barbershops, the old timers seemed like dinosaurs about to go extinct, taking the trade with them. In fact, a lot of the guys featured in this book have passed away since my time with them. Finding a truly old-school shop is getting to be harder and harder. Seems like everywhere I go, everybody says the same thing: "An old barbershop? No, there aren't any of those around here anymore." Fortunately, there has been a resurgence in the barbershop world. As of this writing, barbering has never been so popular. Every other corner you look on, a barbershop has moved in. That's not to say that they are all worth a damn, but that of course goes with any industry. The important thing is that among the vast sea of new barbers, there are those who really care. Those who are doing it for the right reasons and upholding the standards of the guys who came before them. This new class of barbers will never replace the last one, nor should they. It's impossible. The old timers just have such a way about them that couldn't possibly be replicated. And their shops' appearance is something that can be achieved only by genuinely occupying a space for more than fifty years. It's reassuring though that the new guys are taking something that was already great and are expanding on it in their own way.

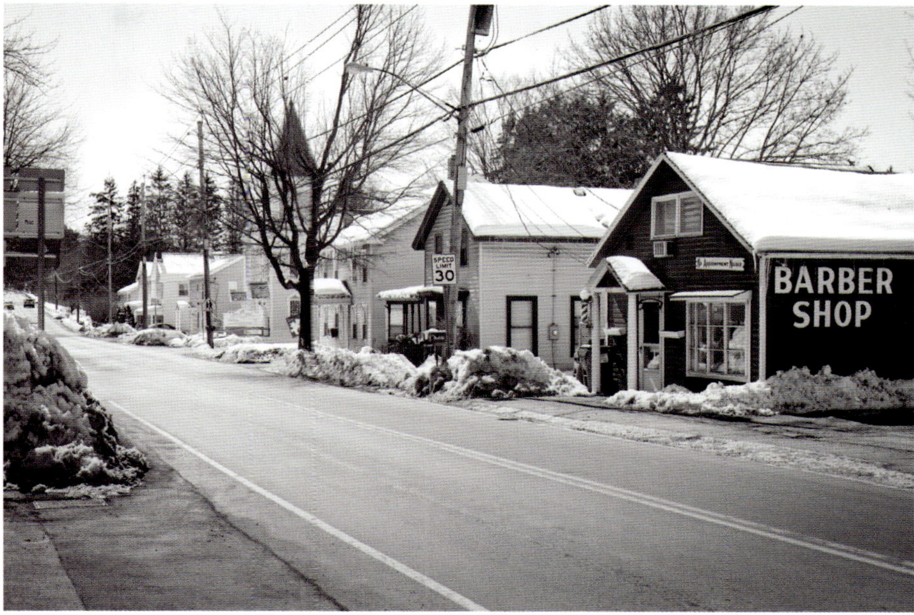

My first barbershop, Bill's Barbershop, West Sand Lake, NY

People always ask if I have a favorite shop, and that can't be answered for a couple of reasons. I've been in well over a thousand, and the truth is, if a shop is in the book, then there is something special about it. That of course is just my opinion. I'm not a barber, so it's really not up to me to say what is good and what isn't. Everything in here is what I consider to be a real barbershop. You see, shops—real shops, that is—are just like people, in that they have a soul. That's why a photograph of an empty shop is just as effective as one with every chair filled. You can just feel what's happened in there.

This project started out of my love for barbershops and the desire to photograph the old timers before they were all gone, but that focus shifted after being introduced to some of the "next generation." So this book is very much about barbering's disappearing past and the stark contrast of its now-vibrant future.

Another thing I feel fortunate about is that you can almost think of this book as a historical document of sorts. A lot of people will never get to experience for themselves what it's like to be in an old shop, but looking through these pages can help them imagine. And as time goes on, and the industry changes, so will barbershops. So what this book as a whole also shows is barbering during what could be its largest boom ever, and the trade's very specific place on the American timeline. Right now we are in a "time," and it all probably seems pretty normal on the surface. Fast forward 25, 50, or 100 years though, and this body of images will look archaic. The clothes, cars, decor, etc. will all seem so foreign. We are in a time, and I'm honored to document it.

OLD SCHOOL

"This place has been a barbershop for about 200 years."

– Felice Garofalo, Tony's Barbershop, Brooklyn, New York

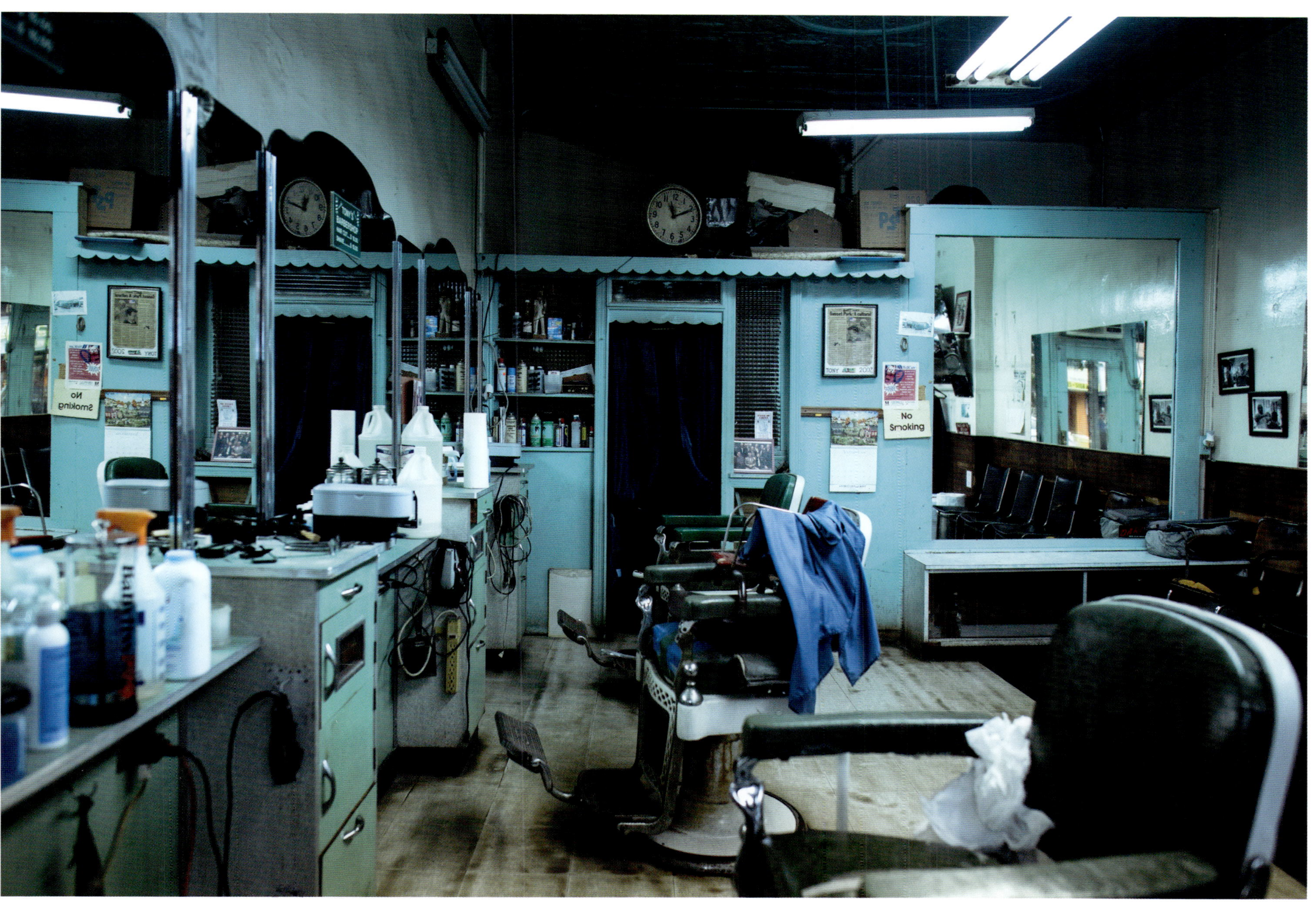

Tony's Barbershop, Brooklyn, New York

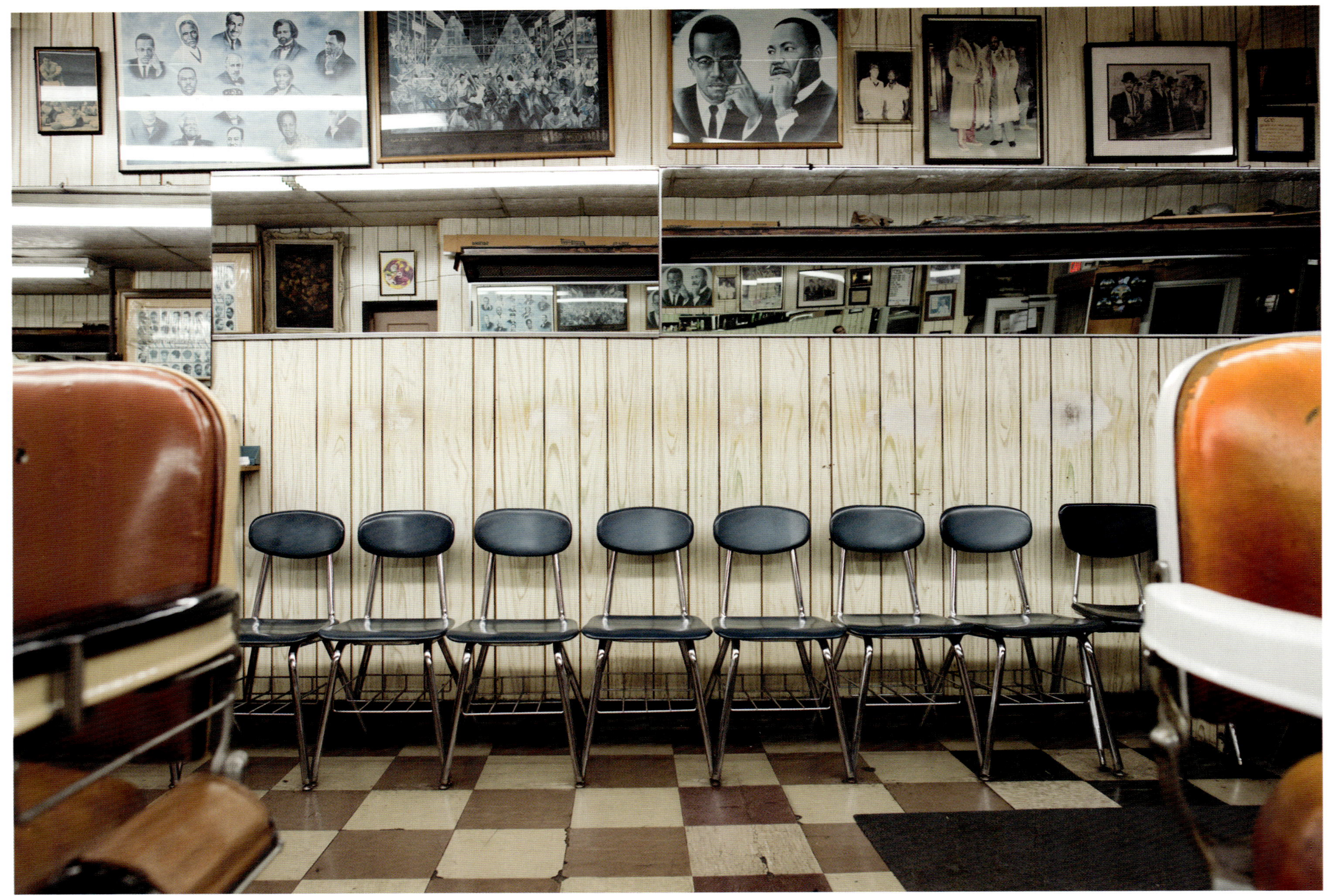

Duckett's Barbershop, Brooklyn, New York

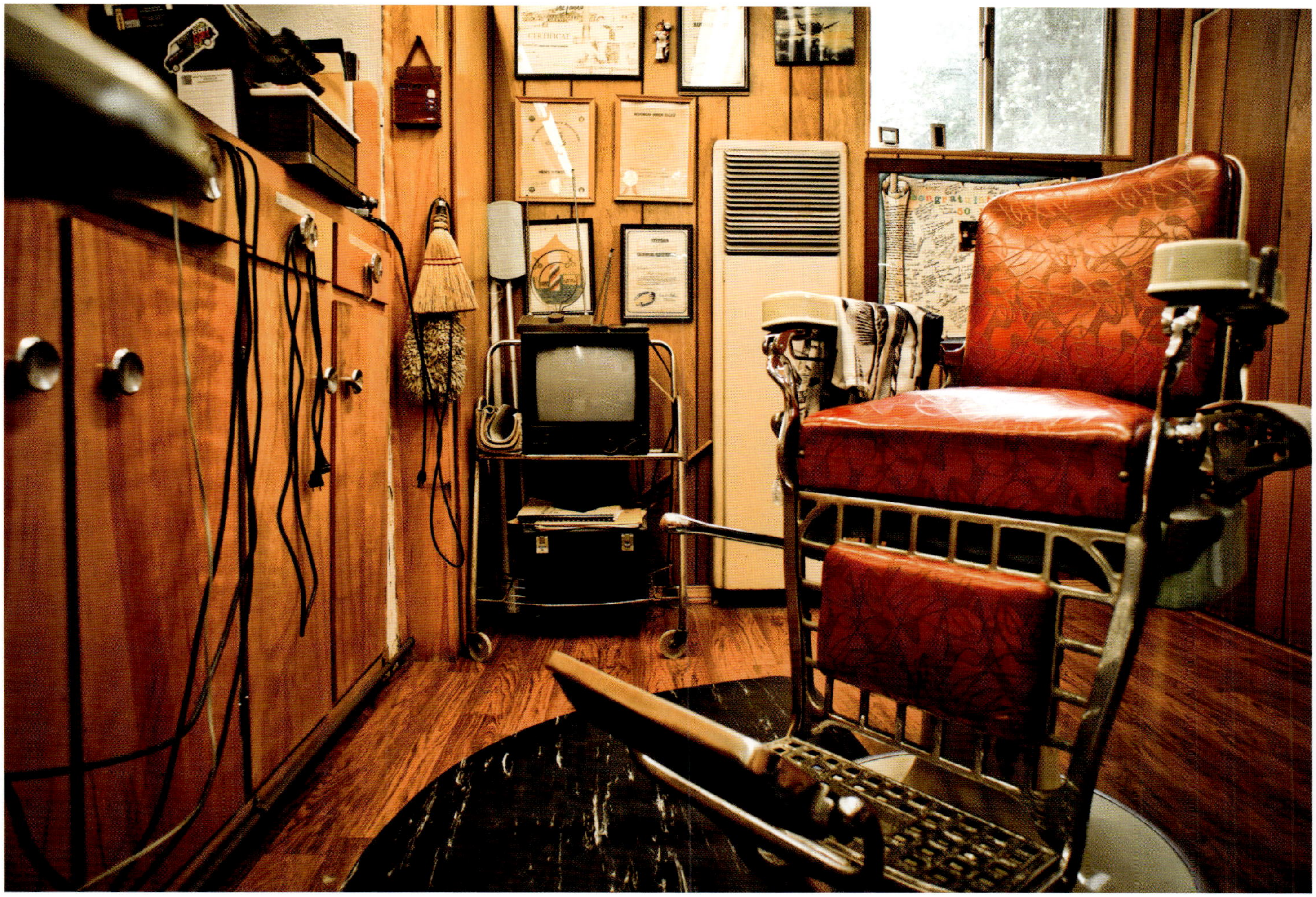

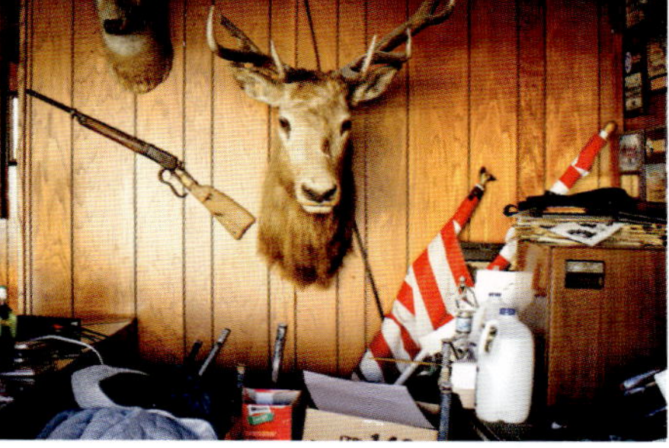

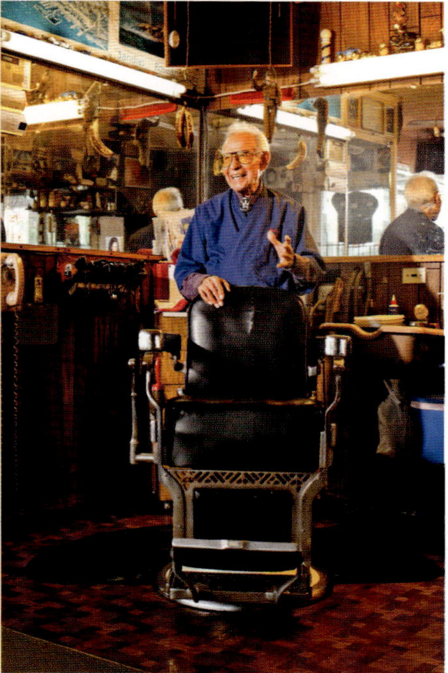

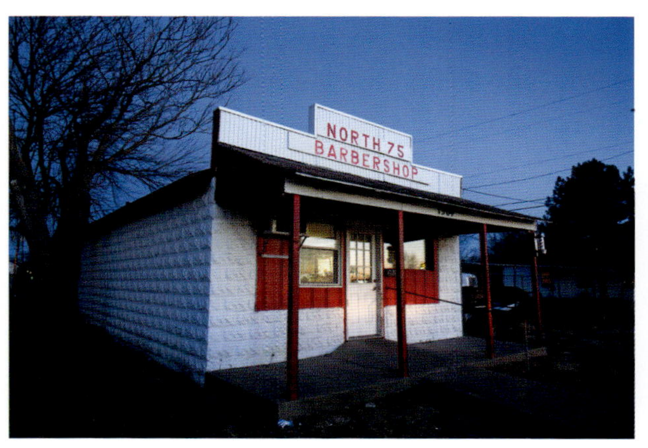
NORTH 75
BARBERSHOP

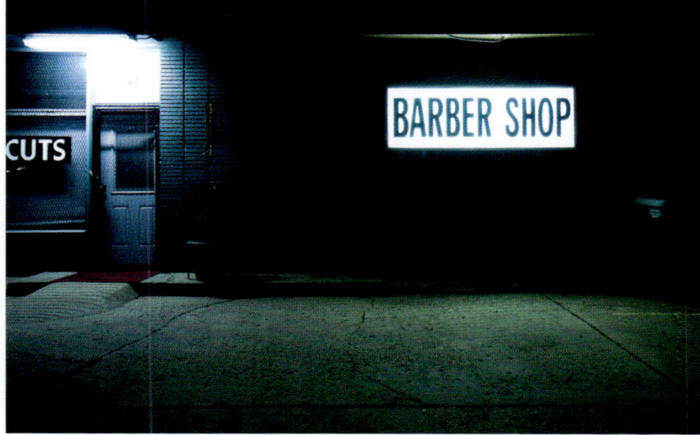
CUTS
BARBER SHOP

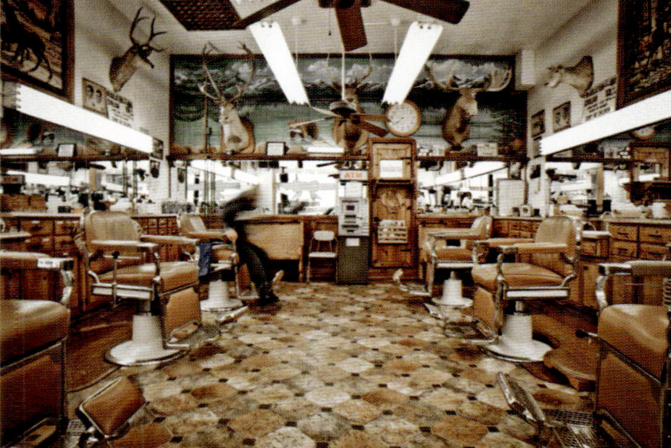

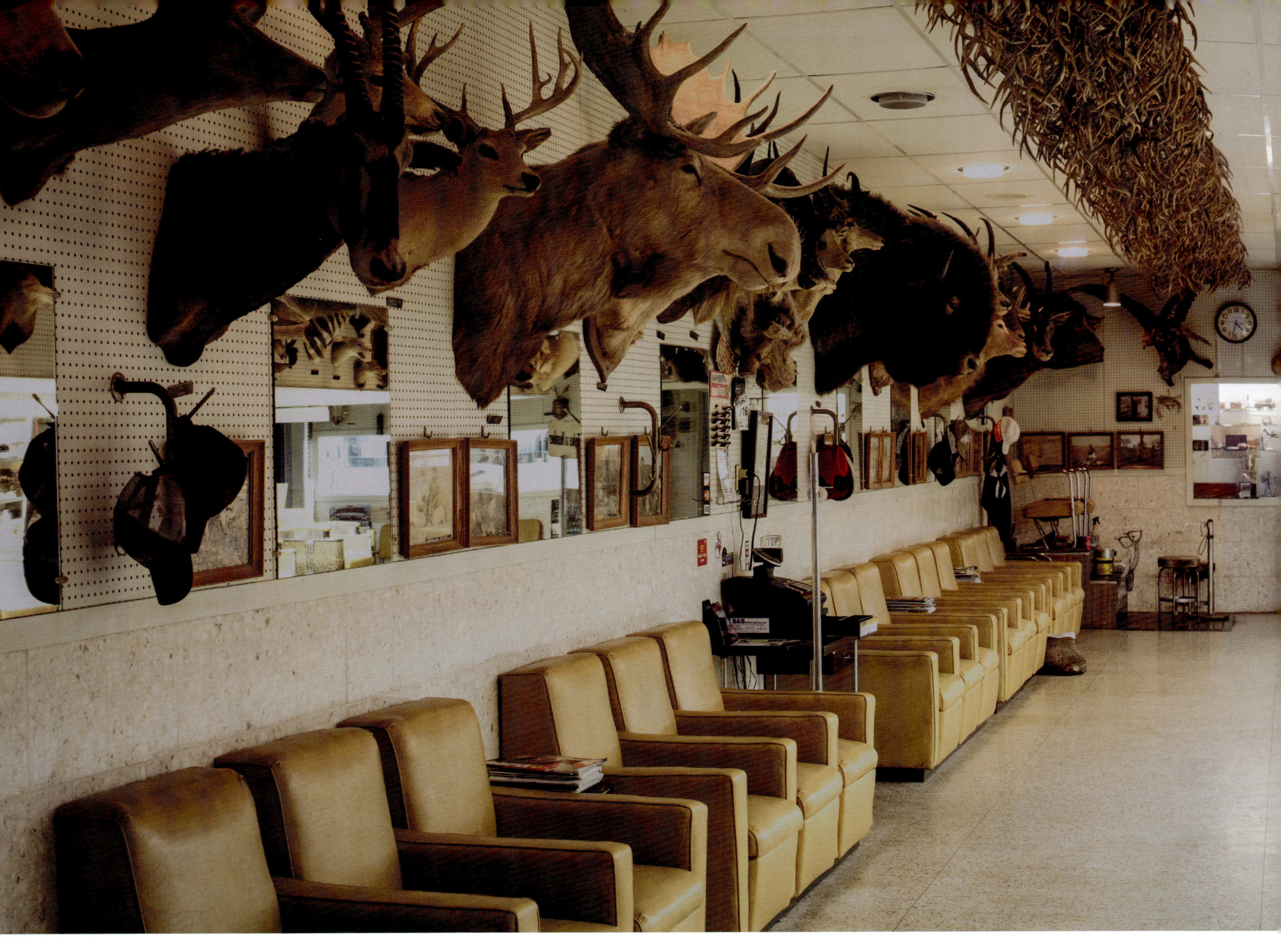

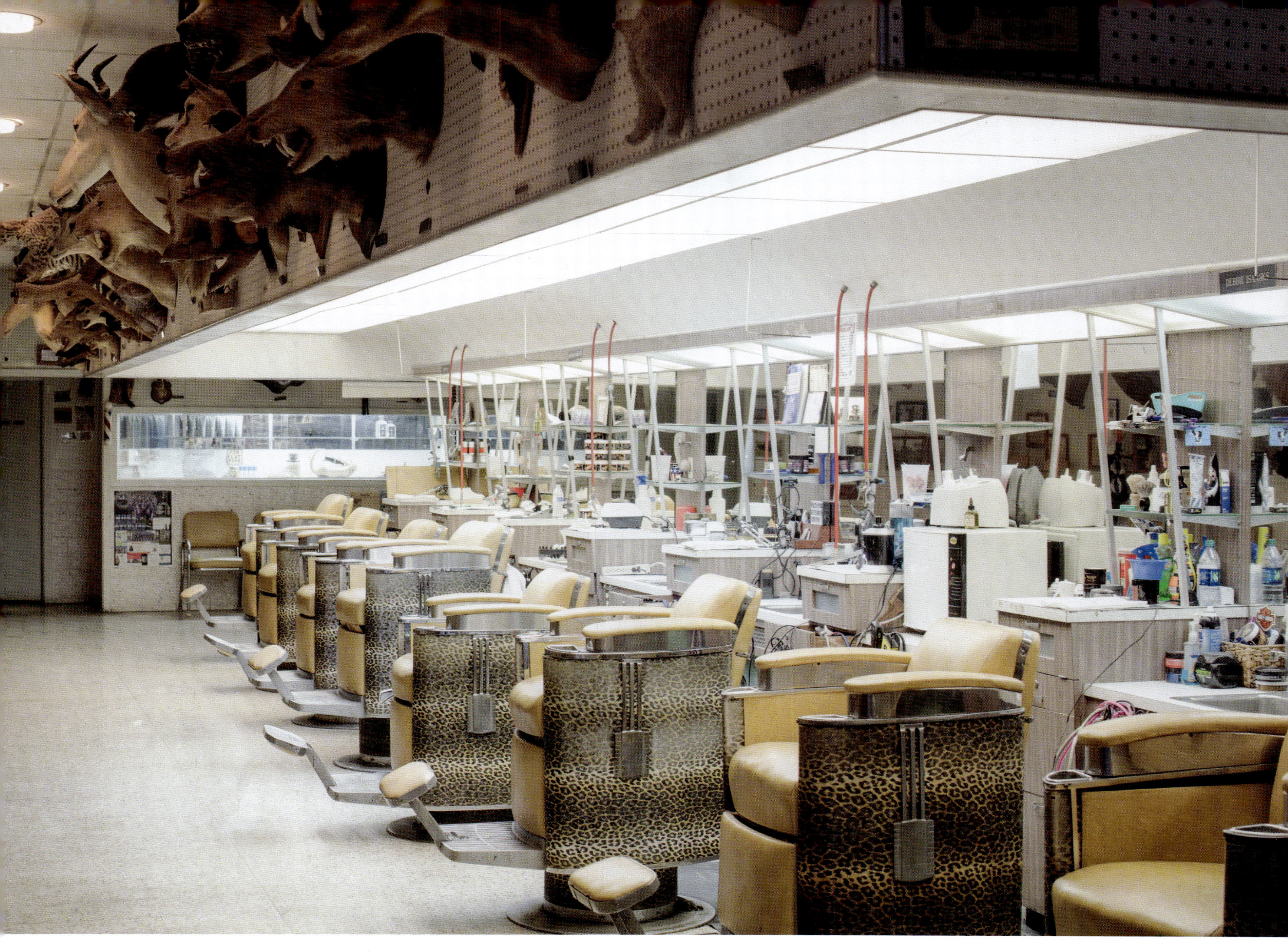

Trophy Barbershop, Baytown, Texas

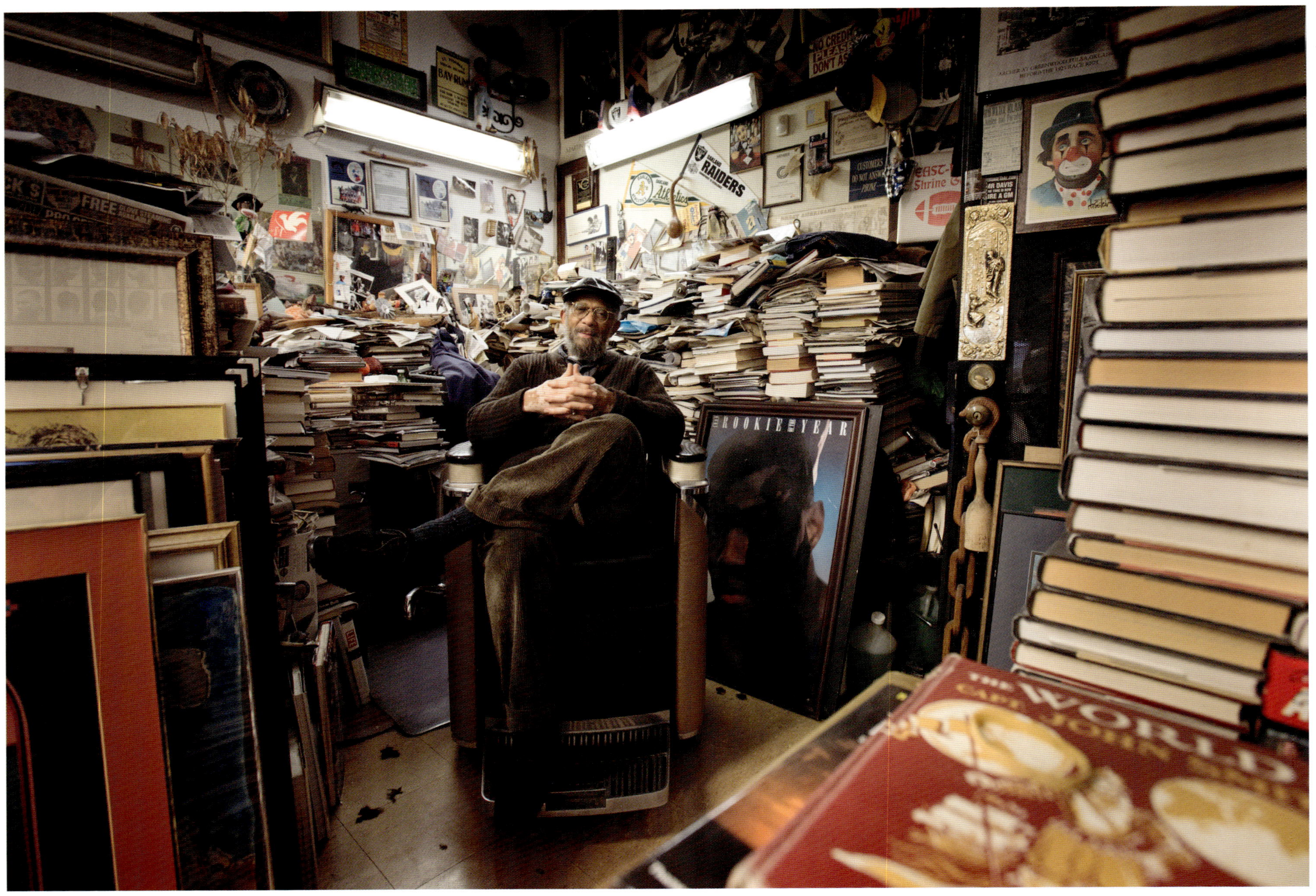

Cuts and Bends, Oakland, California

“I started cutting hair probably about 1954, when I was about the 10th grade—17 years old. Sorta finding my way . . . and . . . I found out I liked it. And I stayed with it. And I guess now I love it. And I hate to give it up . . . and I plan to do it until I can’t do it anymore.”

– Kenneth Hogan Sr., Cuts and Bends, Oakland, California

“What do I know about barbershops? I come here. I go home. And that’s it.”

– John Fiumefreddo, The Park Slope Barber, Brooklyn, New York

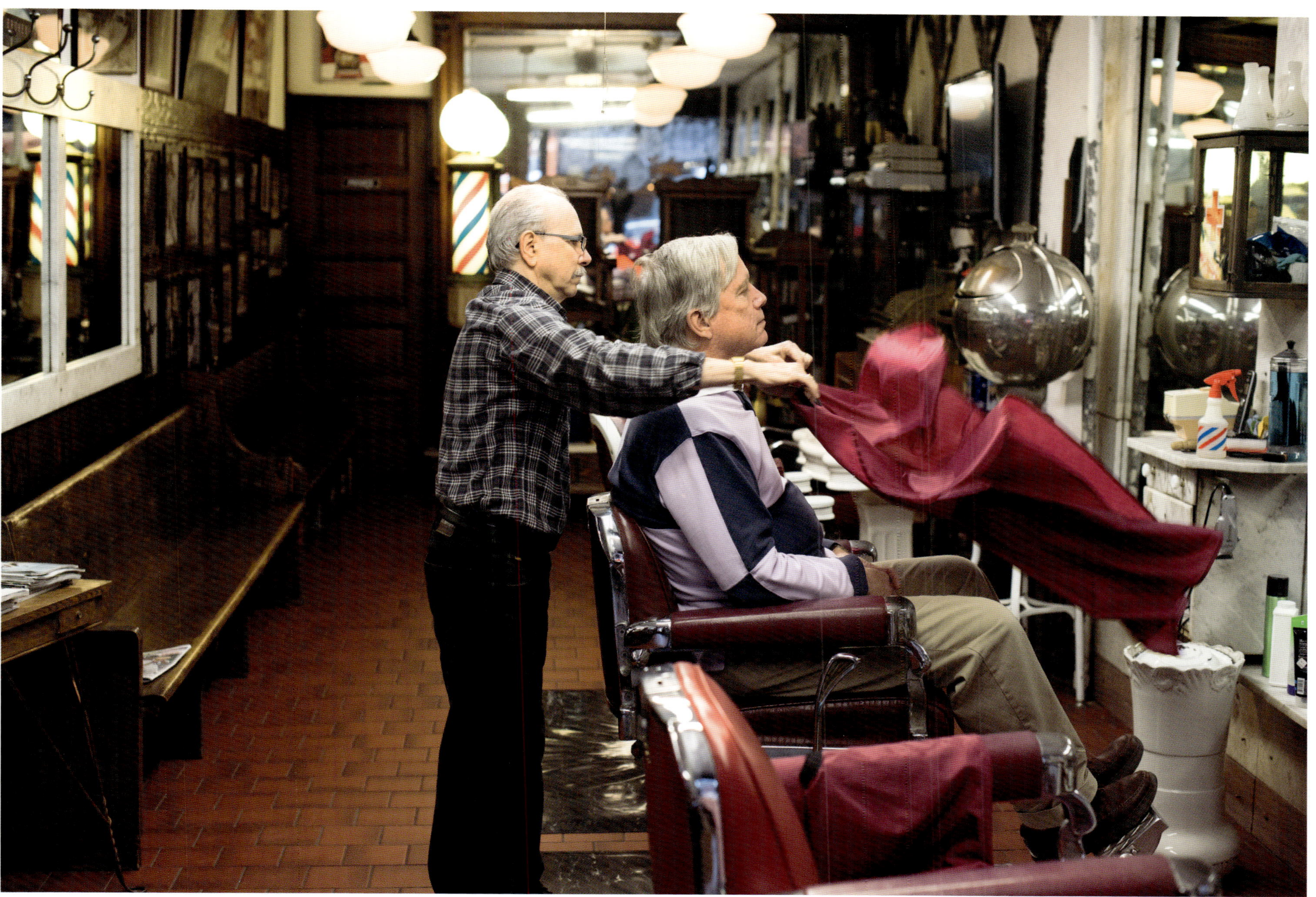

The Park Slope Barber, Brooklyn, New York

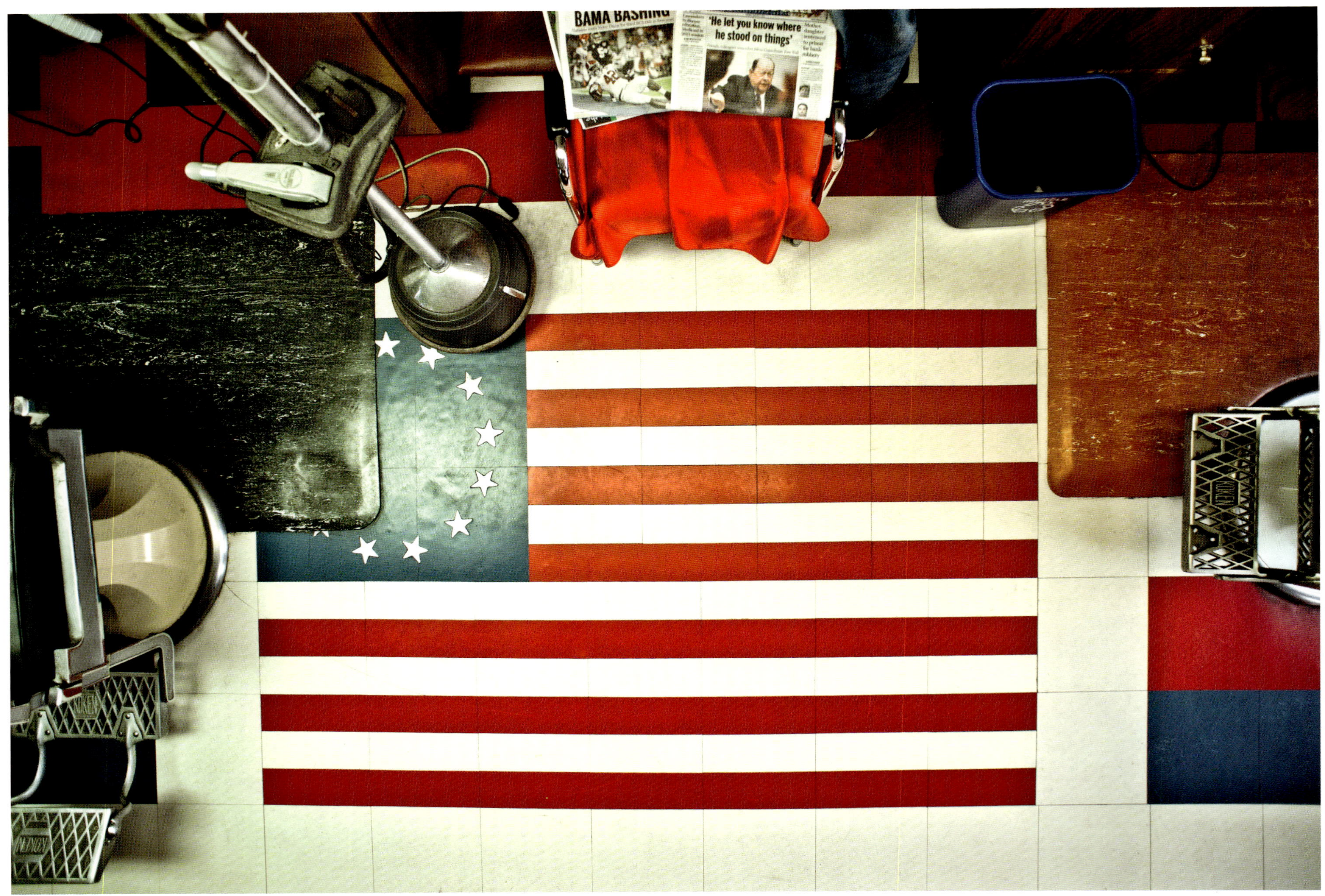

Red's Barbershop, Gulfport, Mississippi

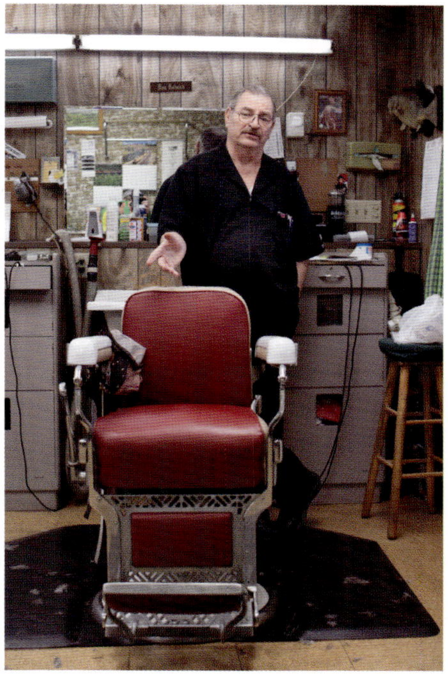

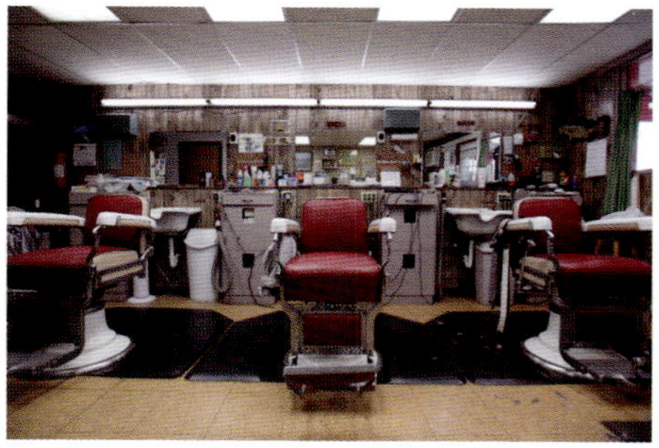

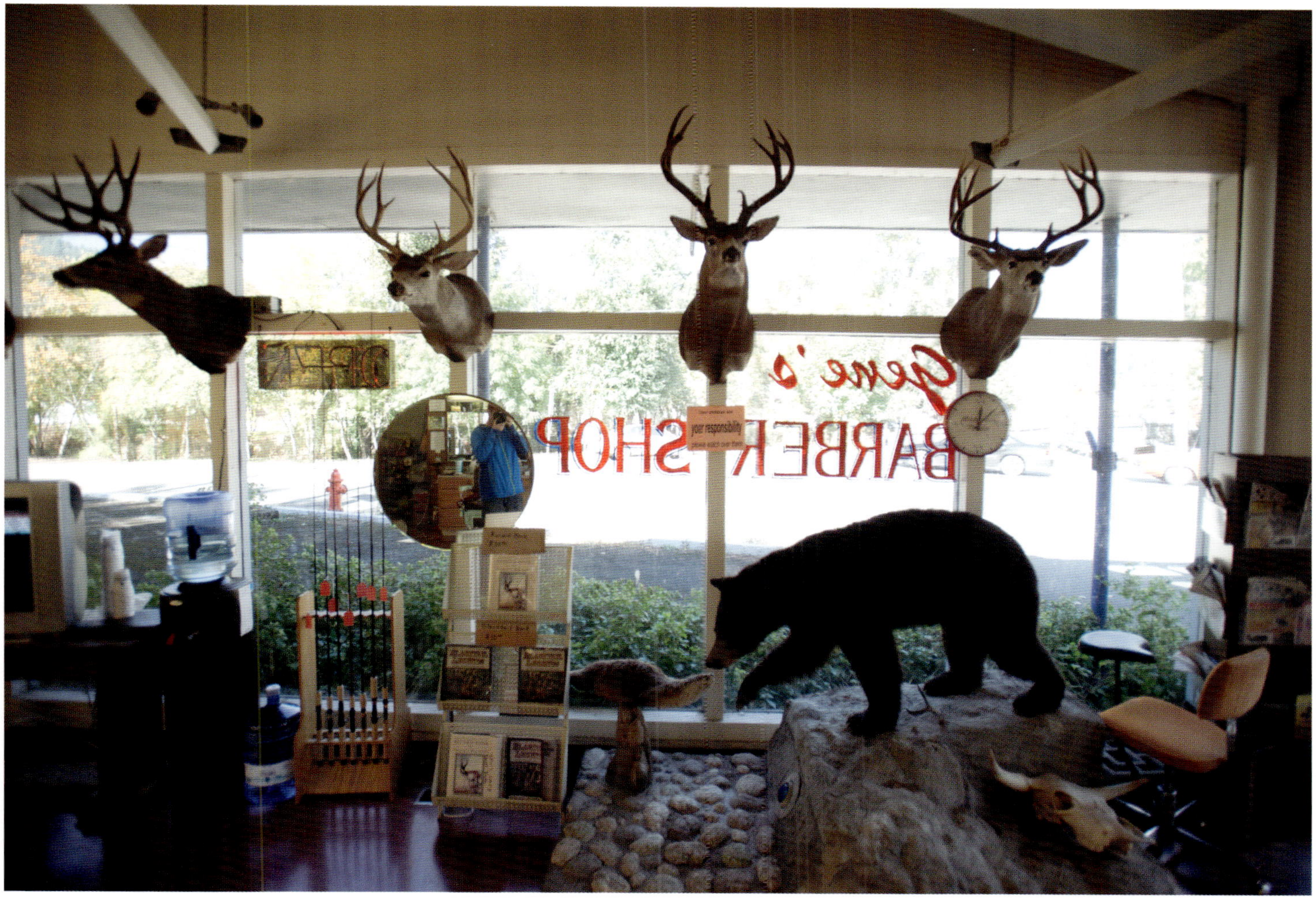

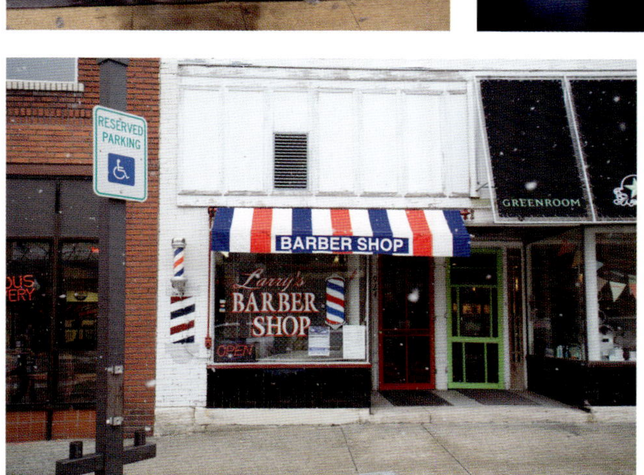
RESERVED PARKING
GREENROOM
BARBER SHOP
Larry's
BARBER SHOP
OPEN

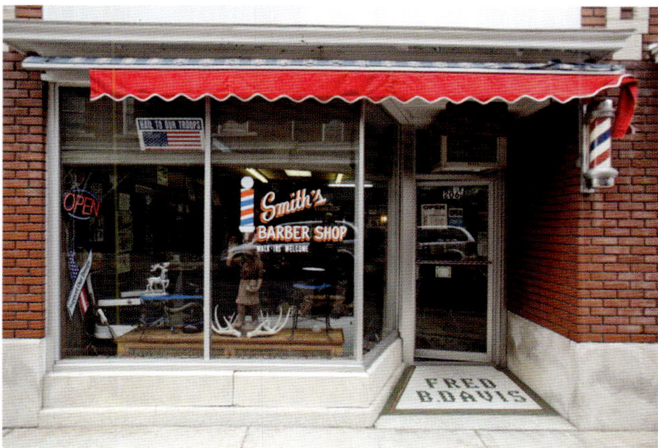
OPEN
Smith's
BARBER SHOP
FRED
B.DAVIS

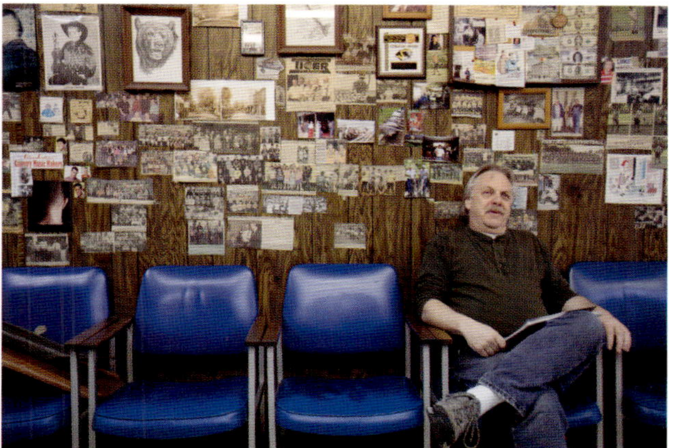

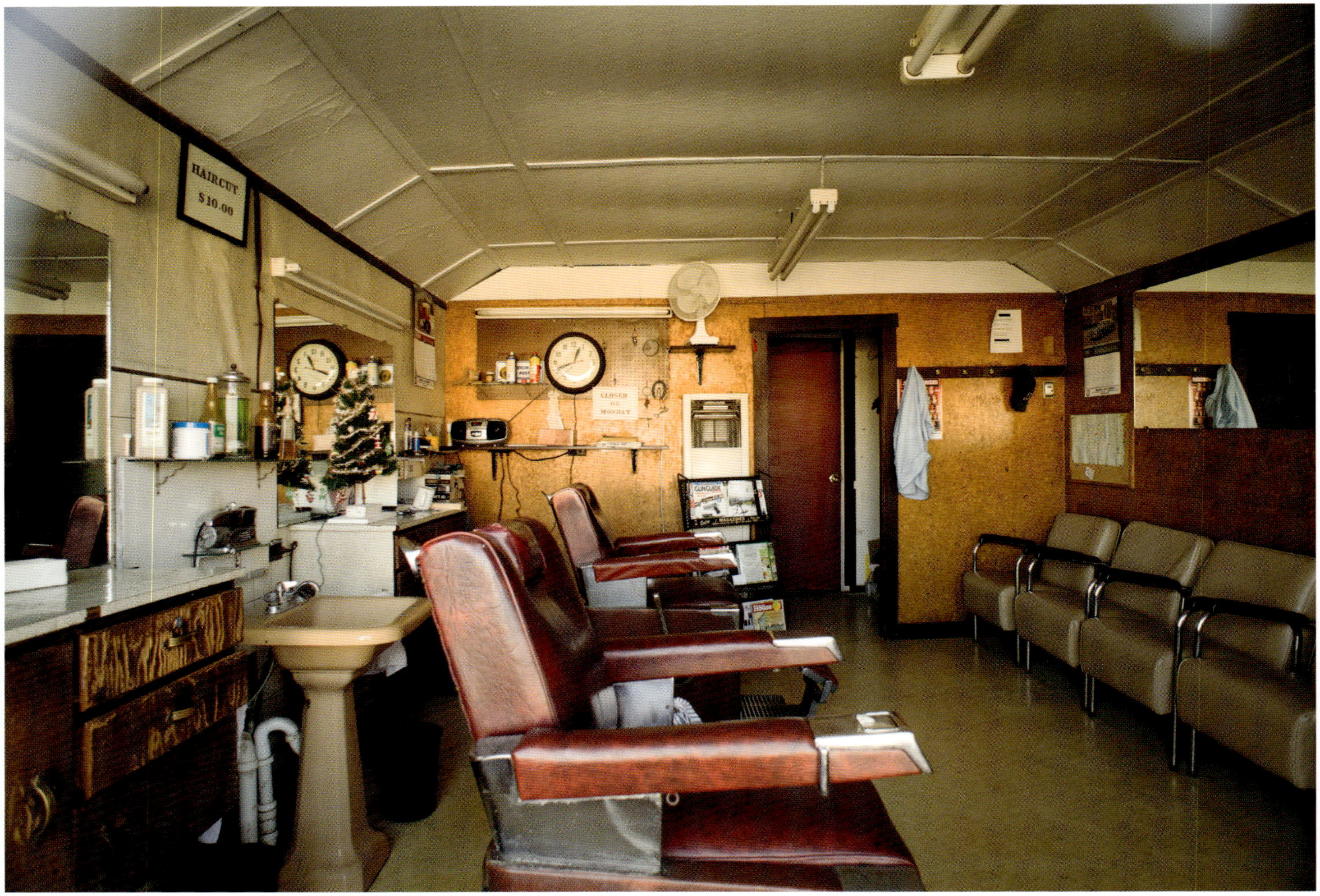

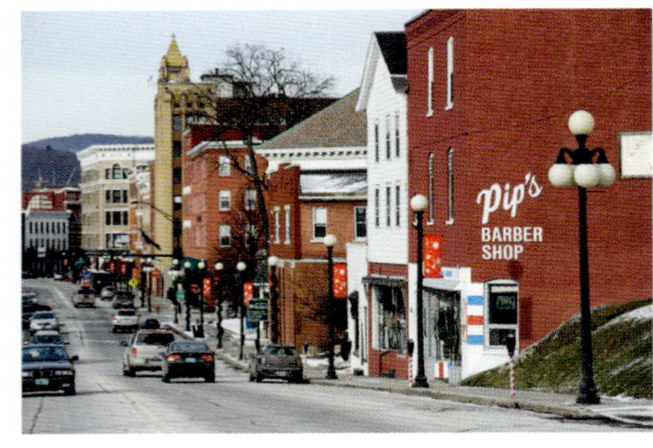
Pip's
BARBER
SHOP

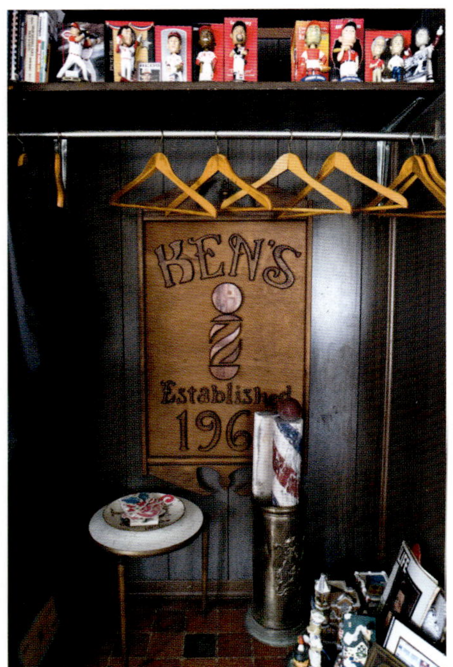
KEN'S
Established
196

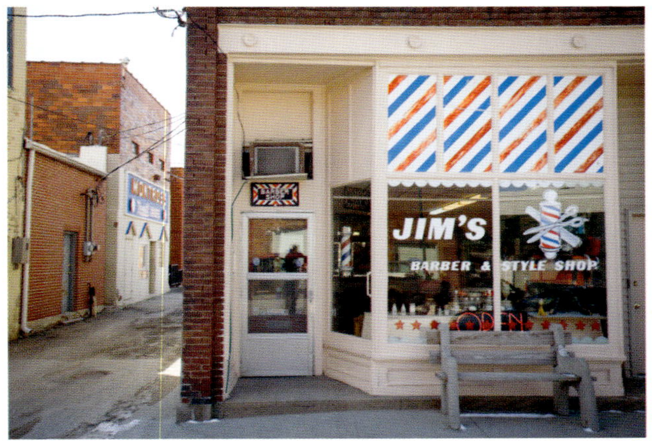
JIM'S
BARBER & STYLE SHOP

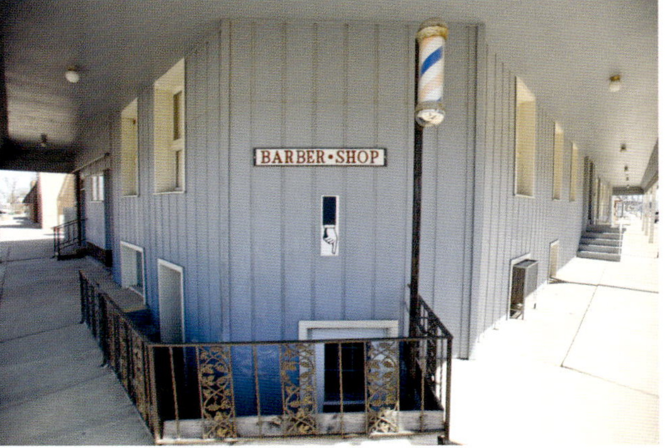
BARBER•SHOP

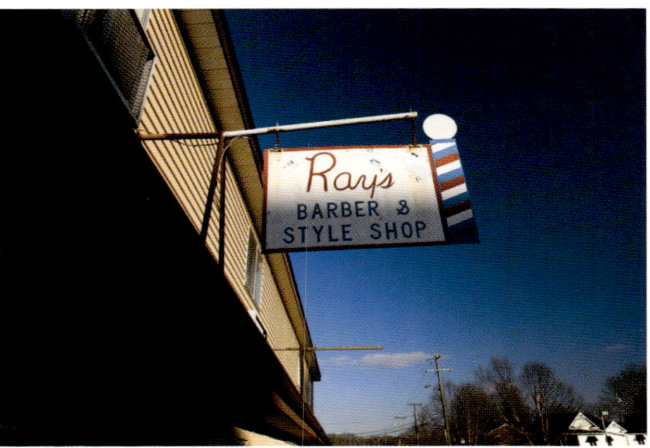
Ray's
BARBER &
STYLE SHOP

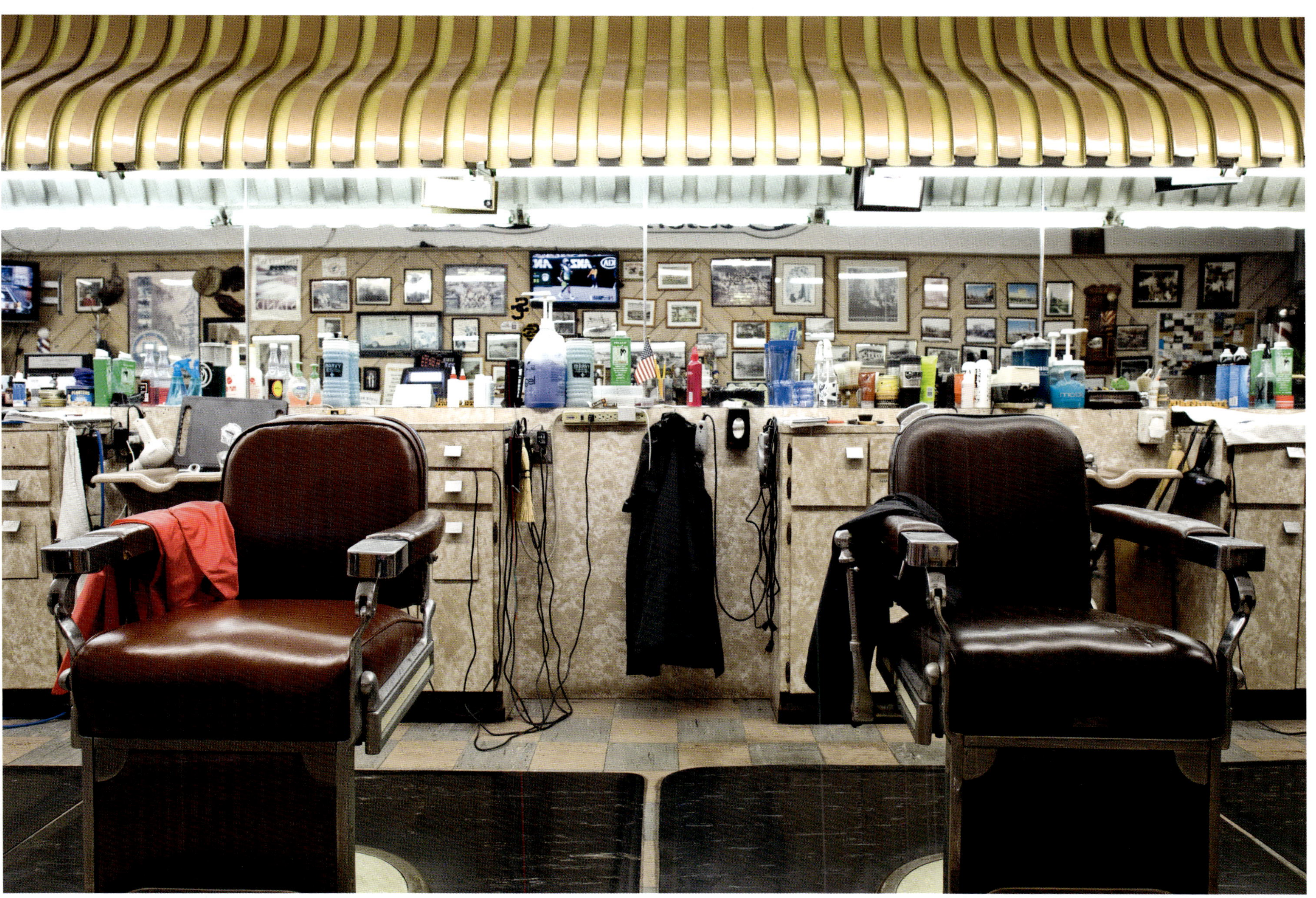

Scissor & Comb Barbershop, Oxnard, California

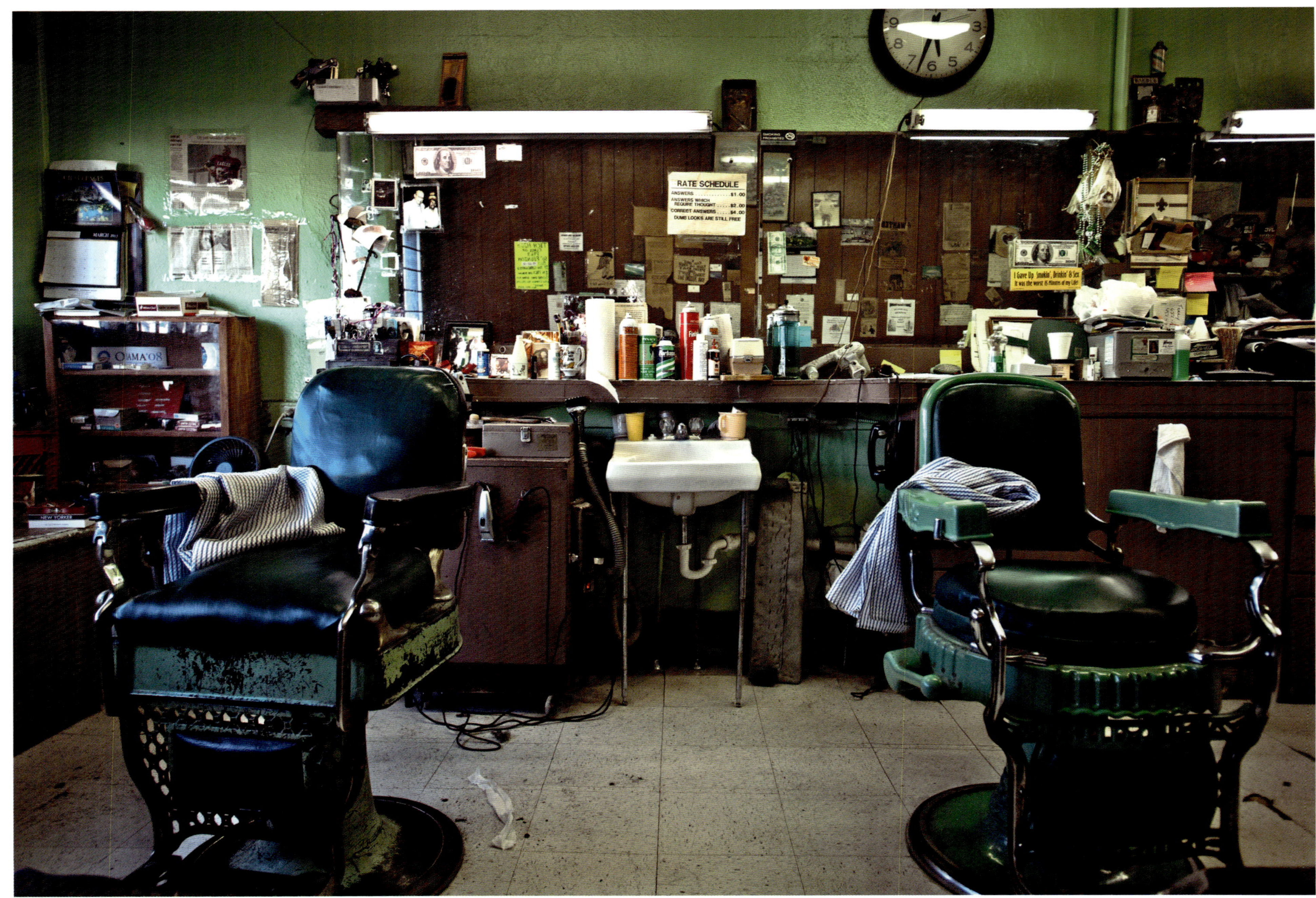

Imperial Barbershop, Omaha, Nebraska

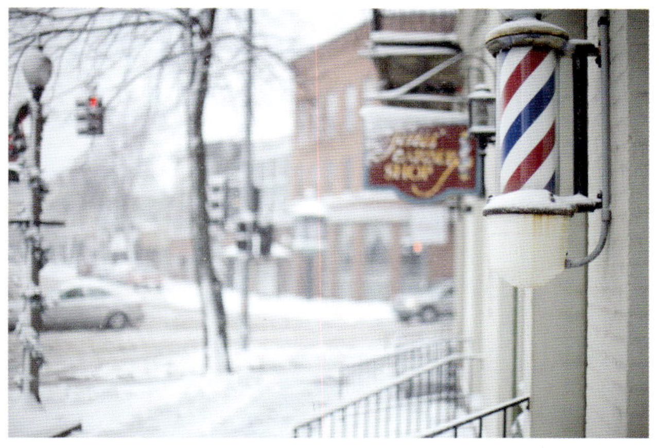

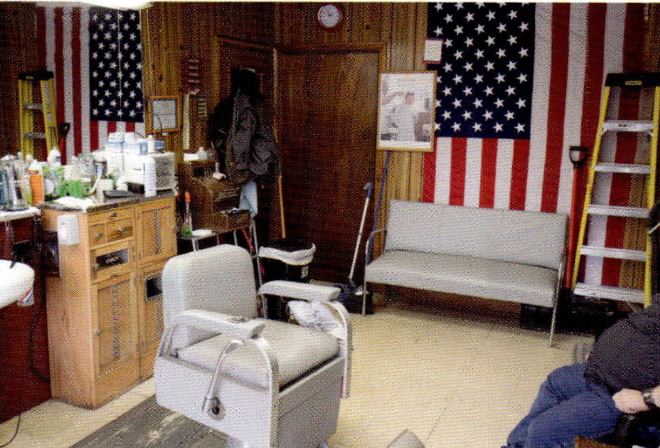

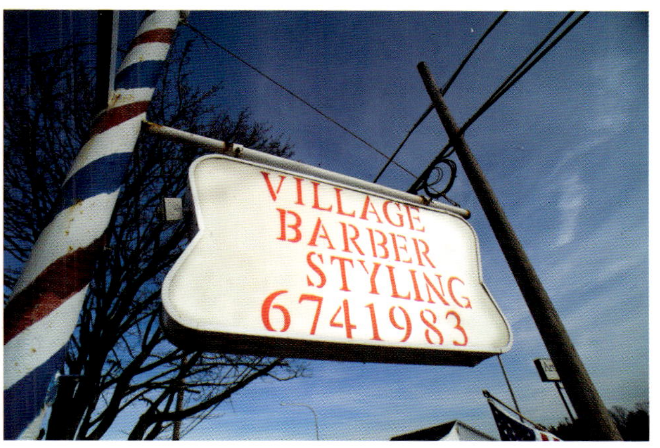
VILLAGE
BARBER
STYLING
6741983

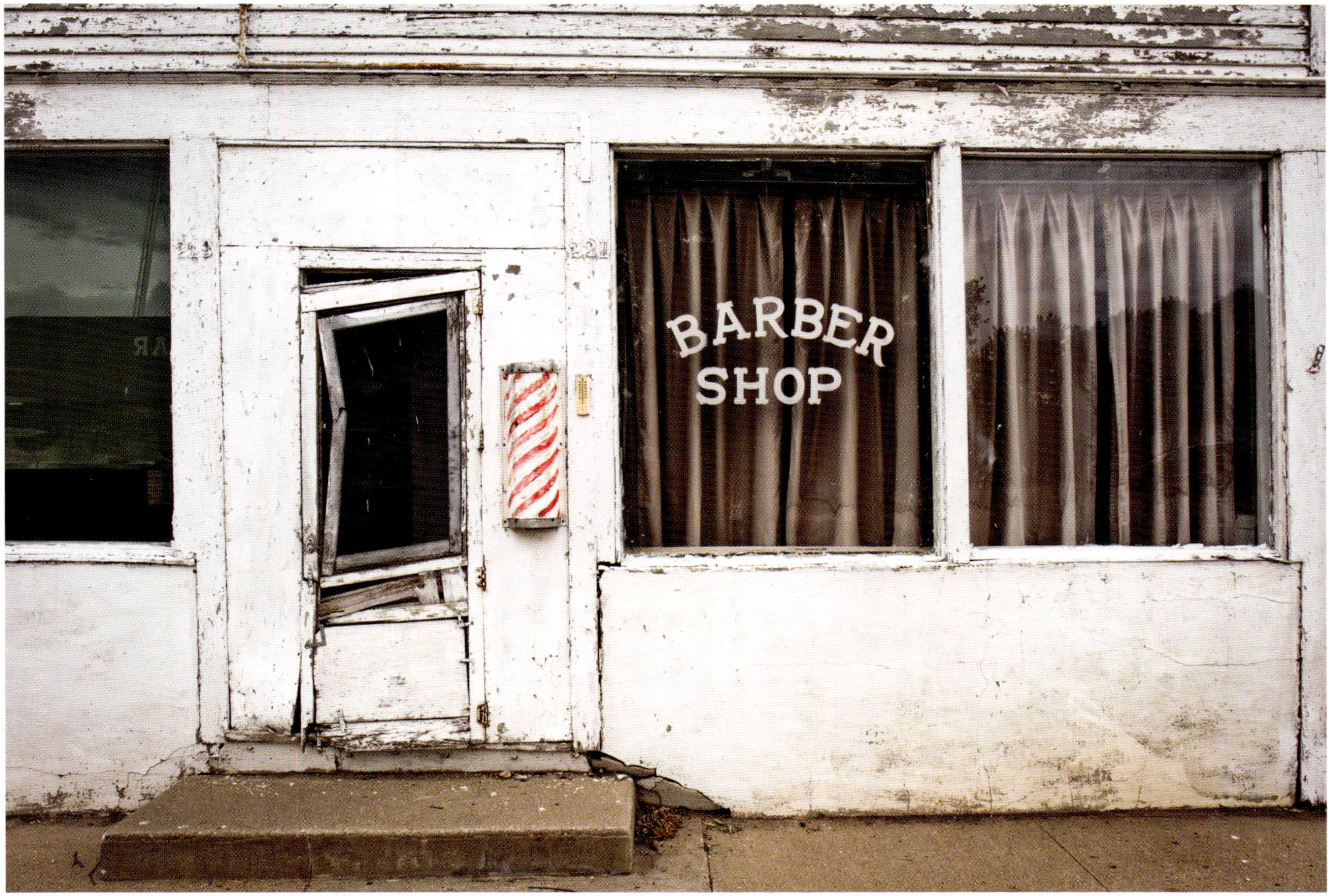

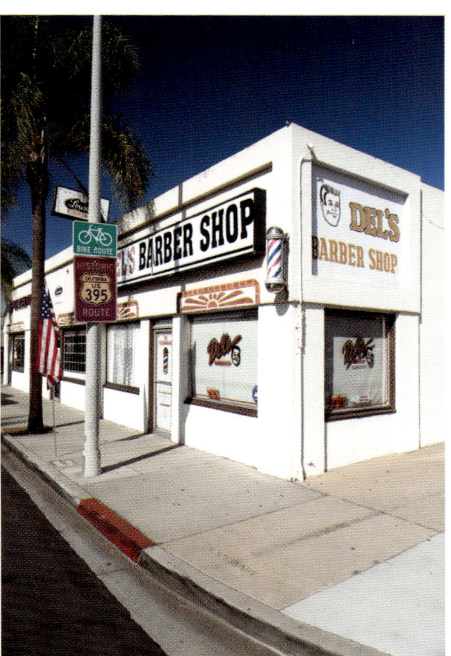
BARBER SHOP
DEL'S
BARBER SHOP
395

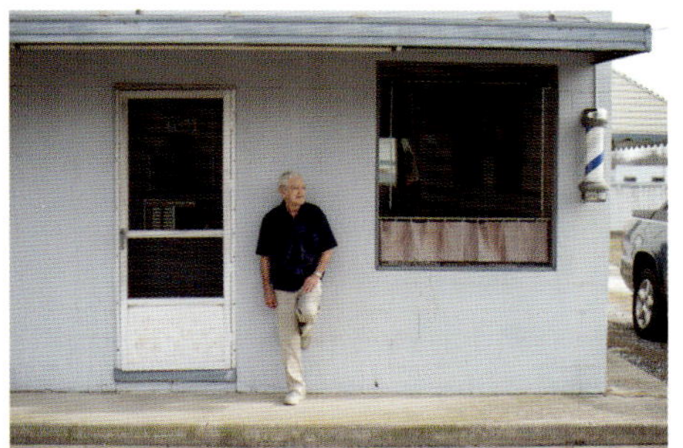

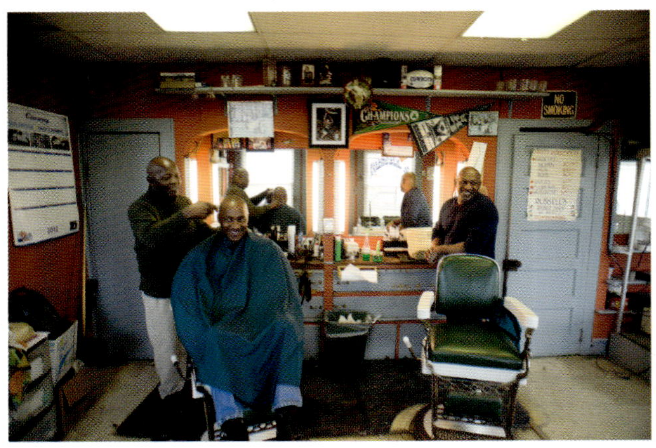
NO SMOKING

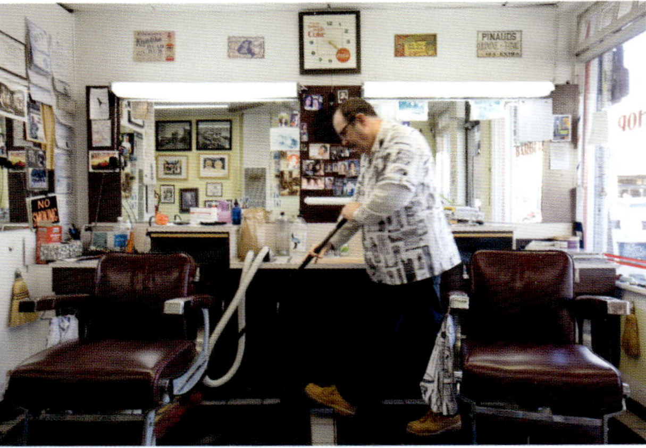

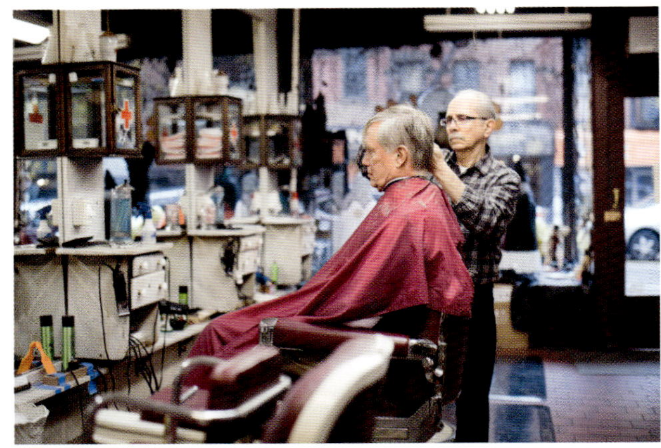

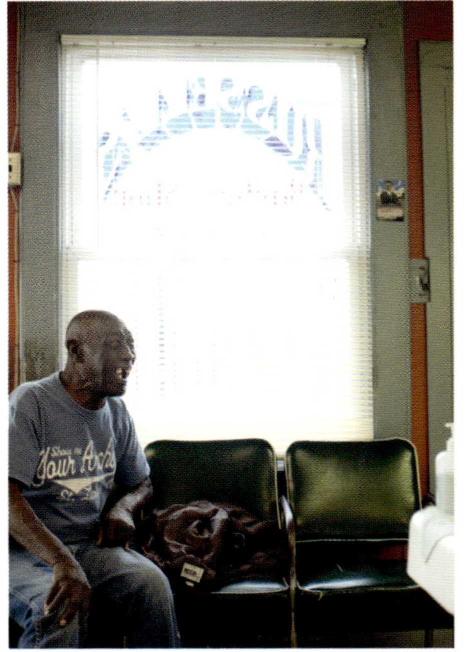

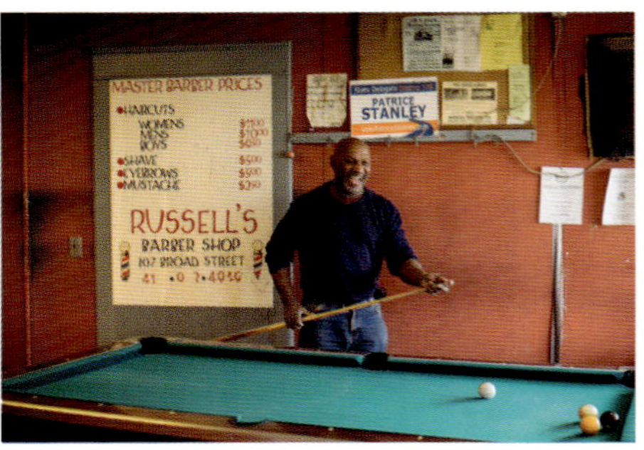
MASTER BARBER PRICES
HAIRCUTS
WOMENS
MENS
BOYS
SHAVE
EYEBROWS
MUSTACHE
RUSSELL'S
BARBER SHOP
107 BROAD STREET
PATRICE
STANLEY

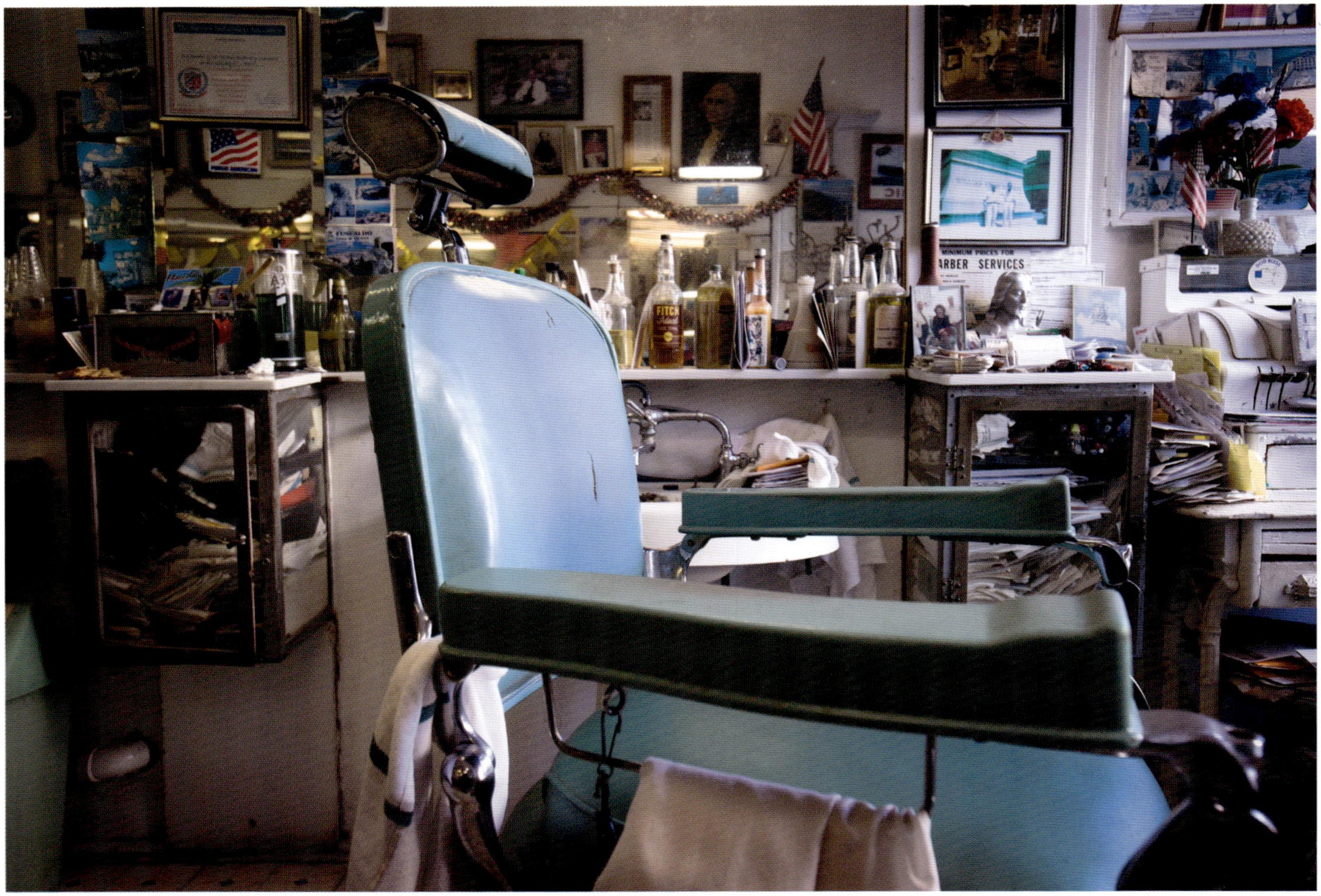

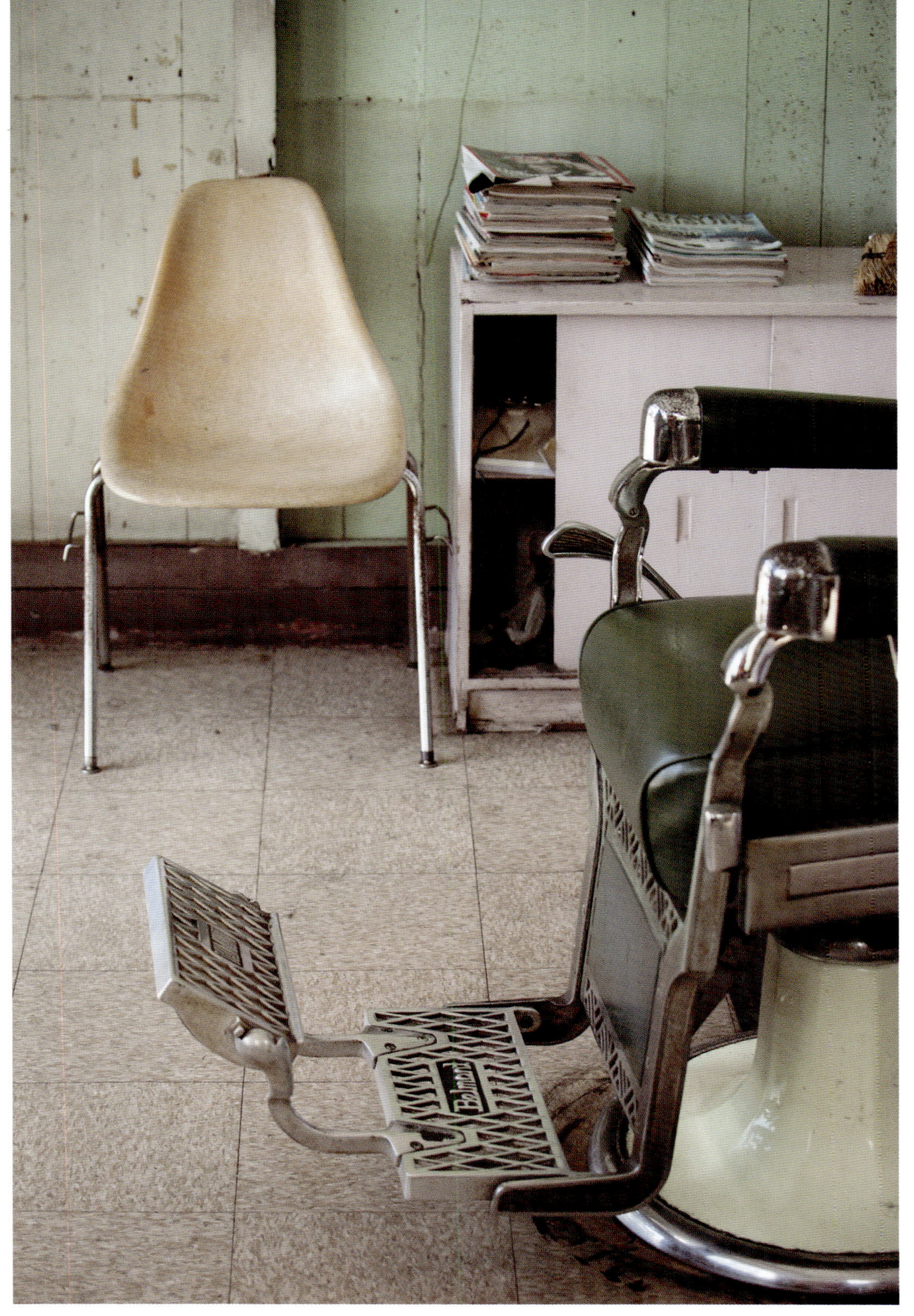

Sue's Barbershop, Maui, Hawaii

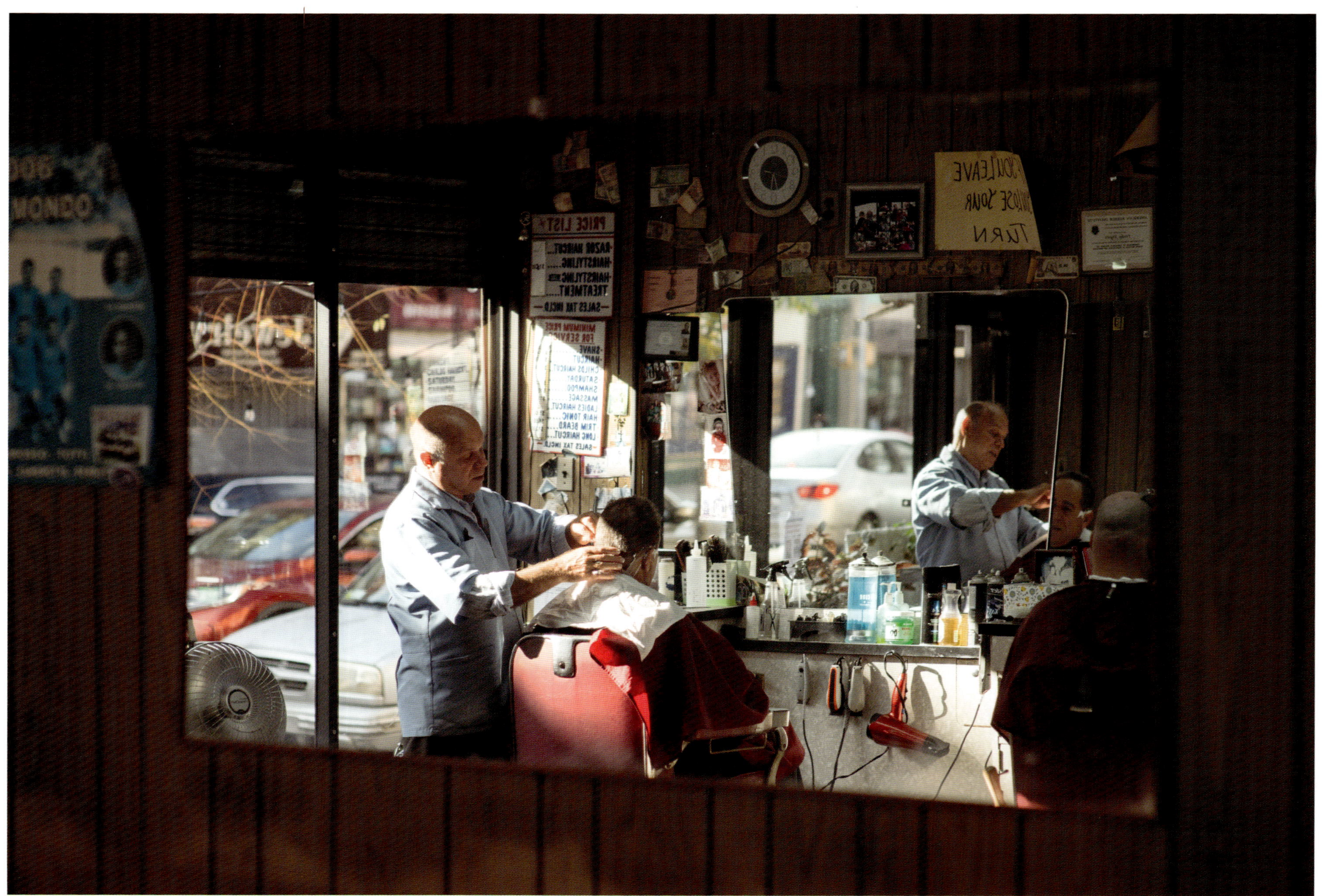

Rome Style Barbershop, Brooklyn, New York

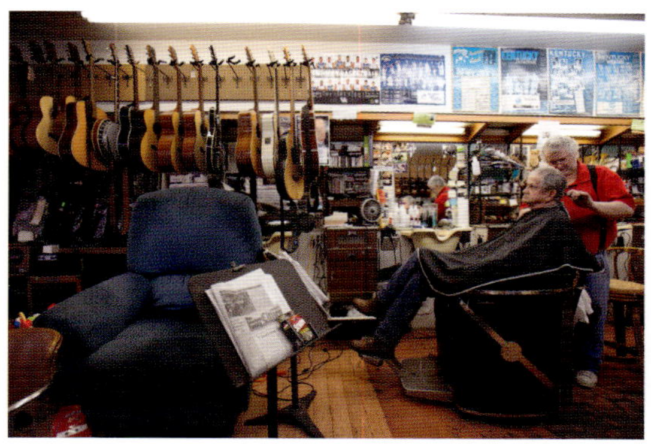
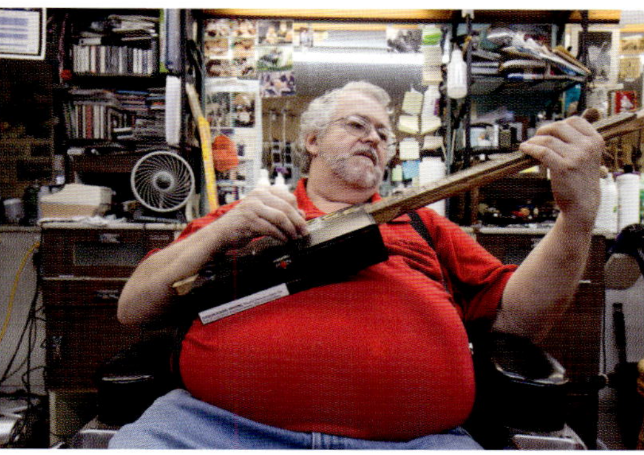
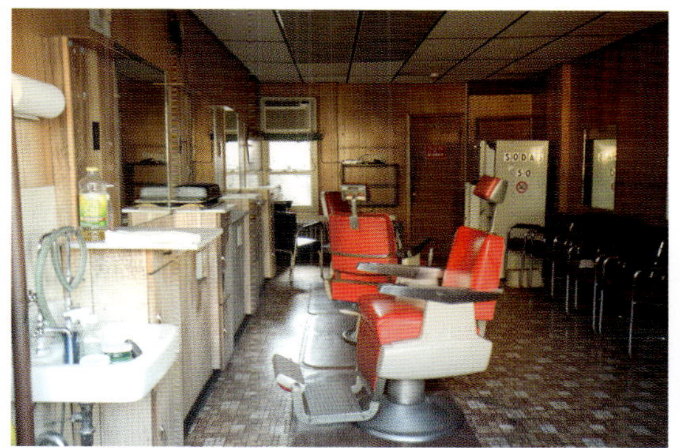
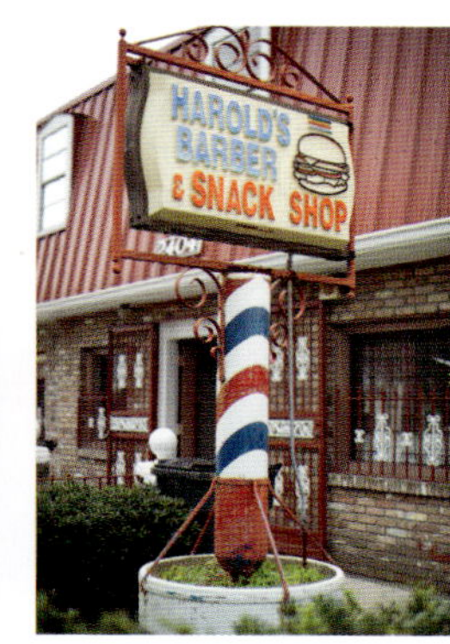
HAROLD'S
BARBER
& SNACK SHOP
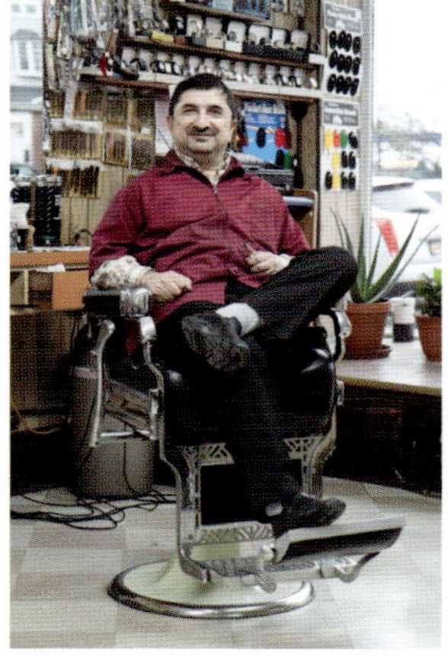
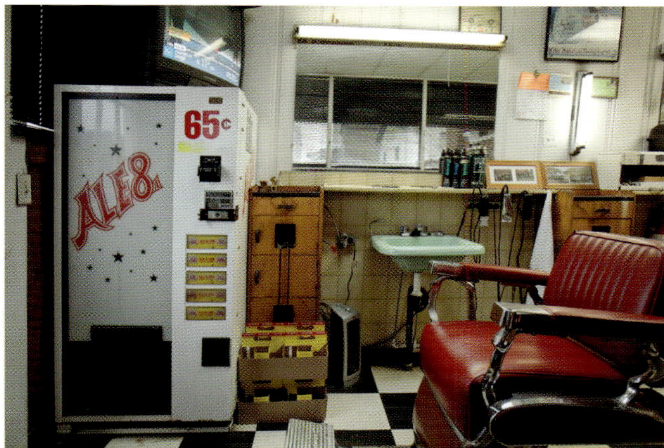
65¢
ALE8
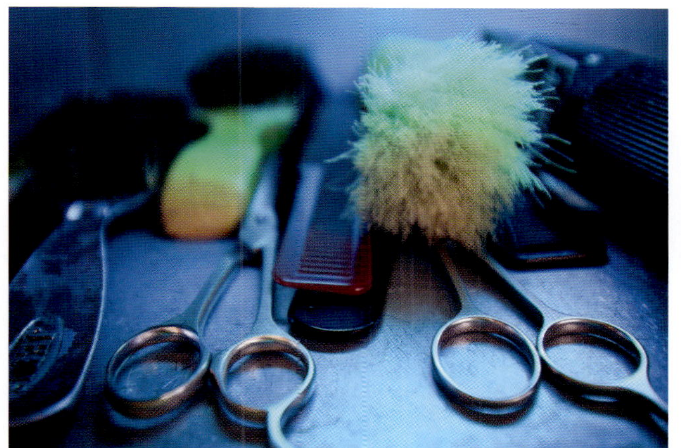
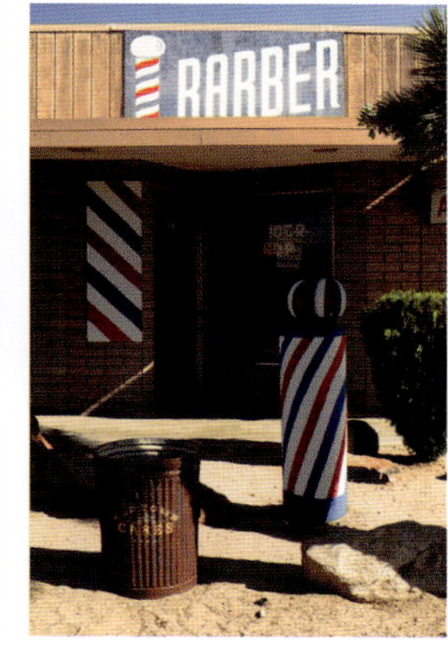
RARBER
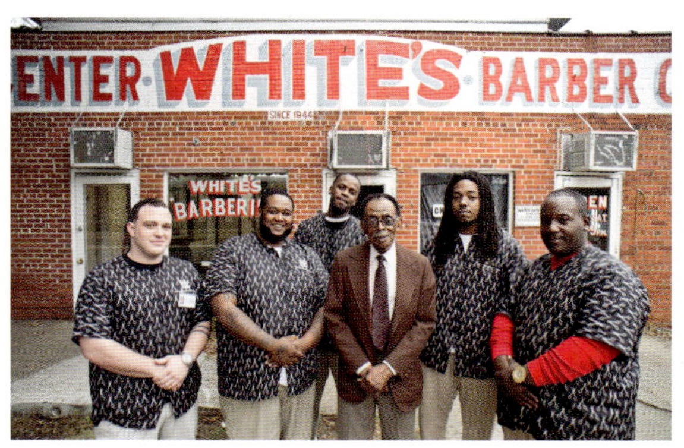
ENTER·WHITE'S·BARBER C
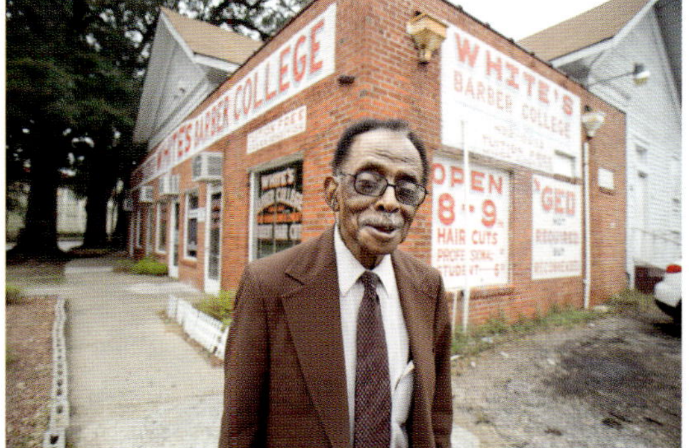
WHITE'S BARBER COLLEGE
OPEN
8 - 9
HAIR CUTS
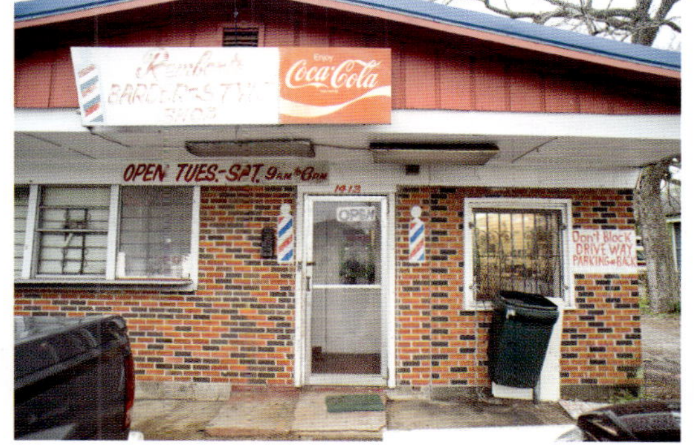
Enjoy Coca-Cola
OPEN TUES.-SAT. 9AM to 6PM
1413
Don't Block
DRIVE WAY
PARKING in BACK
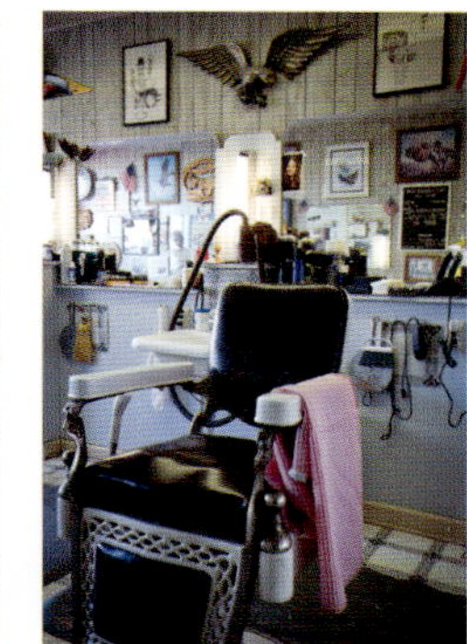

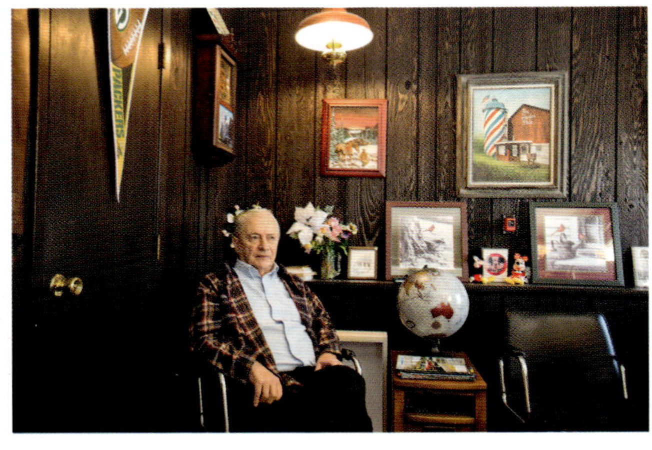

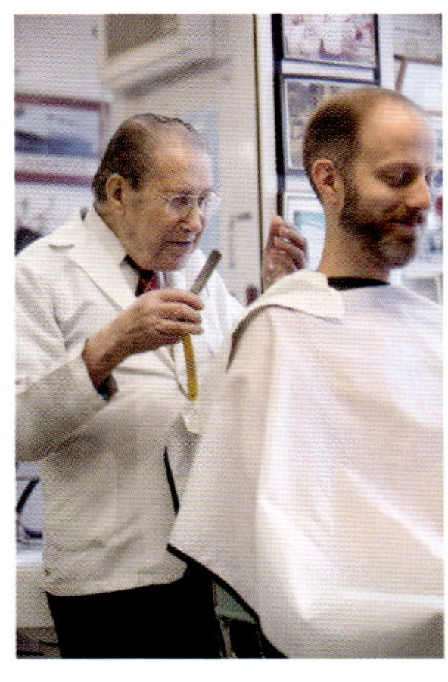

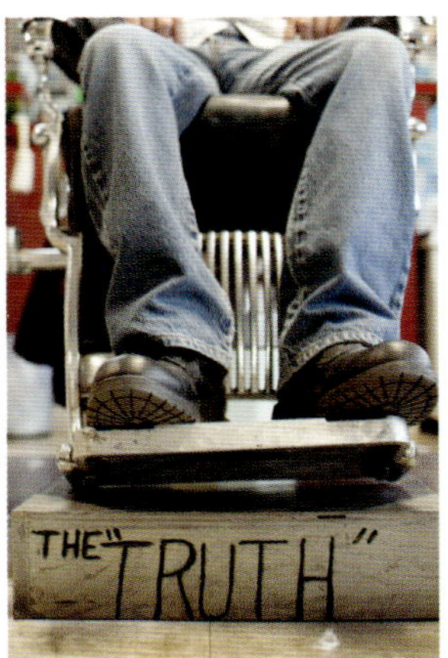

THE "TRUTH"

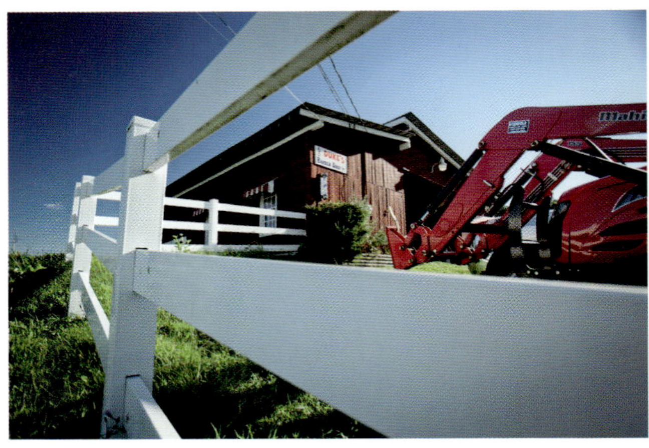

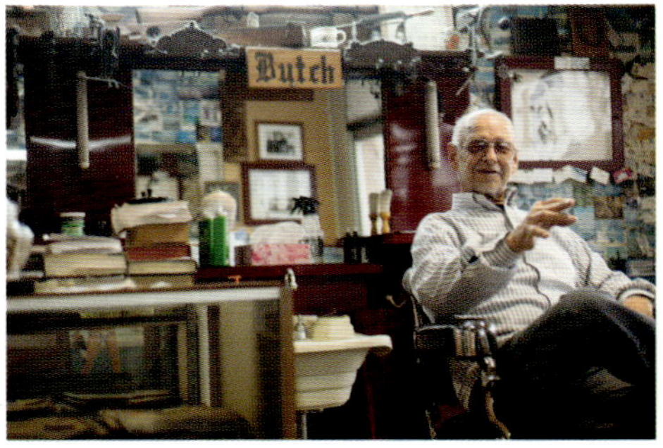

Butch

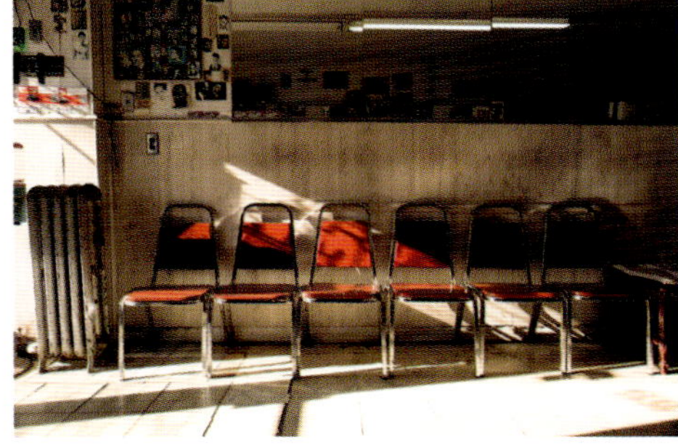

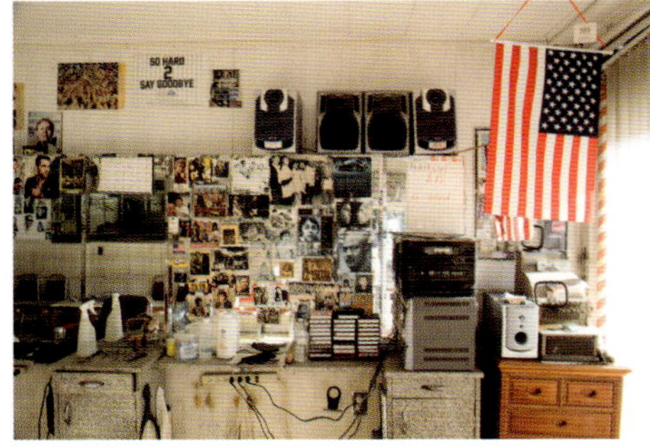

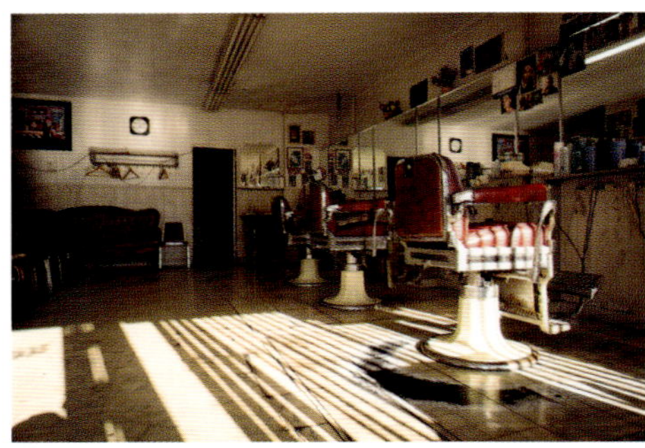

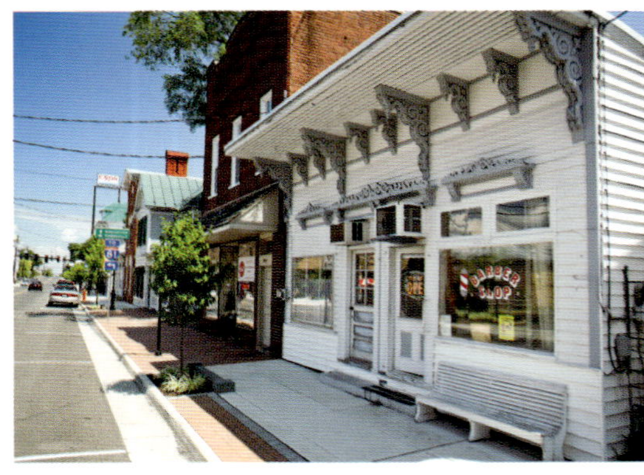

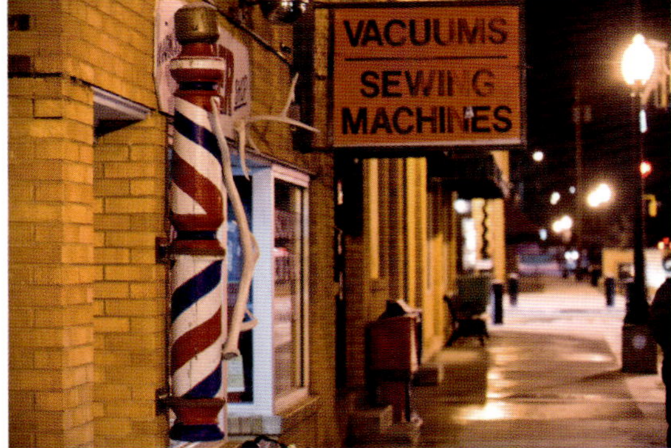

VACUUMS
SEWING
MACHINES

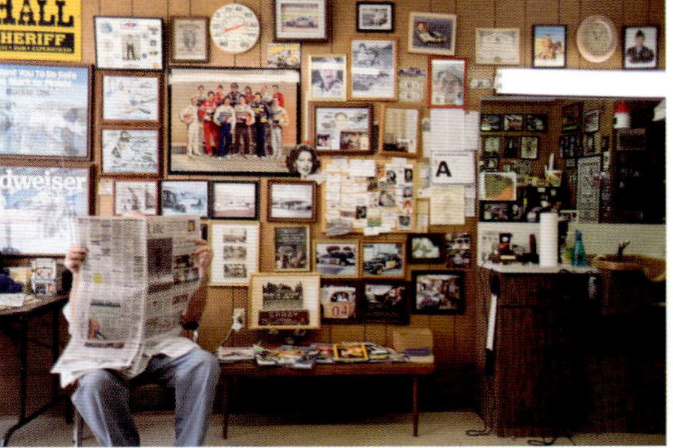

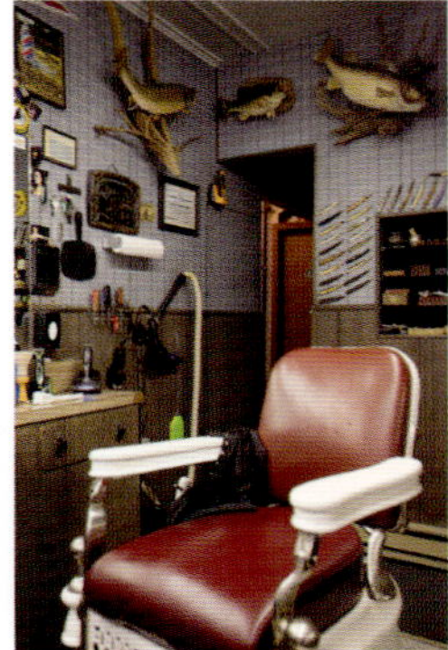

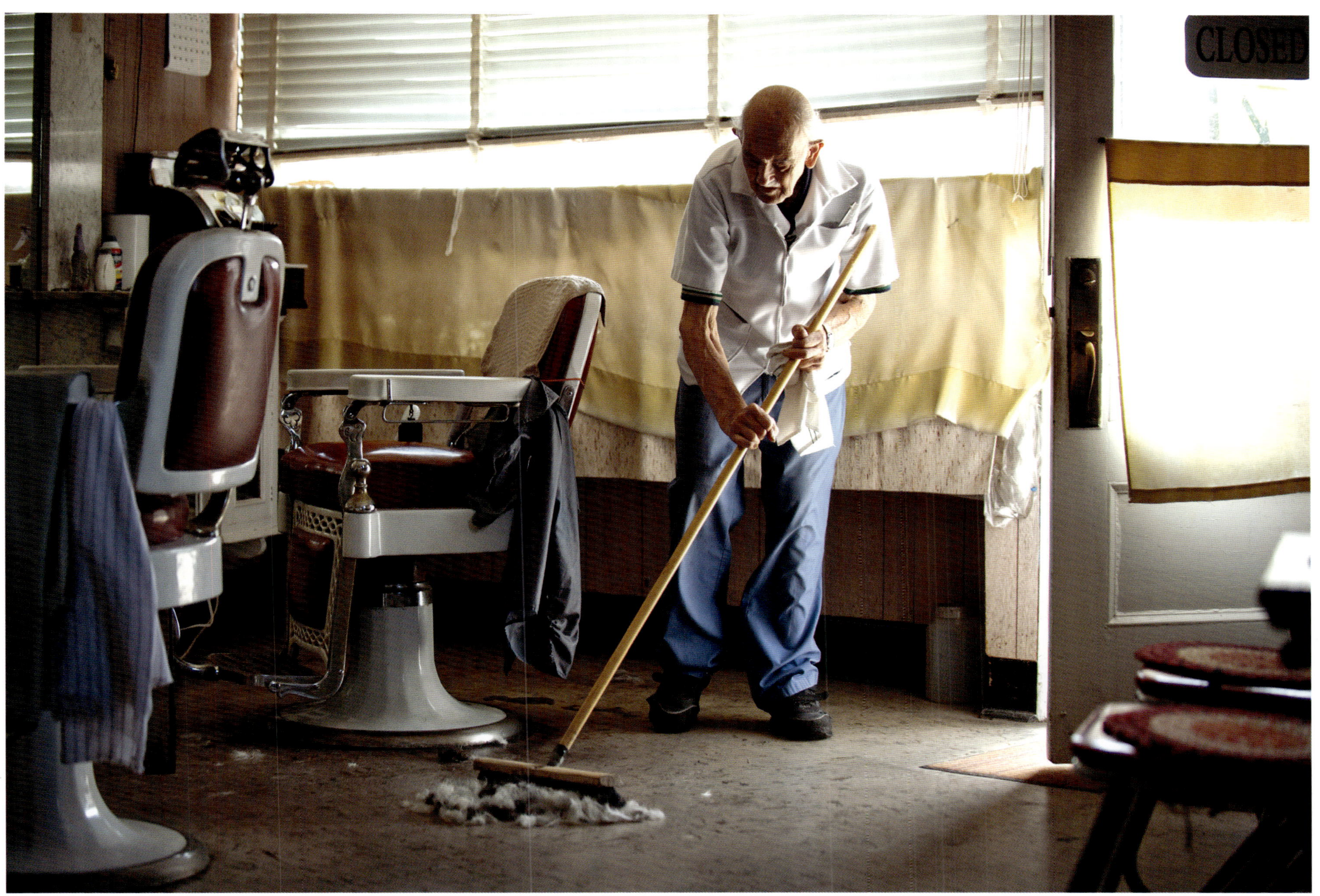

Tony's Barbershop, Greenwich, Connecticut

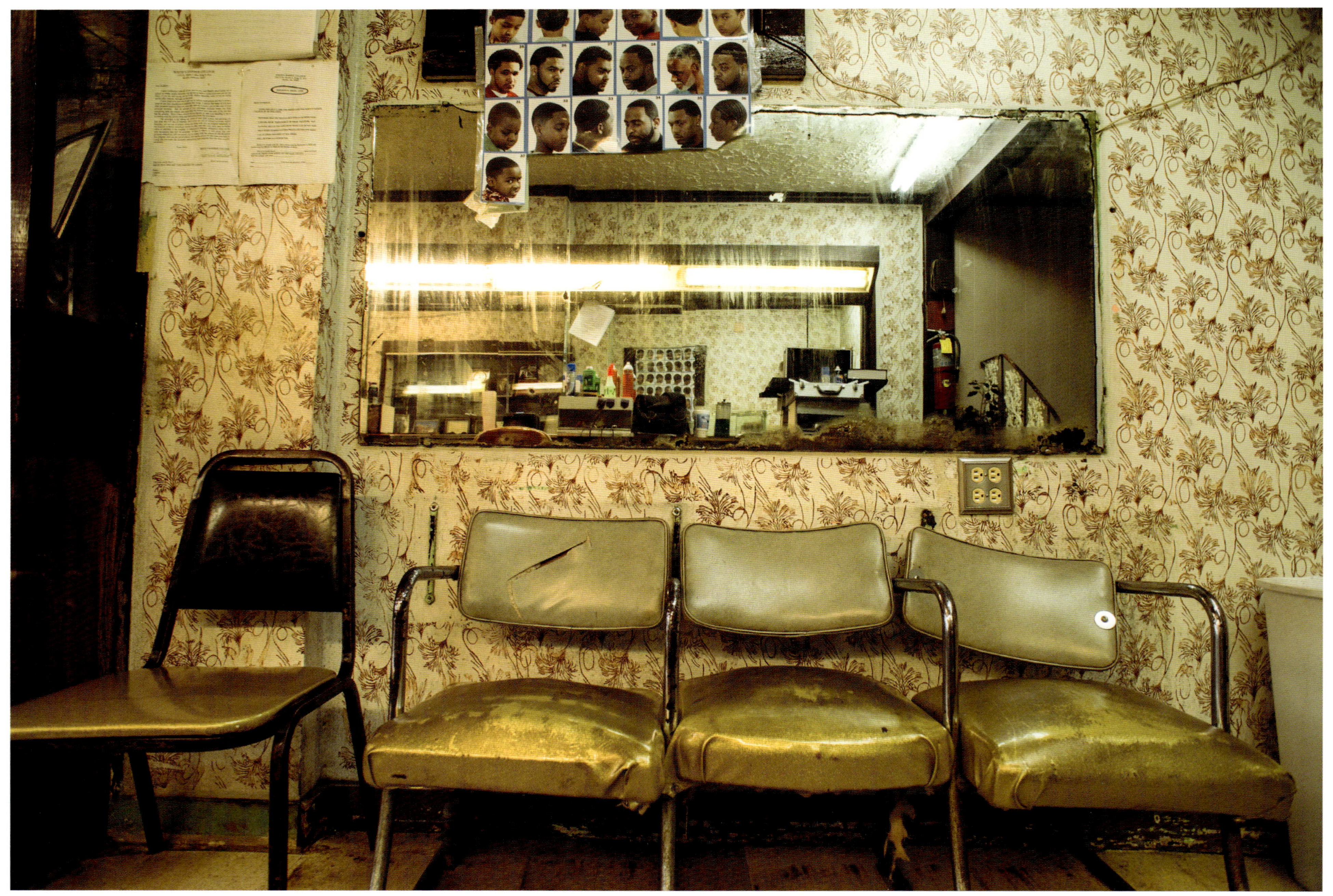

White's Barbershop, Mobile, Alabama

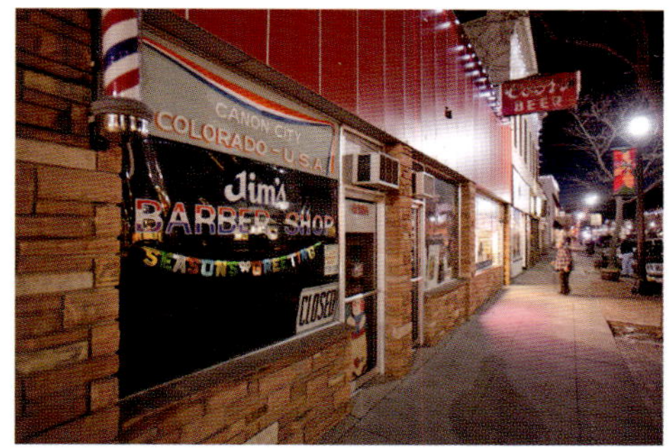
CANON CITY
COLORADO U.S.A.
Jim's
BARBER SHOP
CLOSED
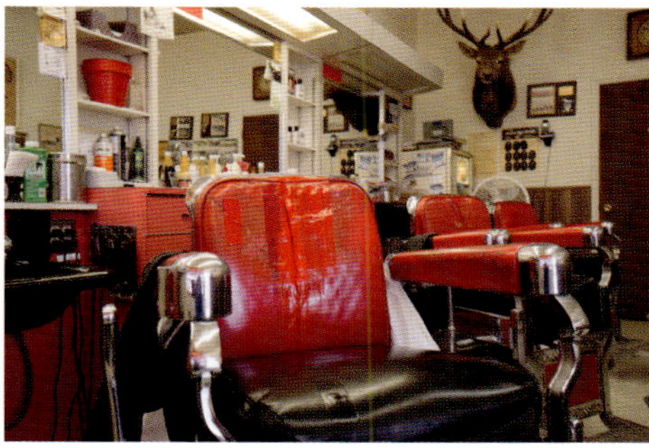
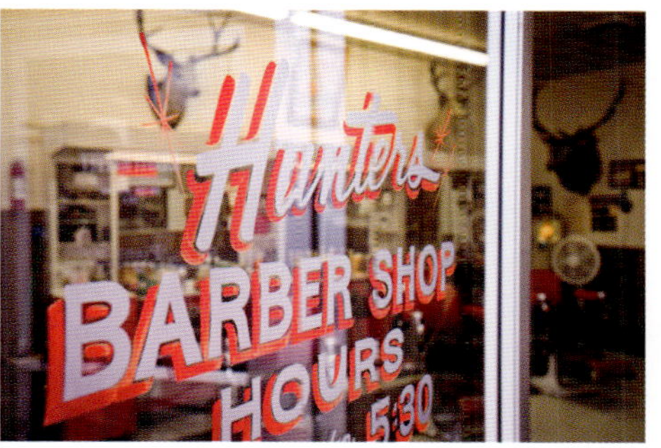
BARBER SHOP
HOURS
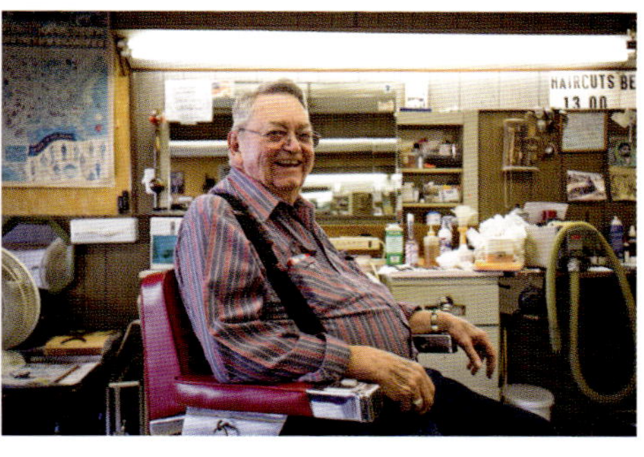
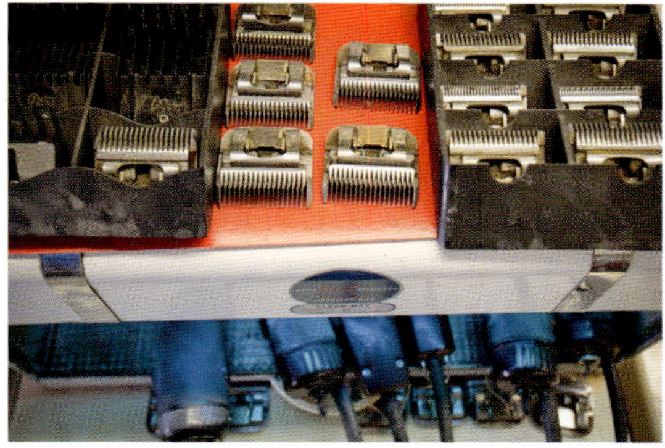
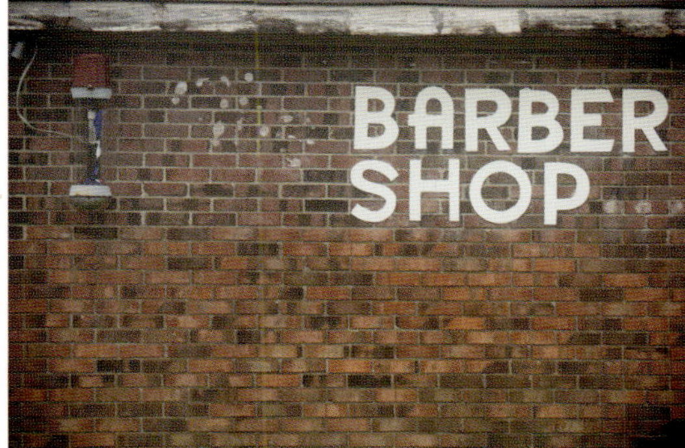
BARBER
SHOP
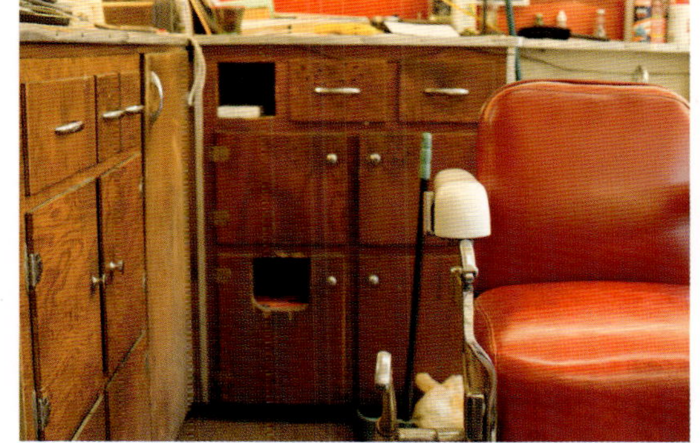
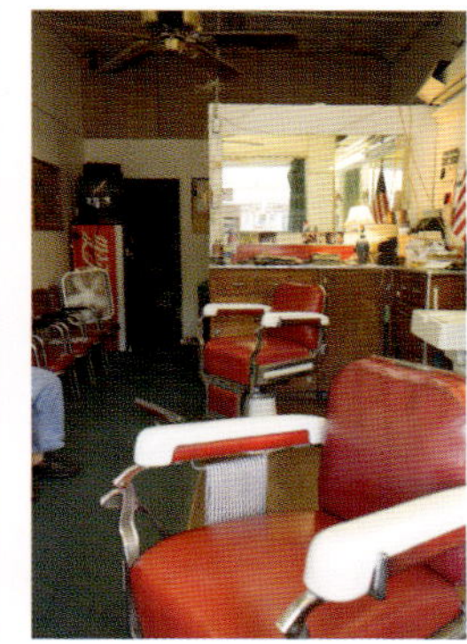
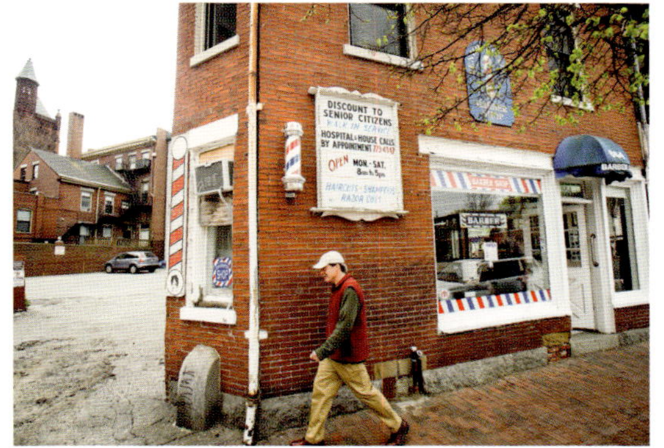
DISCOUNT TO SENIOR CITIZENS
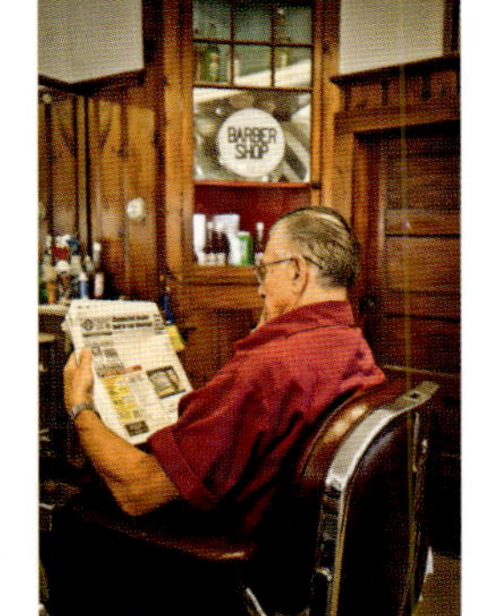
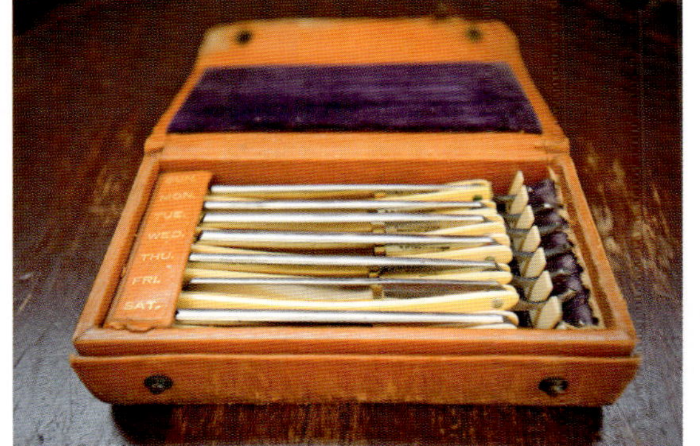
TUE.
WED.
THU.
FRI.
SAT.
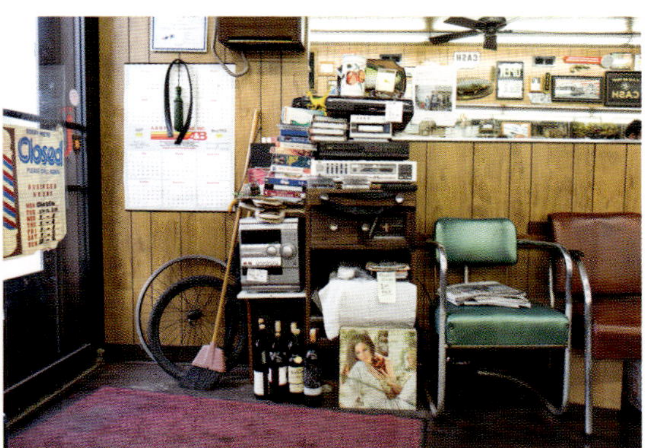
Closed
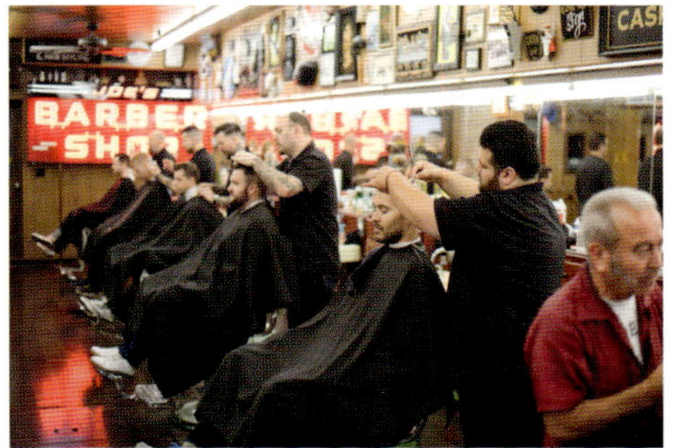
BARBER
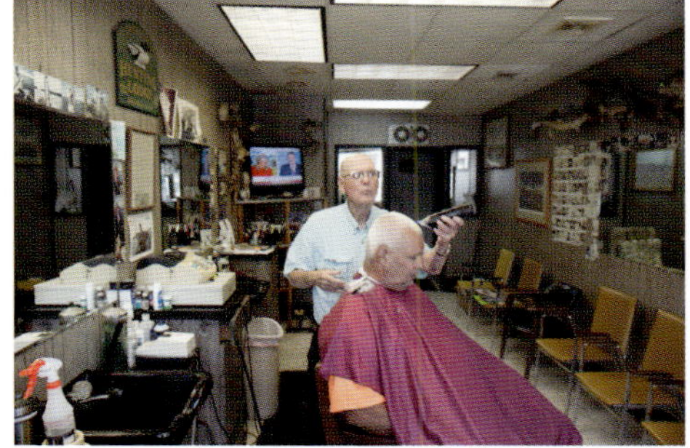
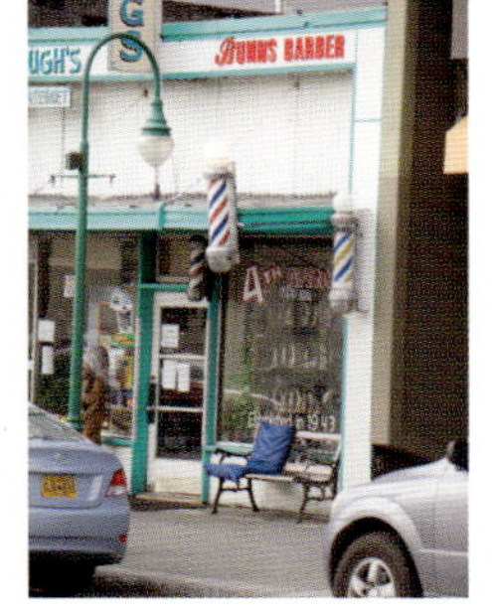
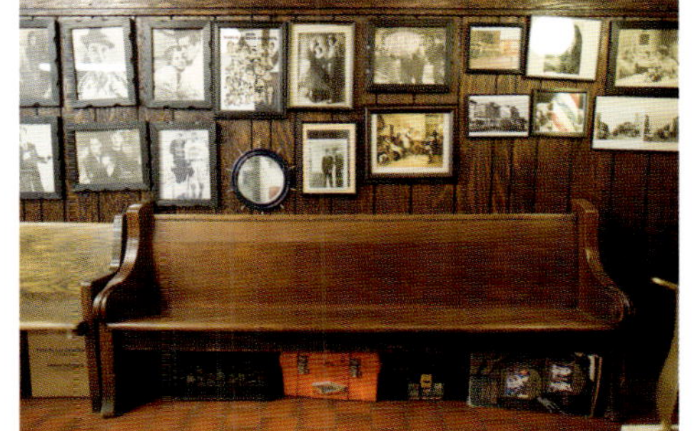
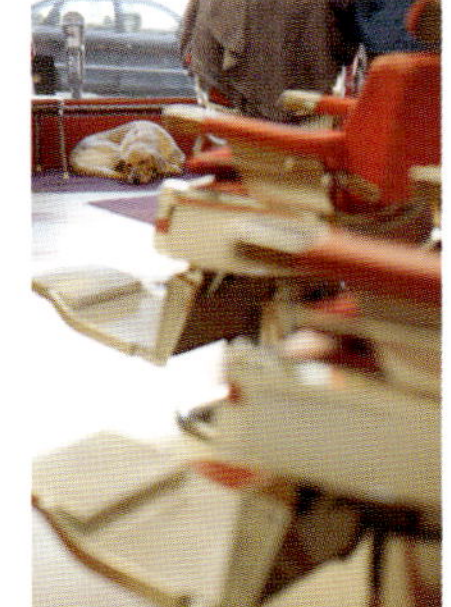

"People left town in the '60s and '70s. Came back and said . . . you mean to tell me this is still Craighead's?"

– Joe, Craighead Barbershop, Nashville, Tennessee

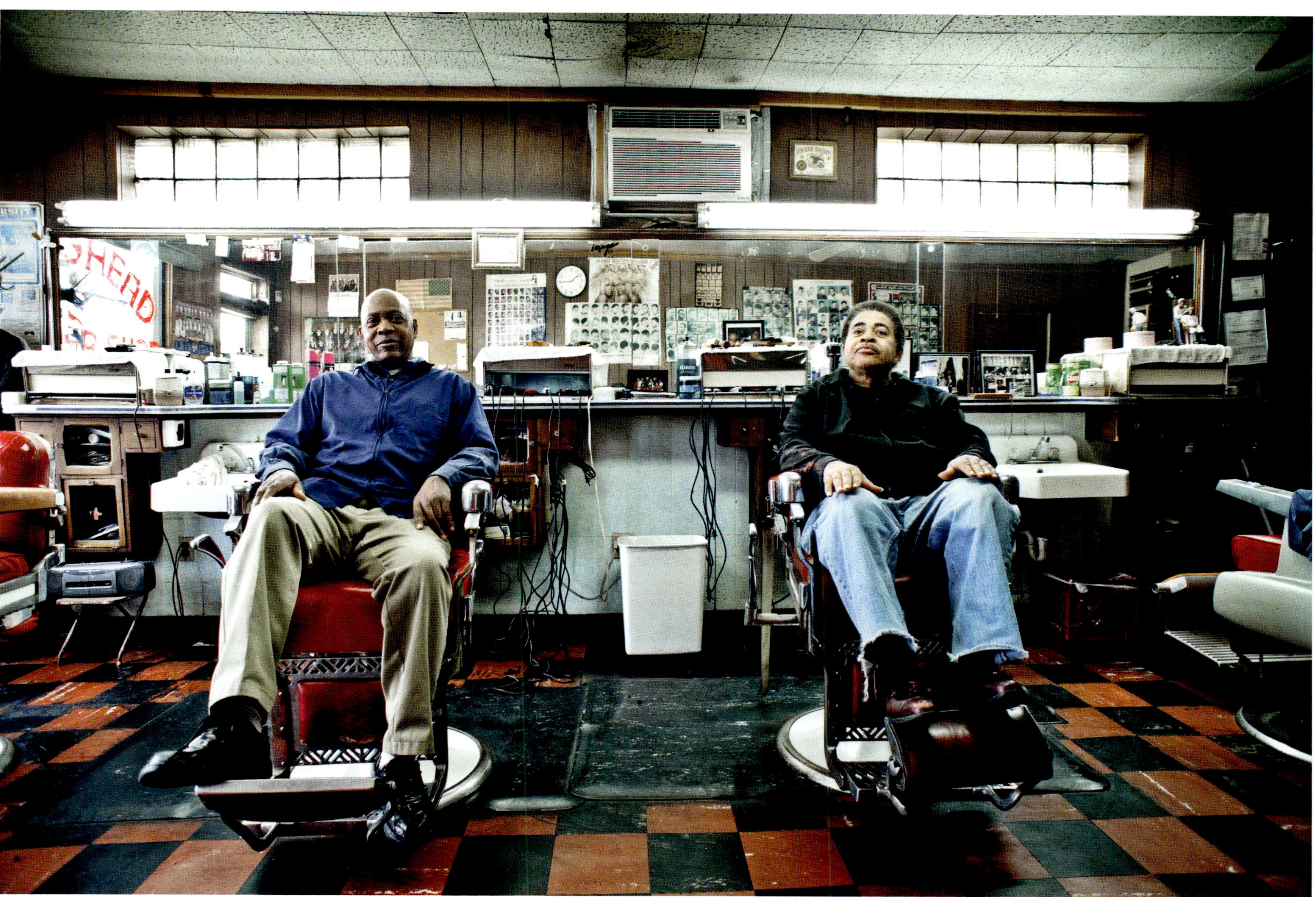

Craighead Barbershop, Nashville, Tennessee

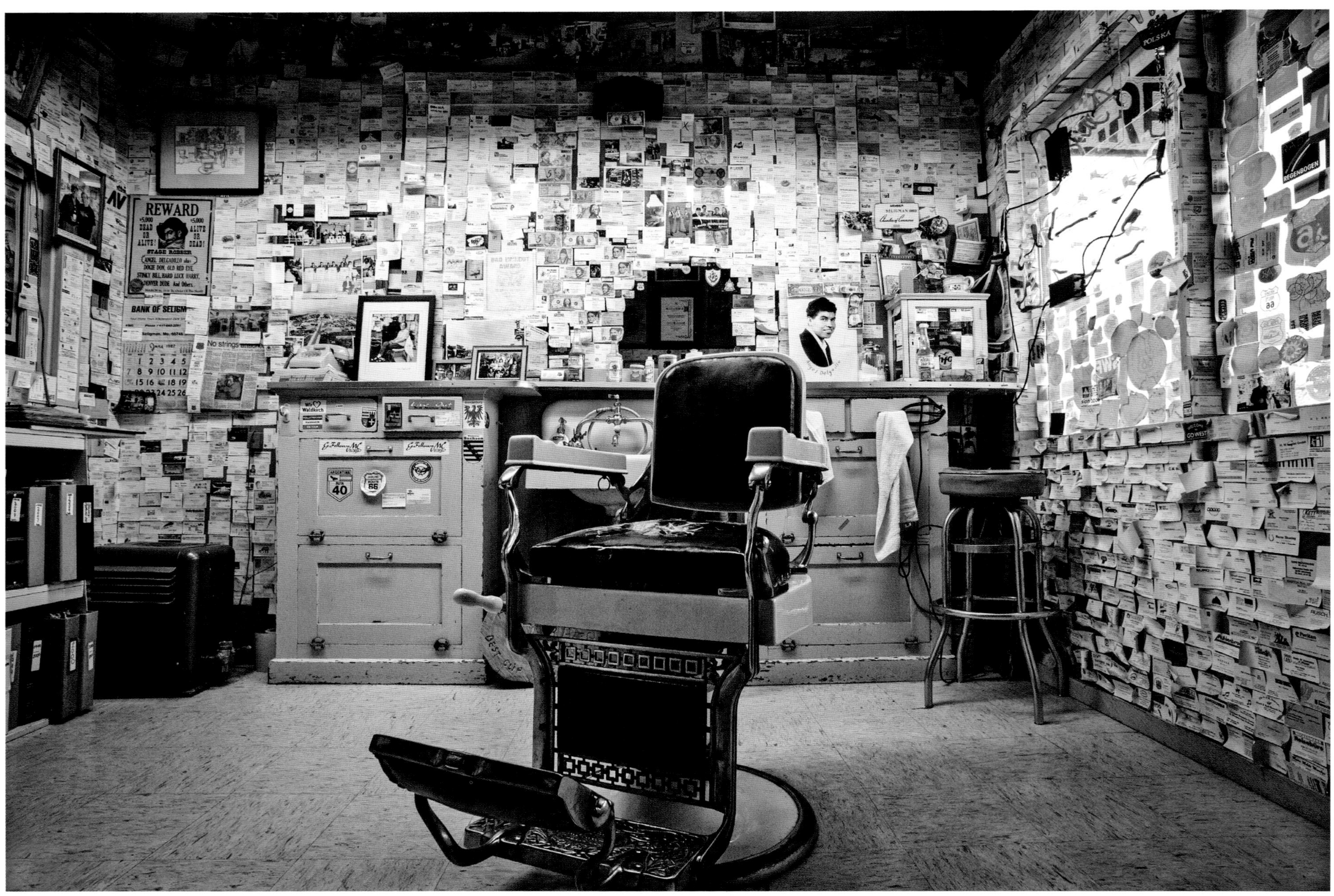

White's Barbershop, Mobile, Alabama

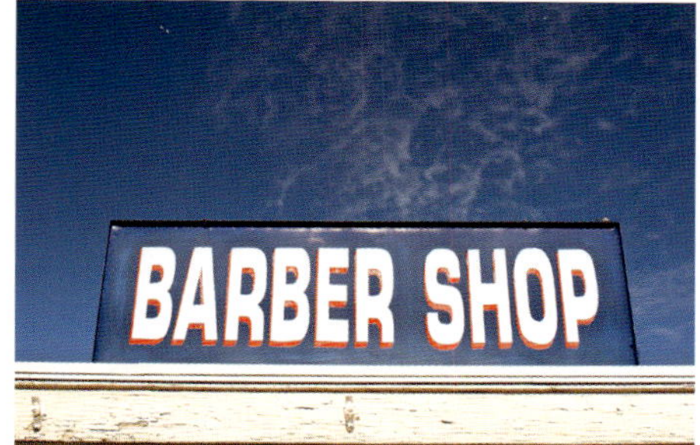
BARBER SHOP

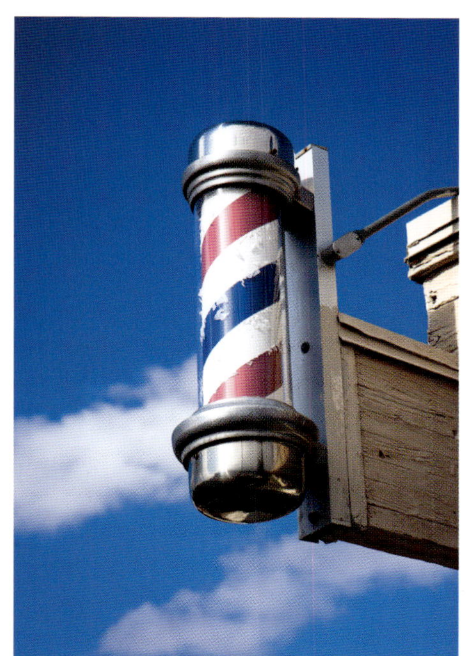

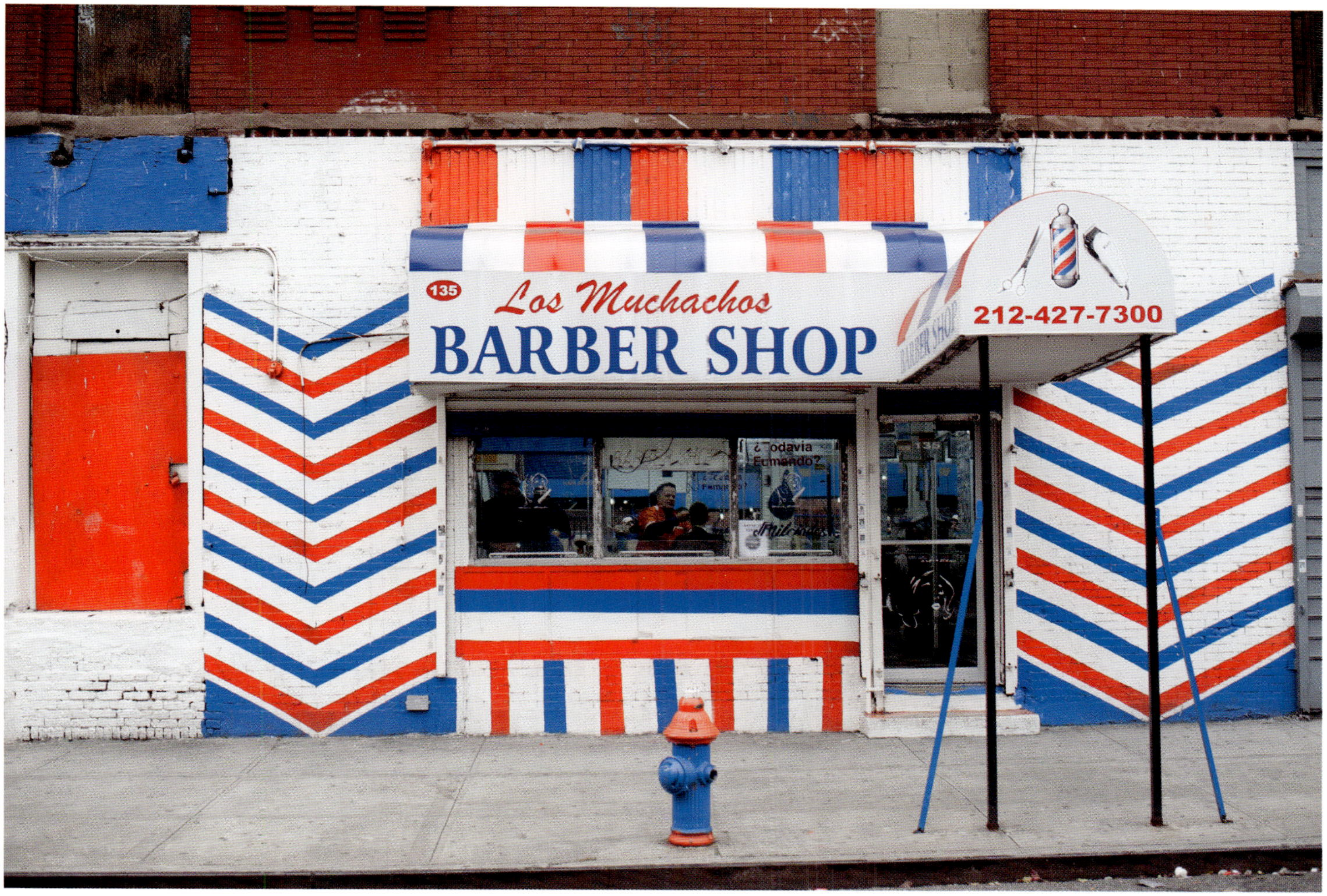

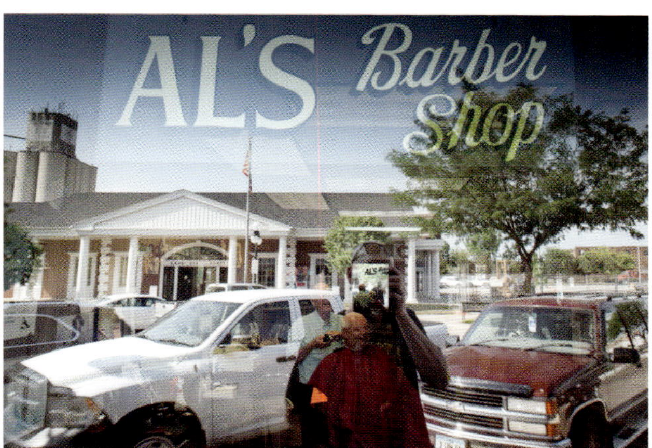
AL'S
Barber Shop

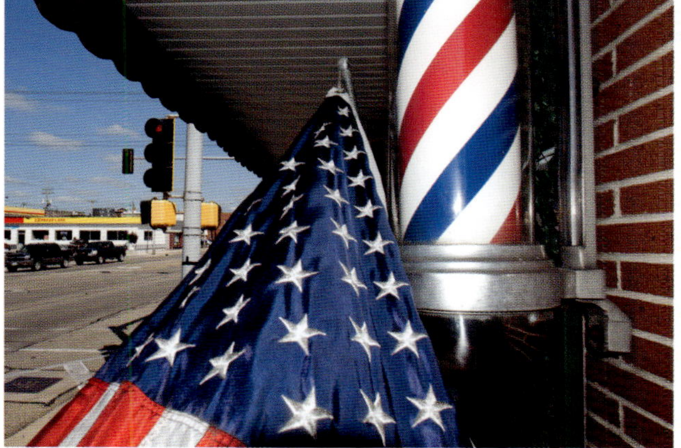

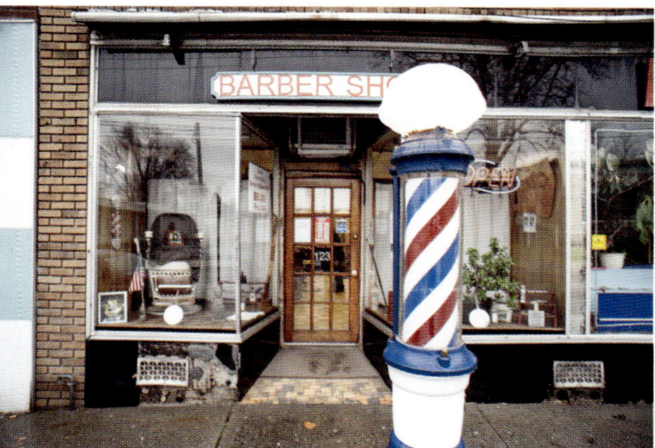

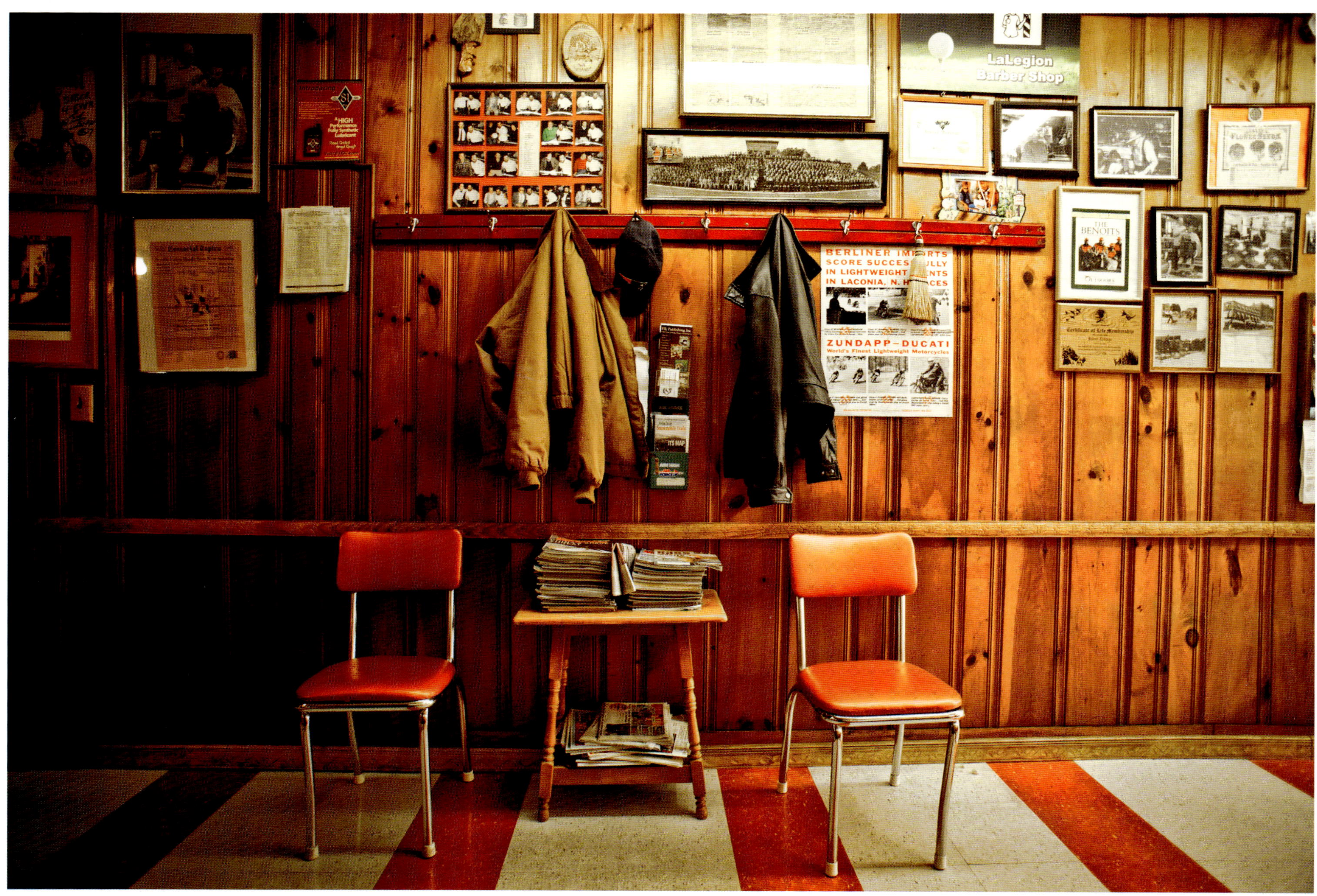

Le Legion Barbershop, Nashua, New Hampshire

"White Russians are for girls. I drink scorpion bowls. They make me steal things I already own."

– La Legion Barbershop, Nashua, New Hampshire

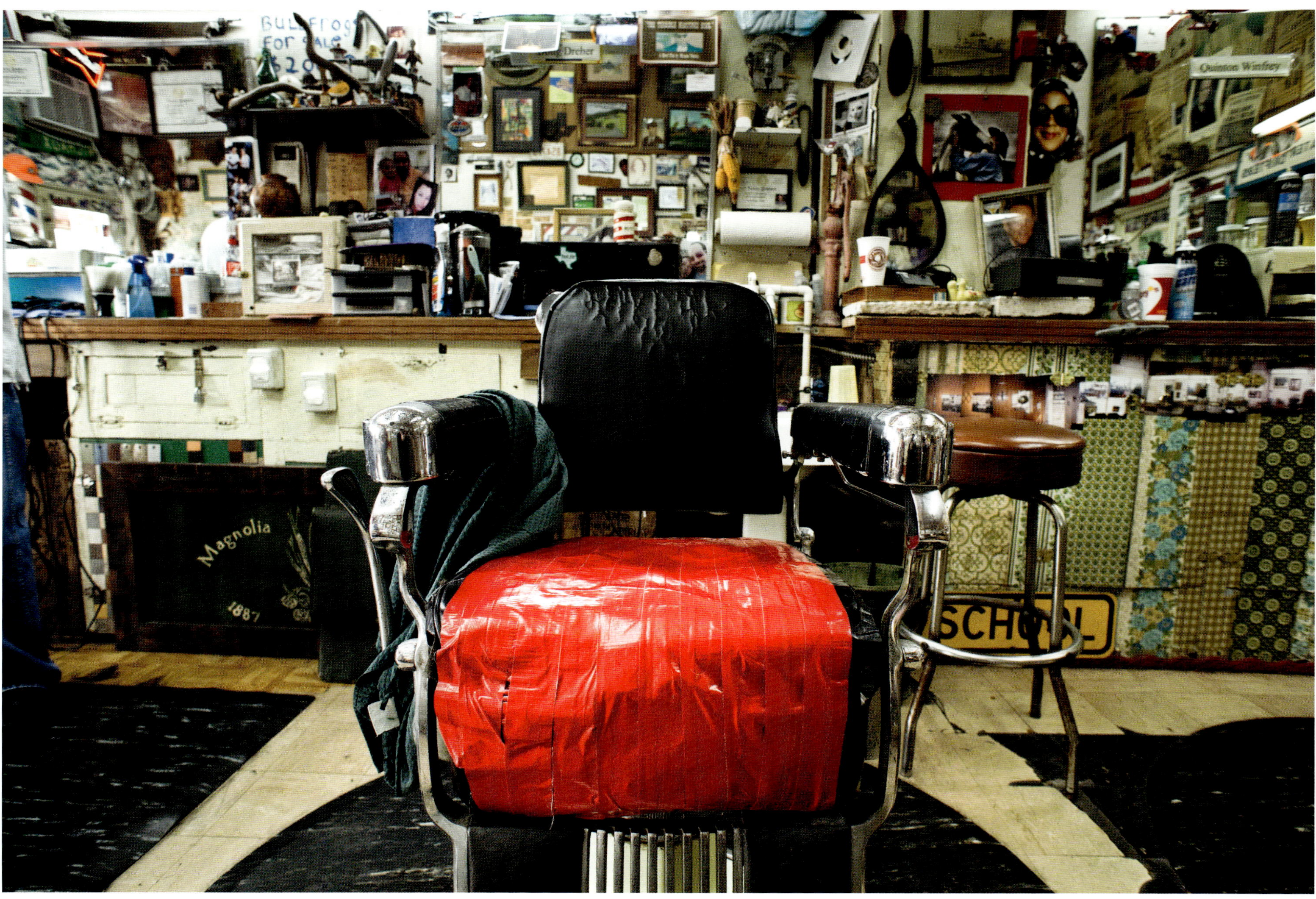

Doug's Barbershop, Houston, Texas

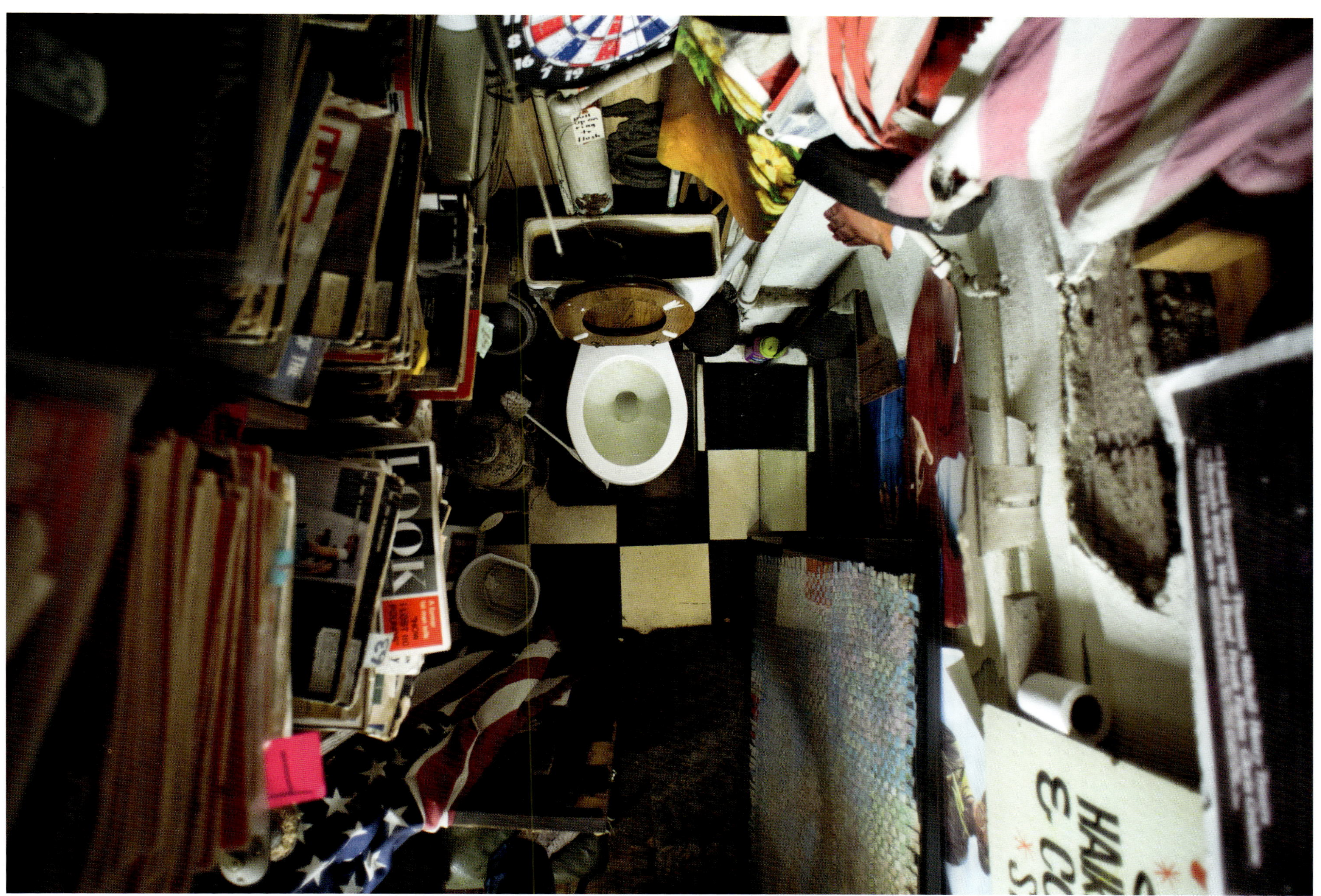

Doug's Barbershop, Houston, Texas

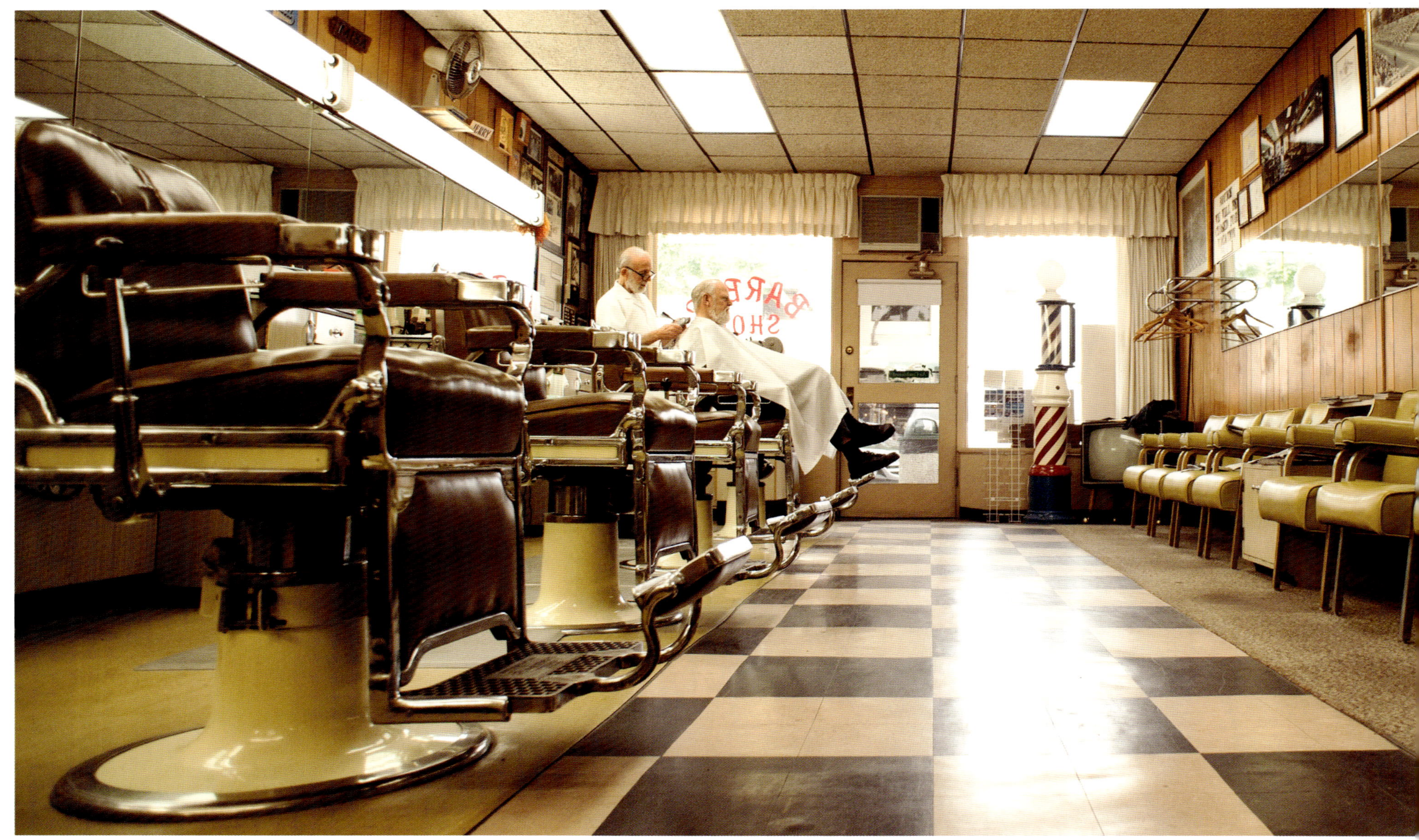

Larchmont Barbershop, Los Angeles, California

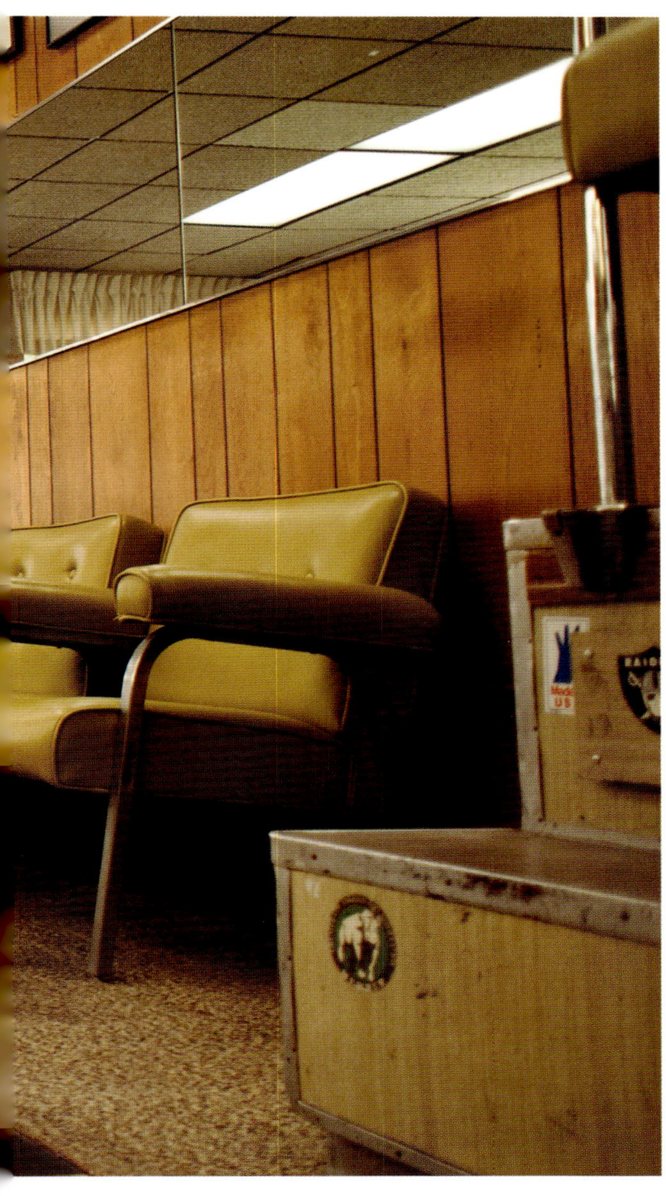

"Fifty-four years in this shop and I've never had a lease."

– Jerry, Larchmont Barbershop, Los Angeles, California

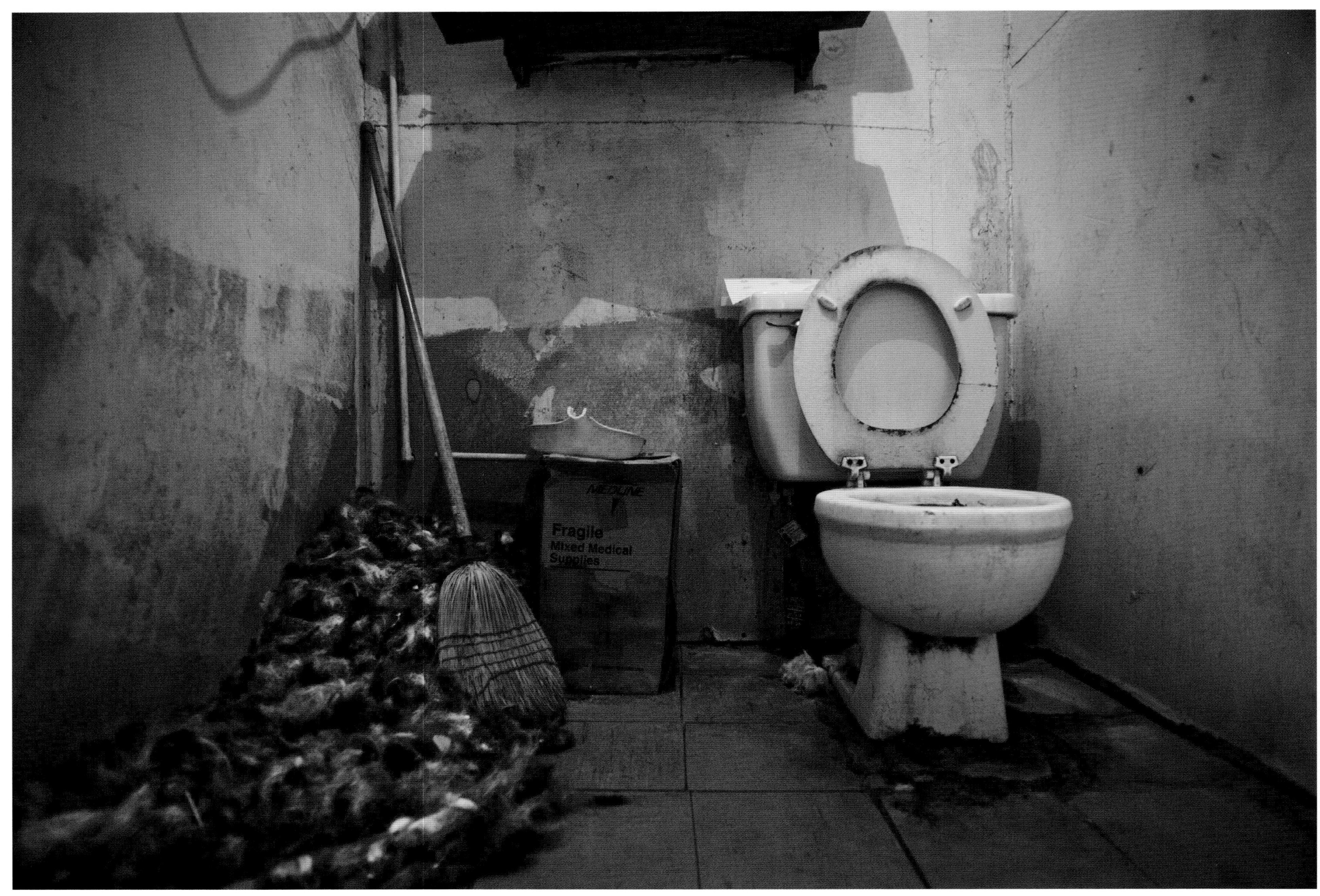

Unknown, Alabama

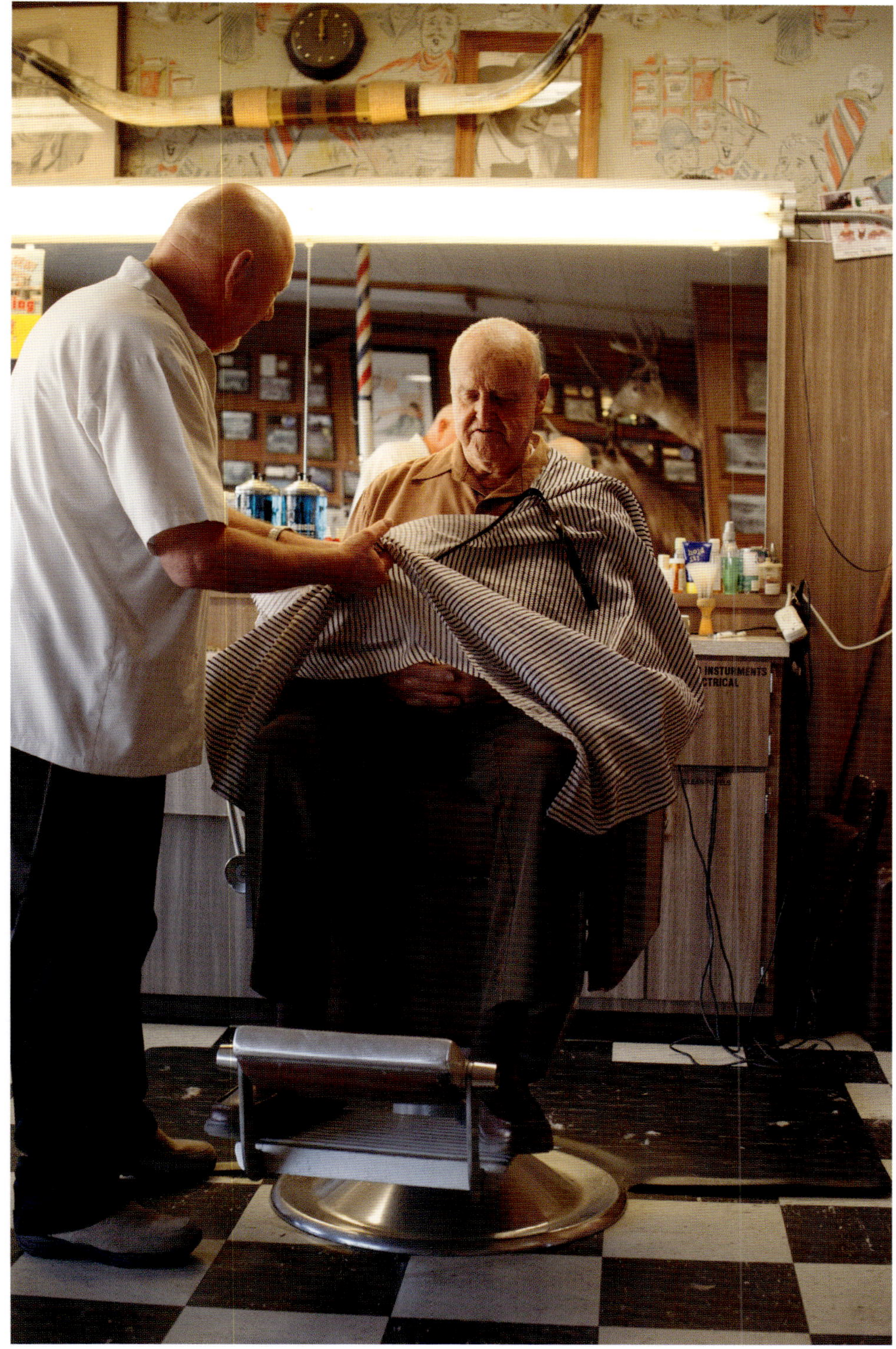

City Barbershop, Ramona, California

"It's getting harder and harder getting into your chair."

"You should have taken better care of yourself when you were younger."

"Well, I'm glad I didn't."

– Customer and Wayne Shannon, City Barbershop, Ramona, California

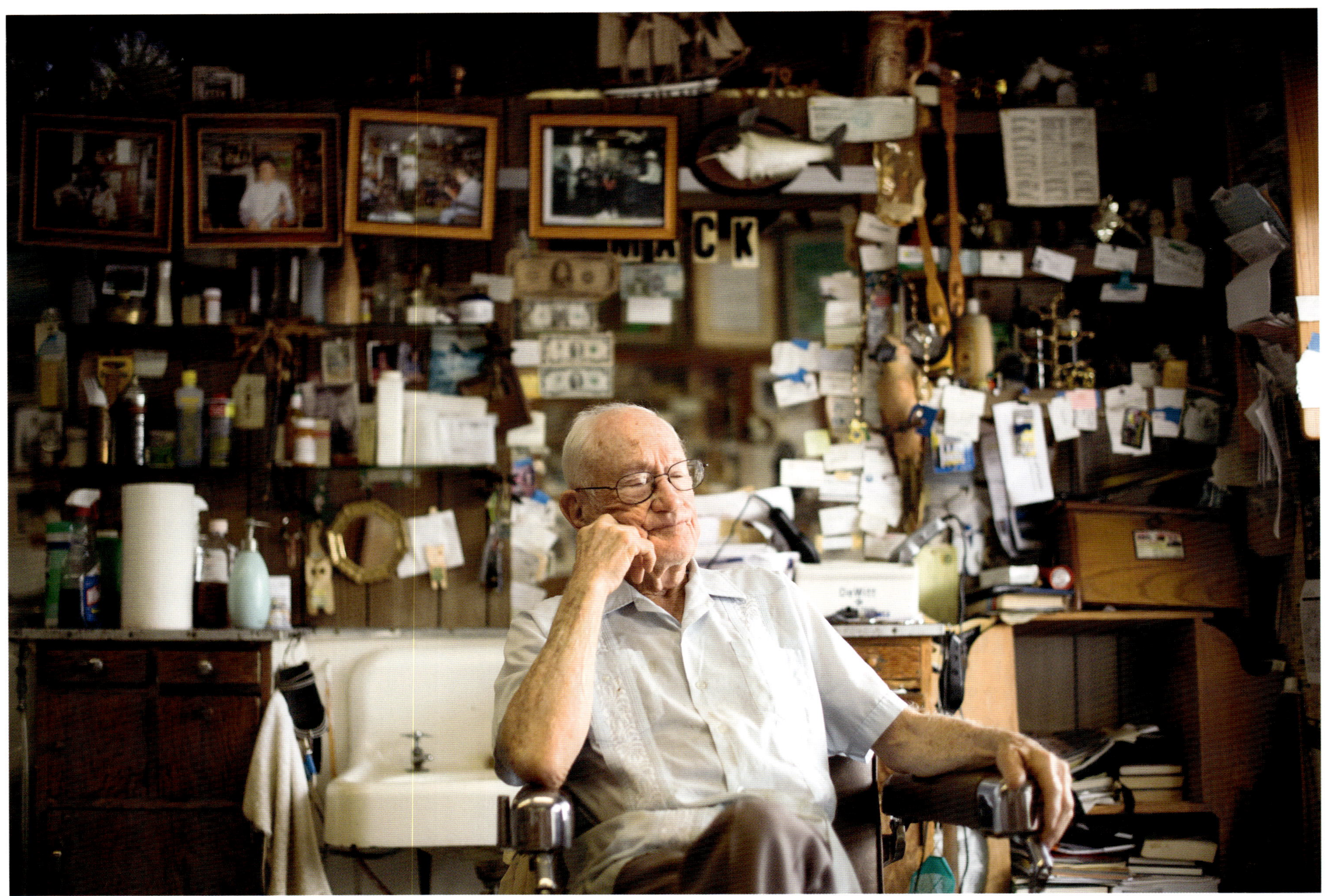

Mack Brooks Barbershop, Crestview, Florida

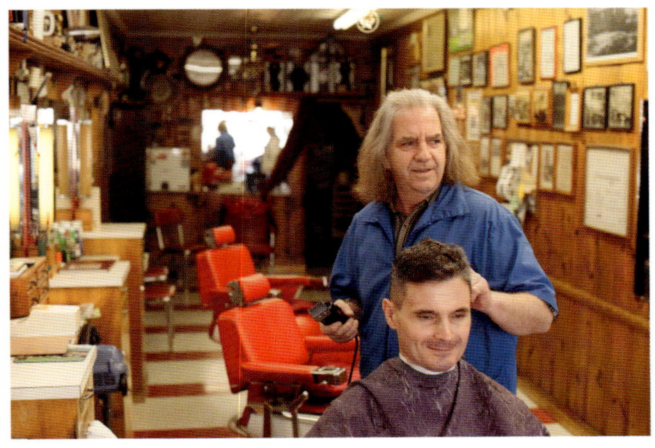

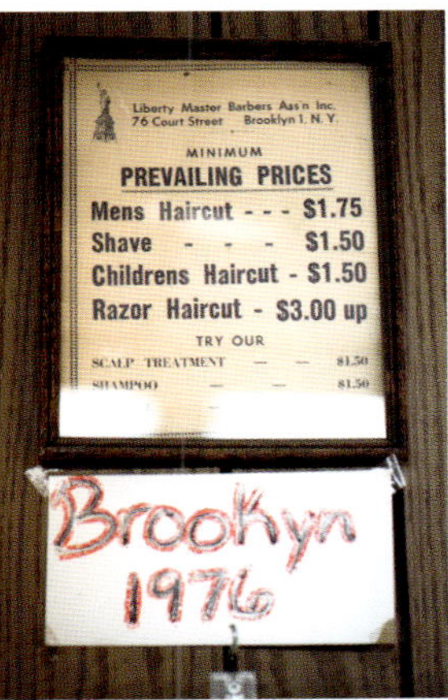
Liberty Master Barbers Ass'n Inc.
76 Court Street Brooklyn 1, N. Y.
MINIMUM
PREVAILING PRICES
Mens Haircut - - - $1.75
Shave - - - $1.50
Childrens Haircut - $1.50
Razor Haircut - $3.00 up
TRY OUR
SCALP TREATMENT — — $1.50
SHAMPOO — — $1.50
Brookyn
1976

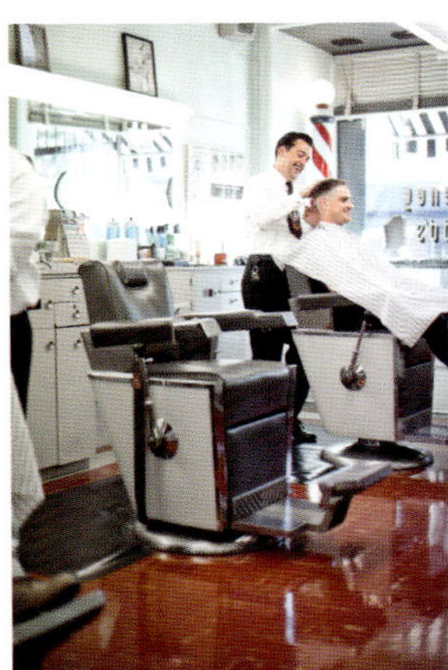

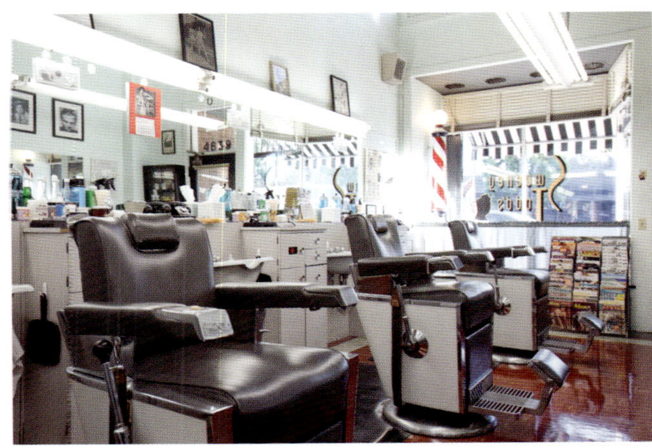

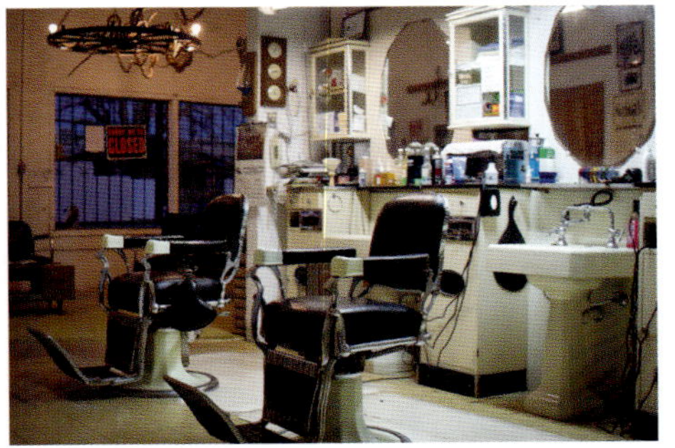

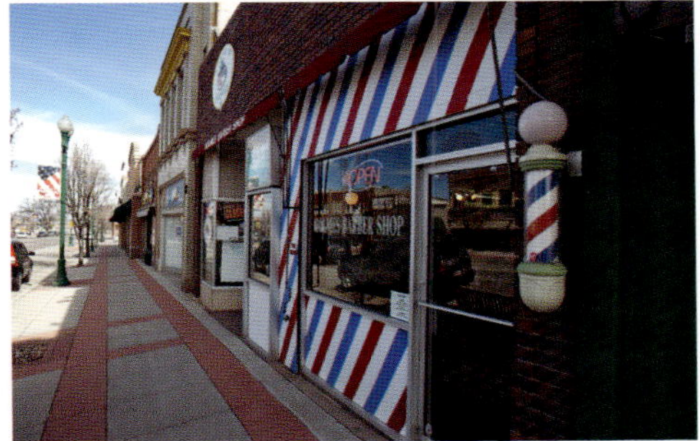

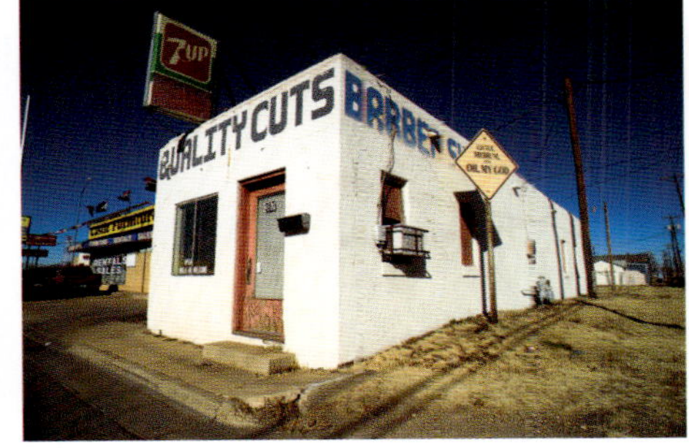
7UP
QUALITY CUTS

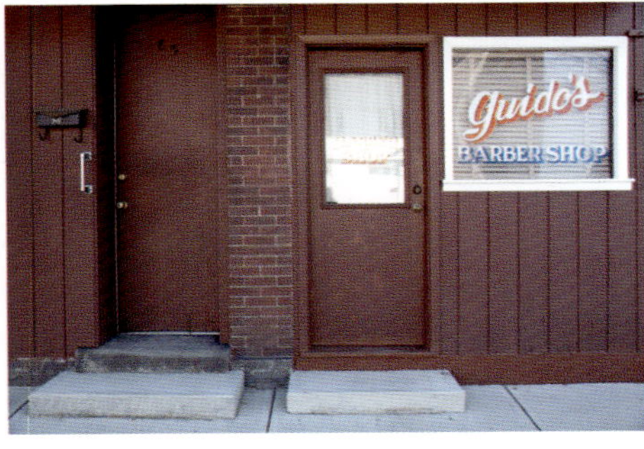
Guido's
BARBER SHOP

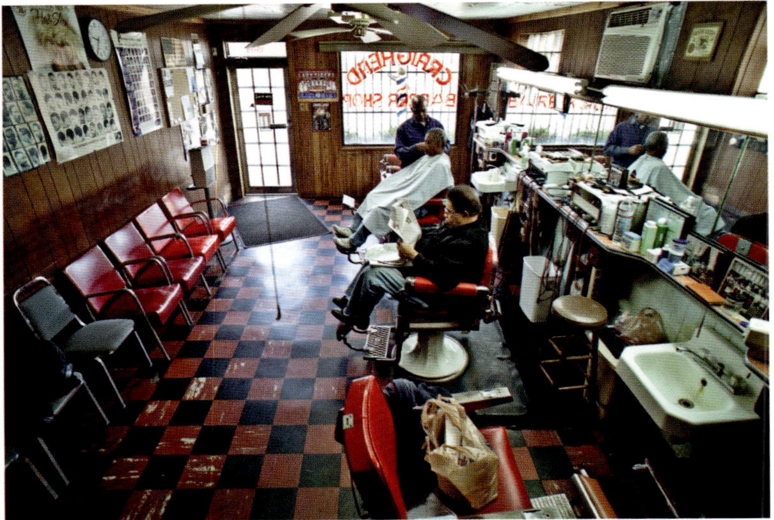

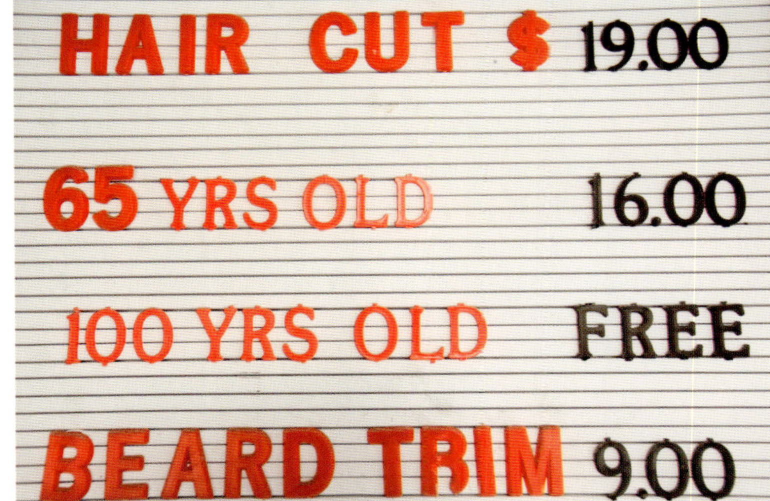
HAIR CUT $ 19.00
65 YRS OLD 16.00
100 YRS OLD FREE
BEARD TRIM 9.00

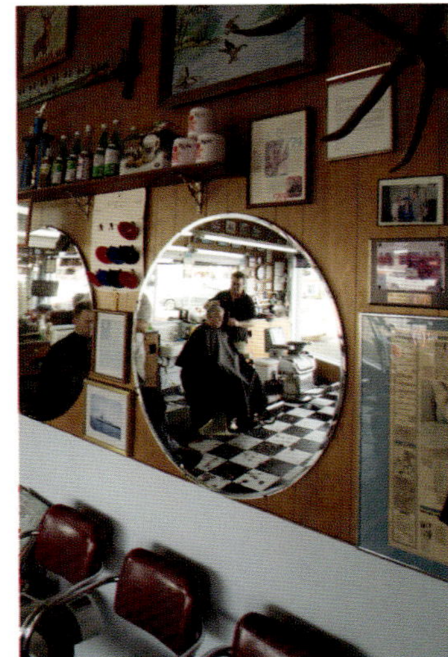

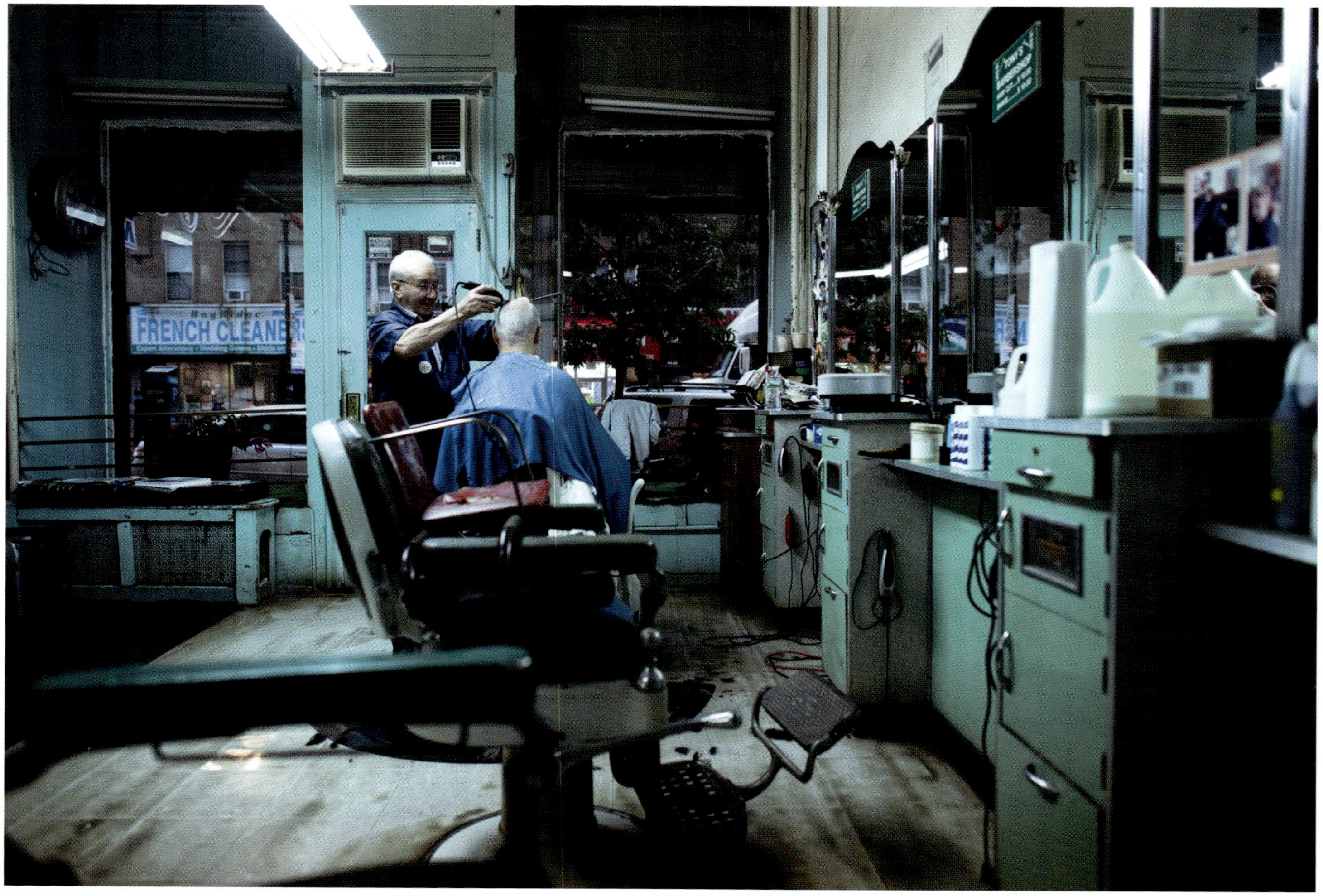
FRENCH CLEANERS

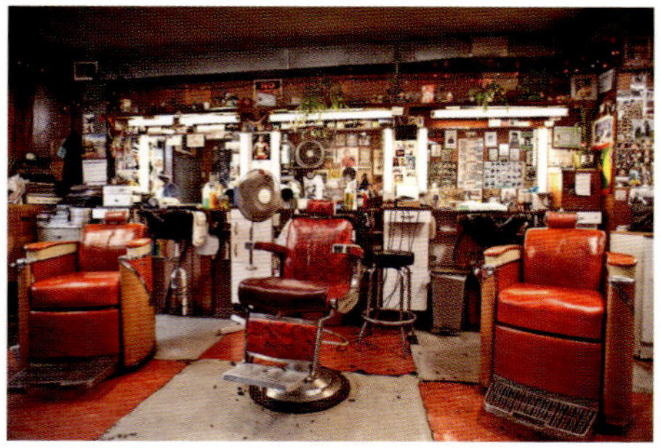

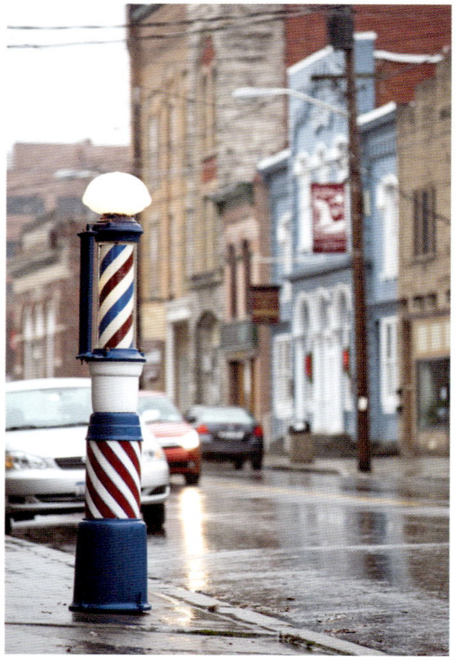

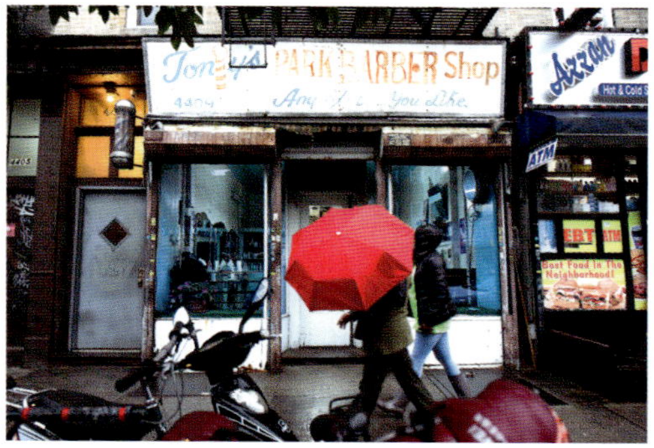
BARBER Shop
ATM

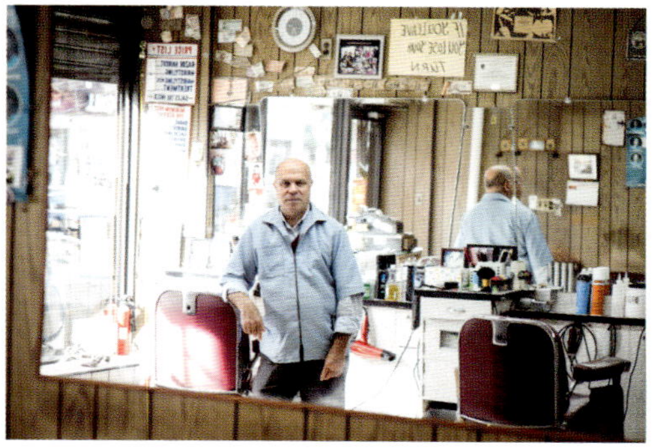

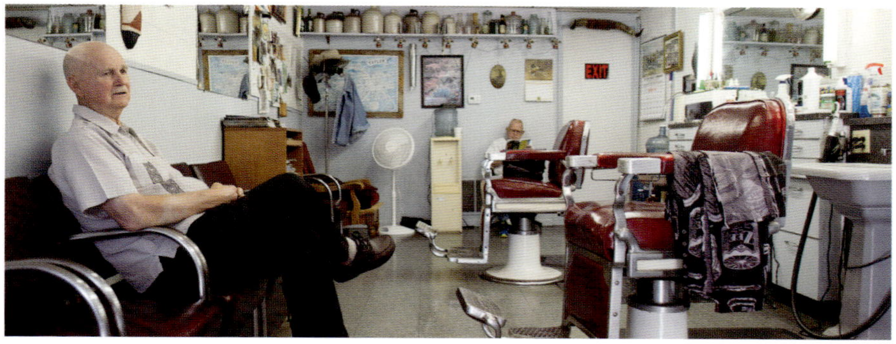
EXIT

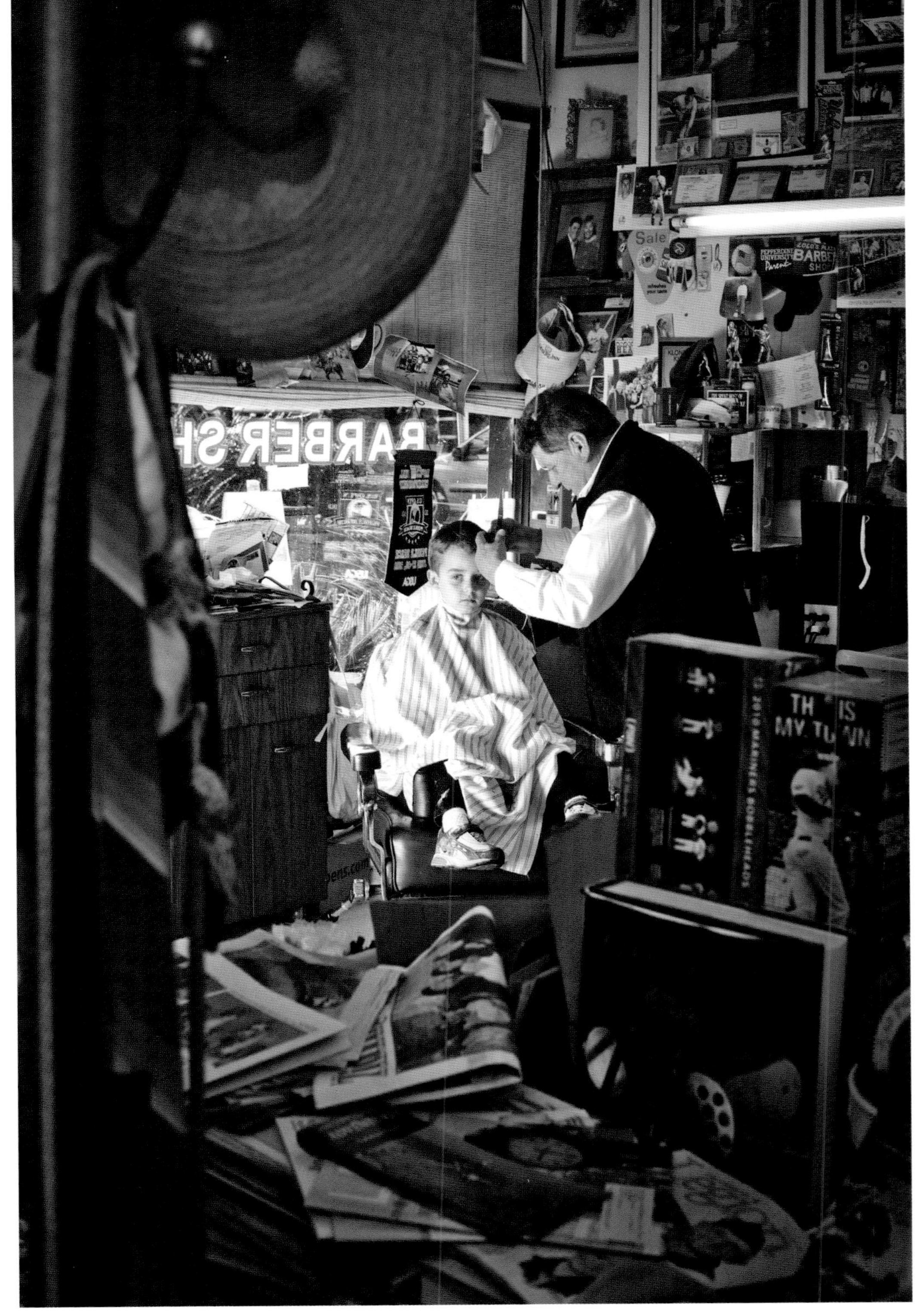

Lolo's Barbershop, Catalina Island, California

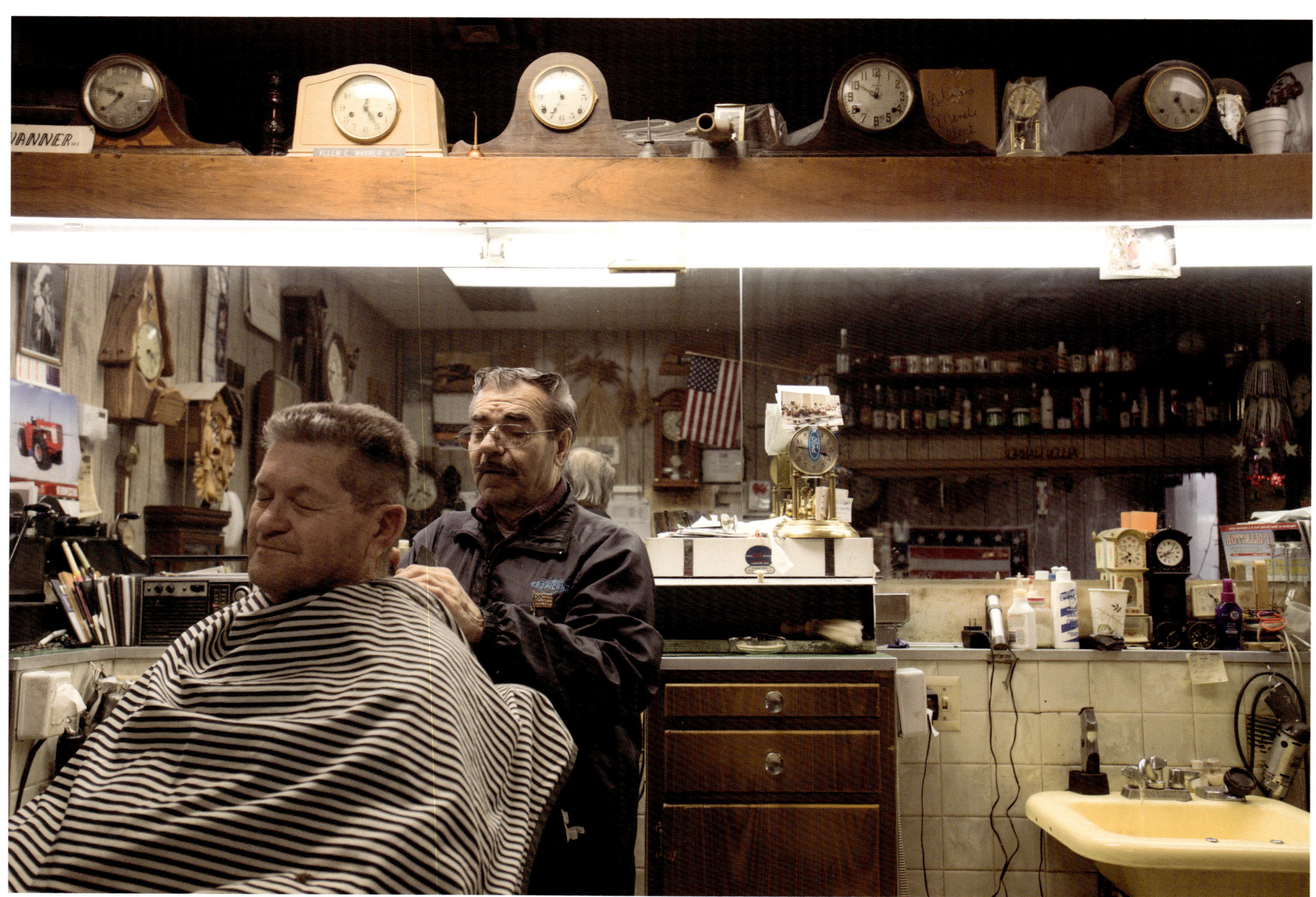

Deluxe Barbershop, Mandan, North Dakota

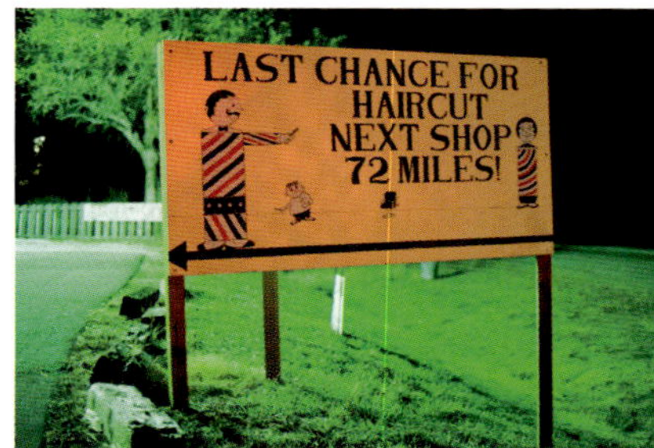
LAST CHANCE FOR
HAIRCUT
NEXT SHOP
72 MILES!

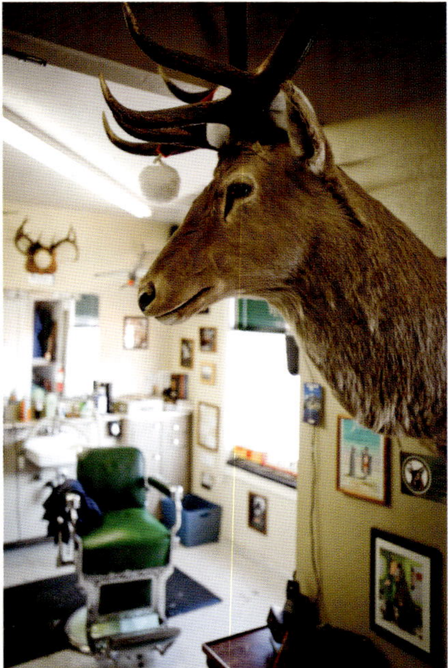

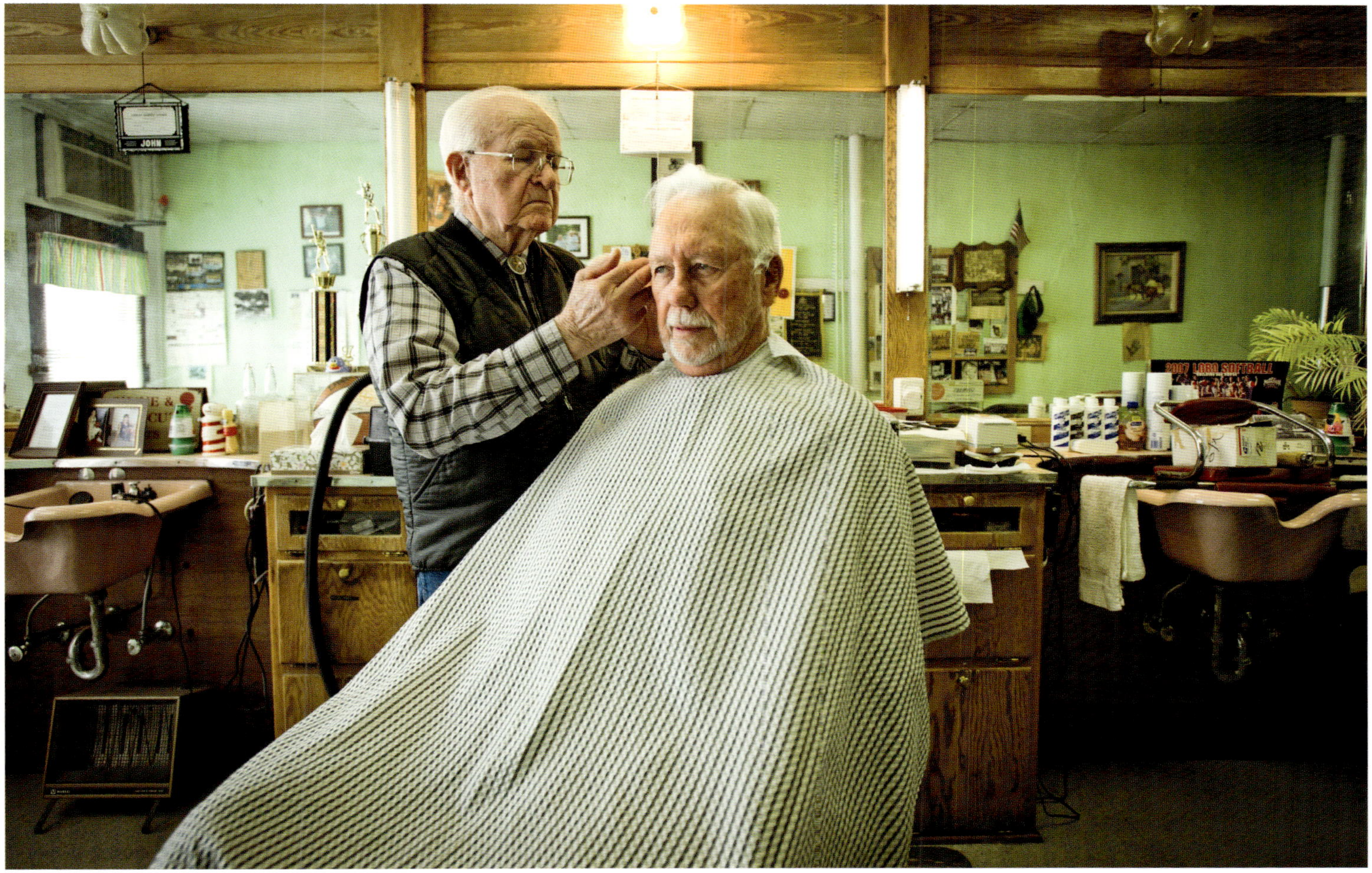

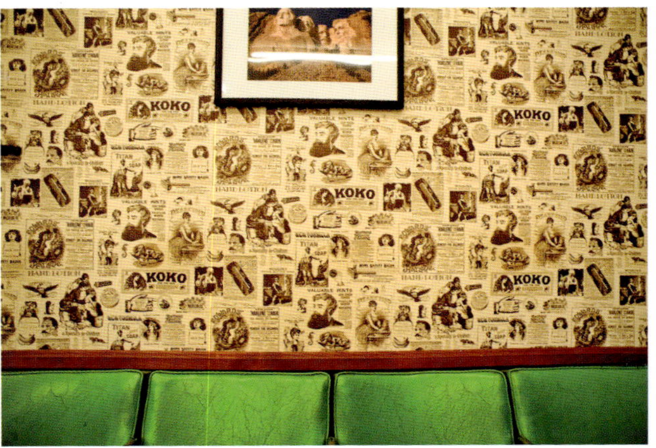
KOKO

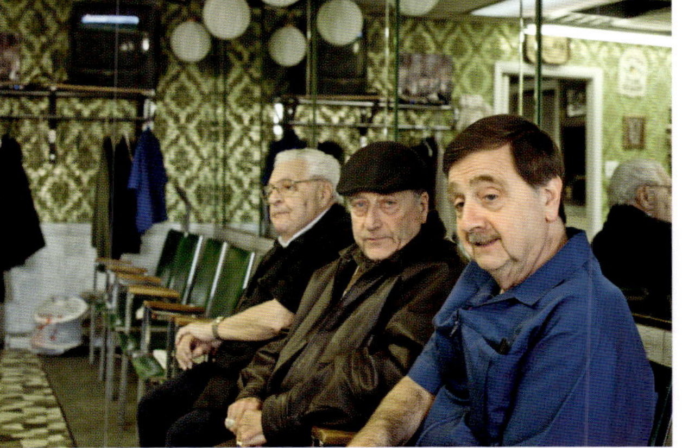

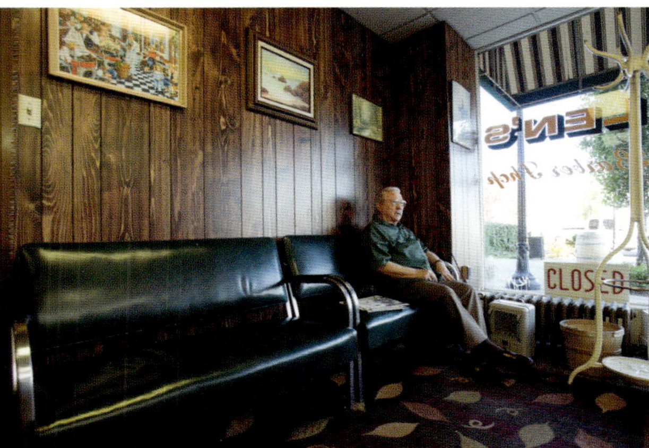

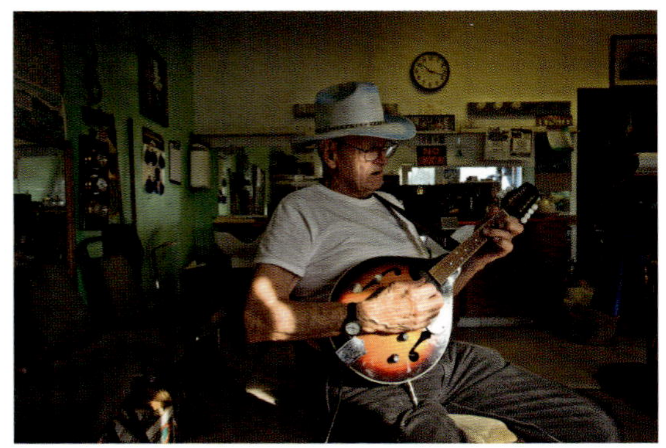

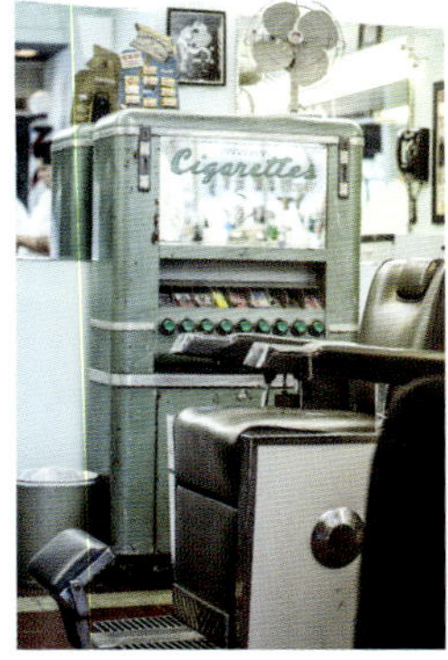
Cigarettes

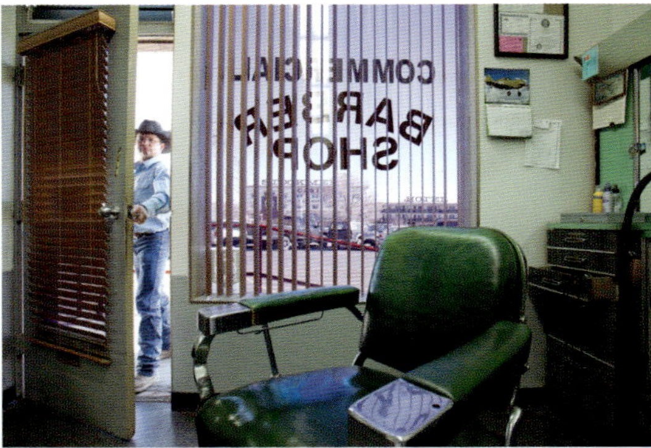

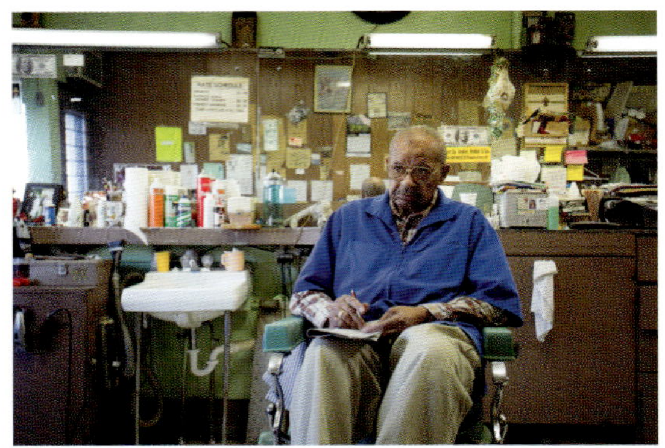

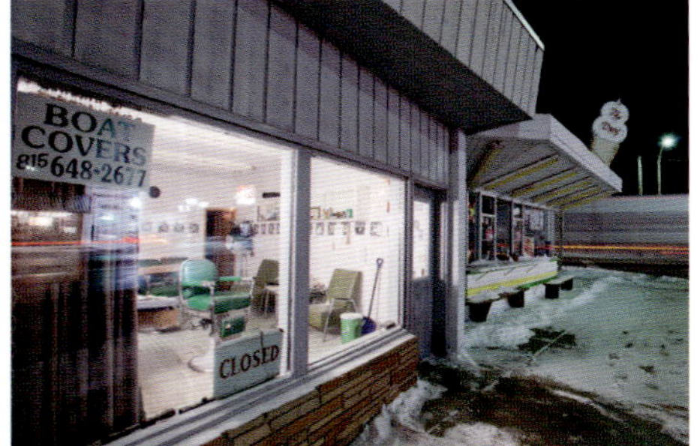
CLOSED

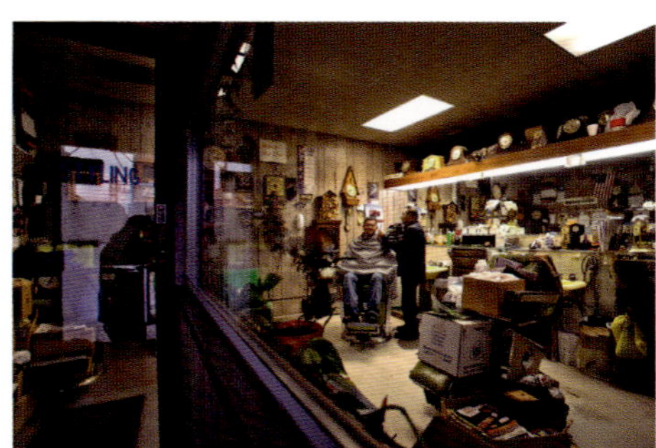

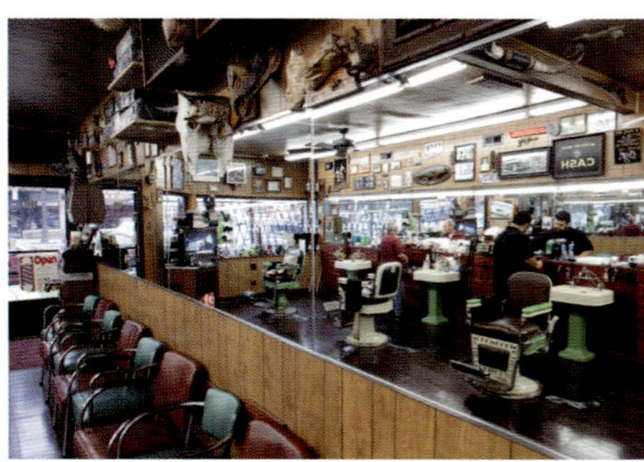

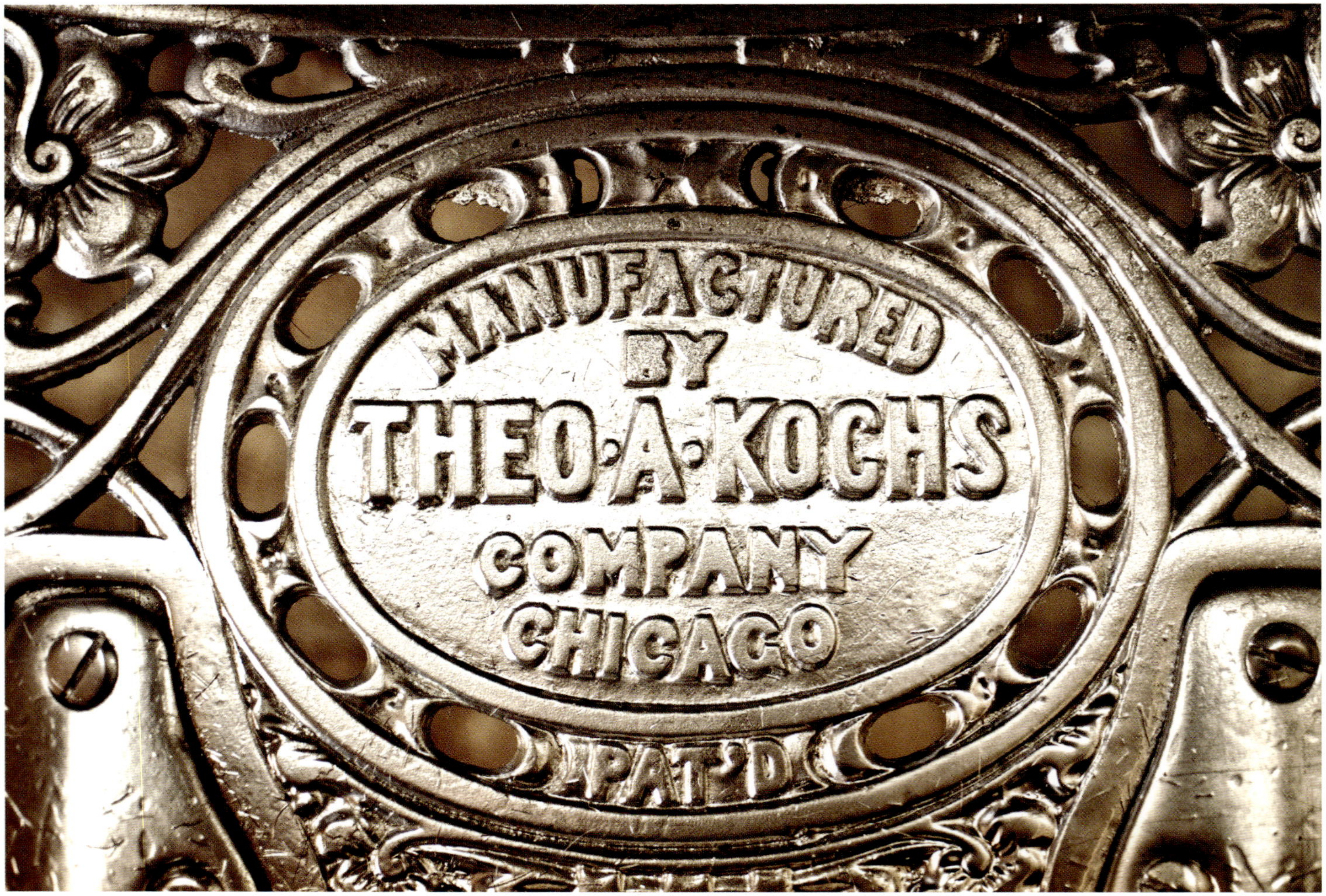

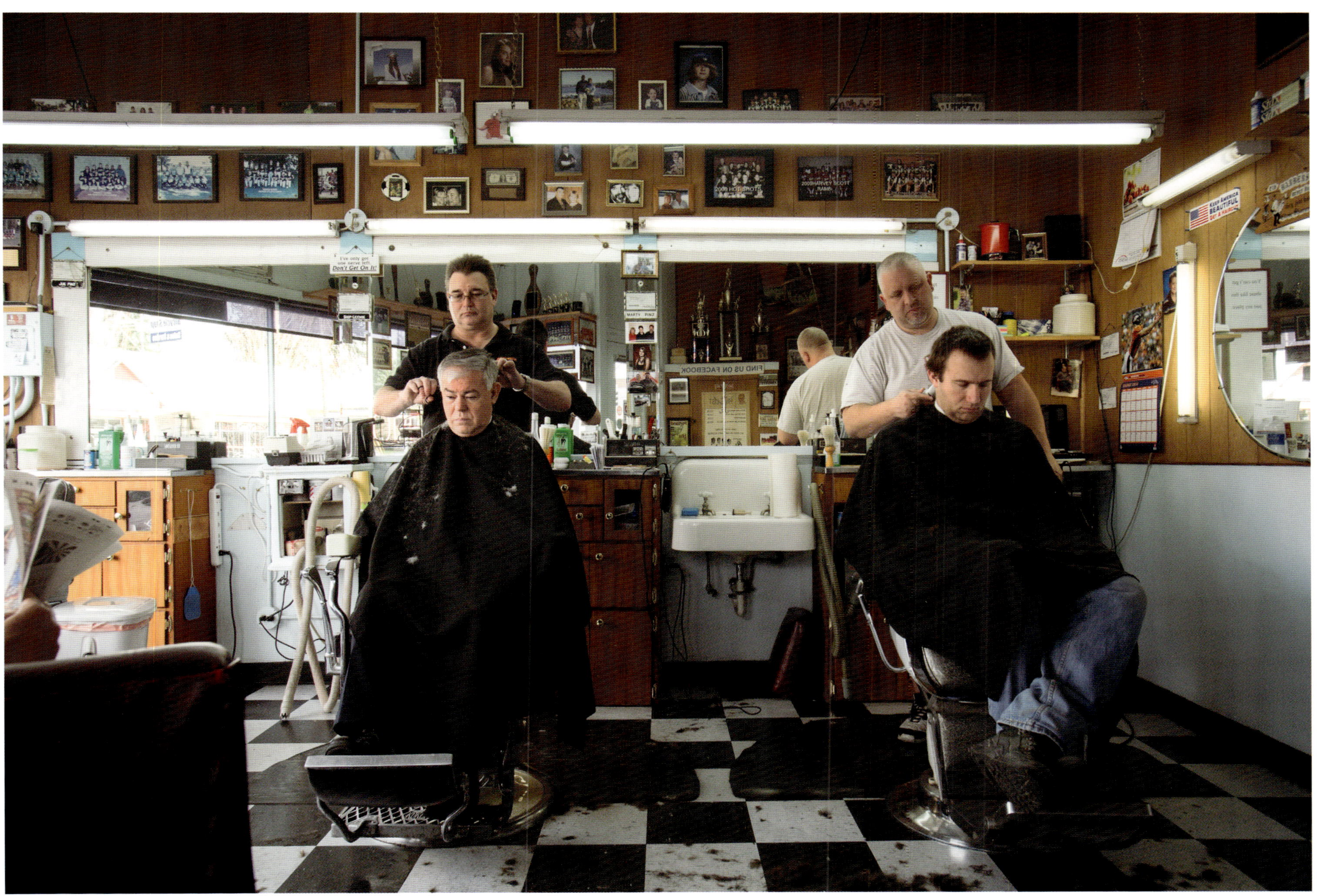

Roseway Barbershop, Portland, Oregon

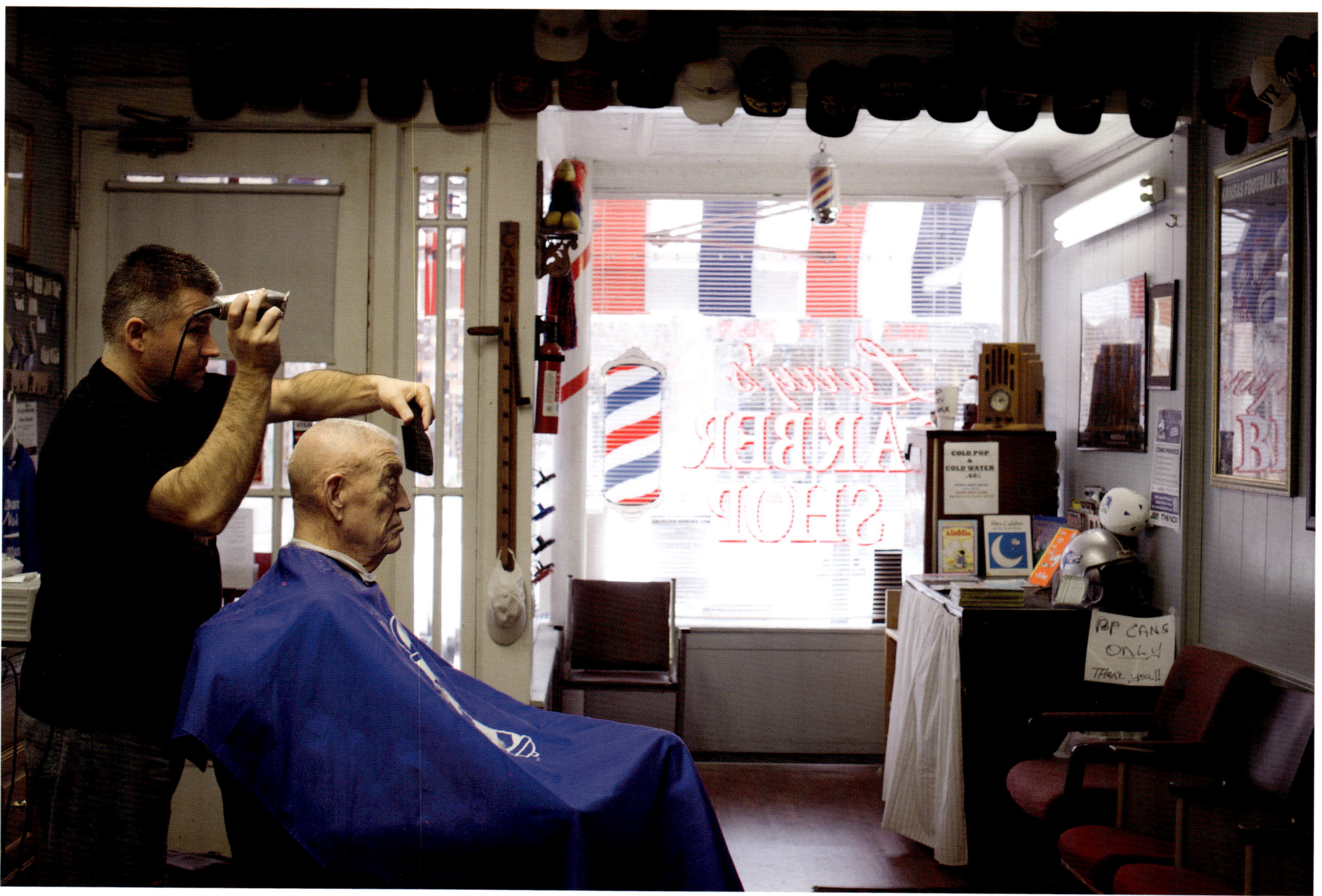

Larry's Barbershop, Lawrence, Kansas

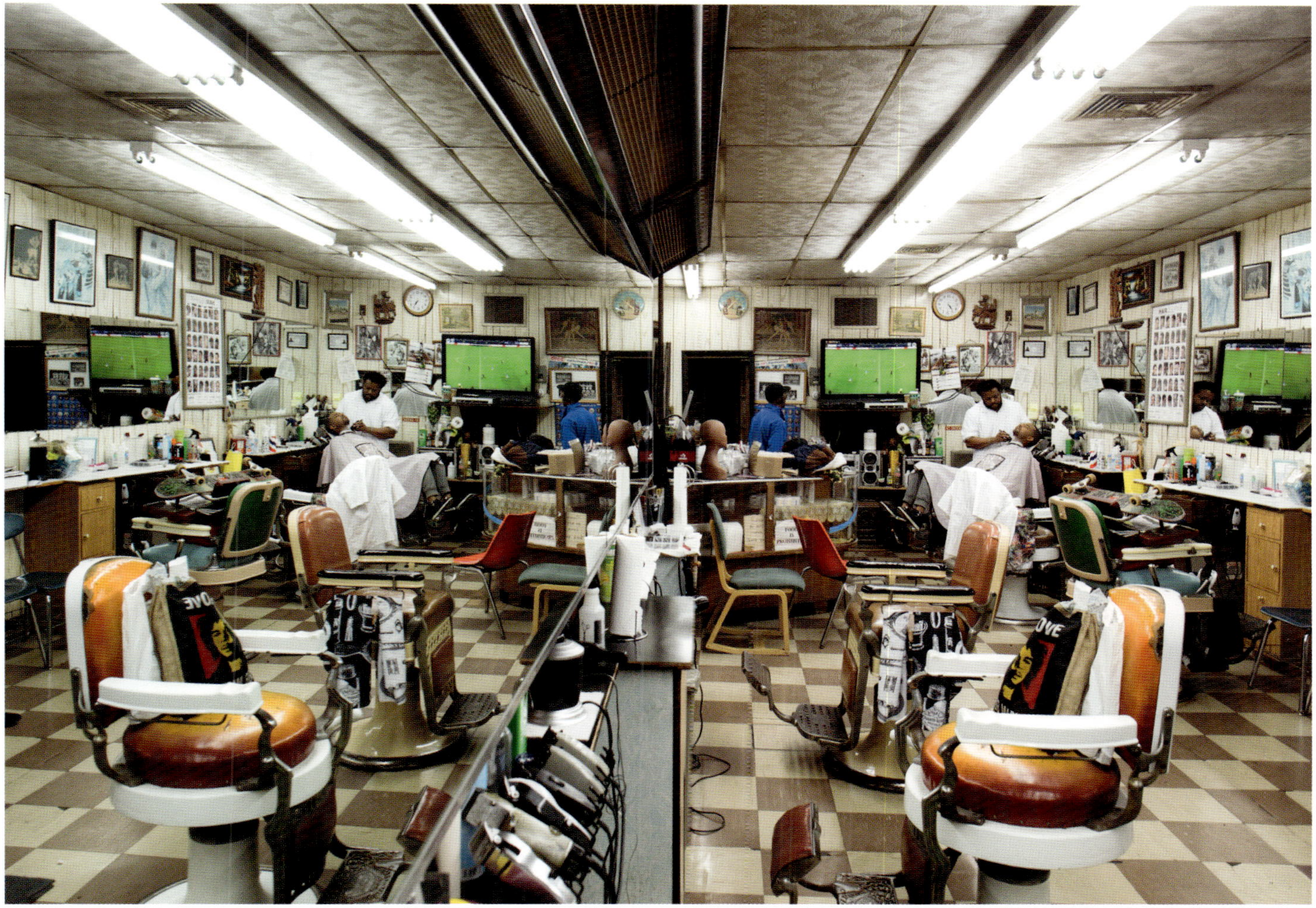

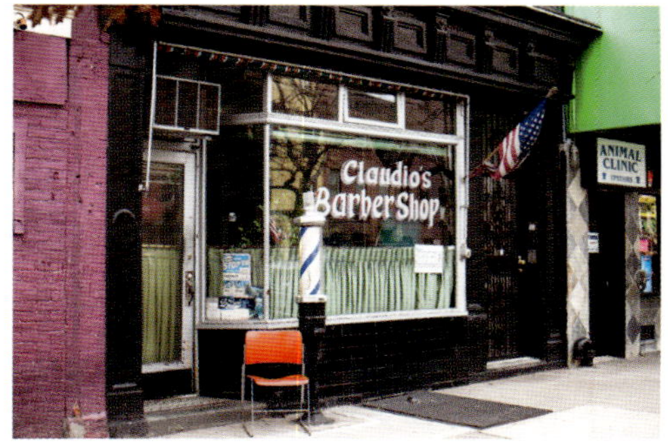
Claudio's
Barber Shop
ANIMAL
CLINIC
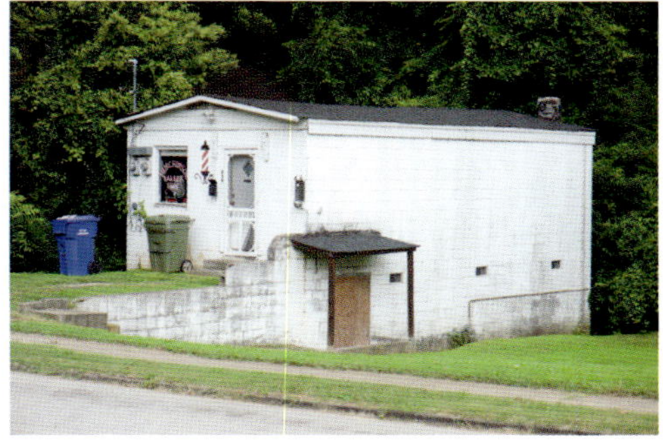
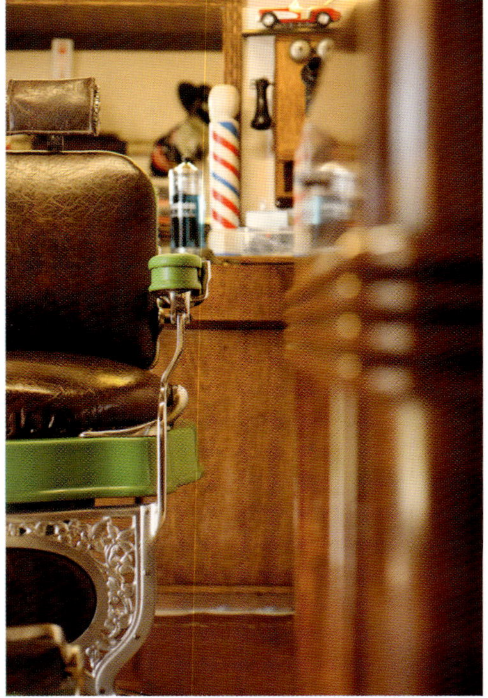
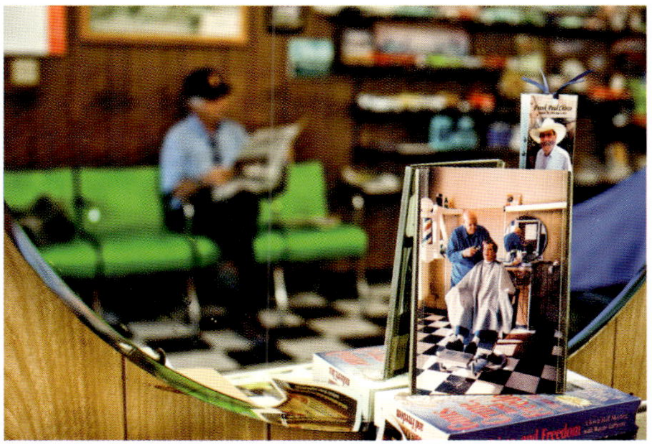
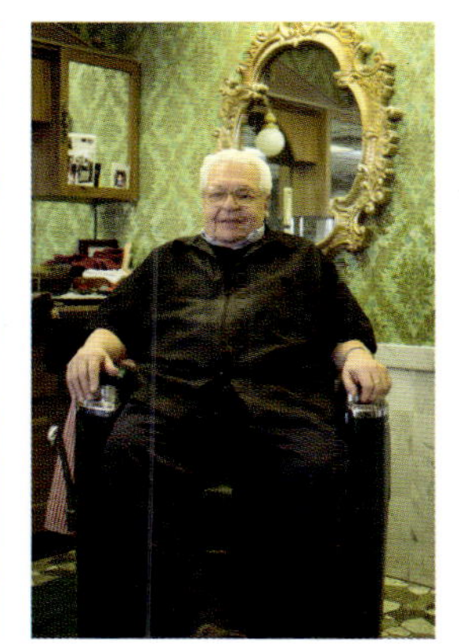
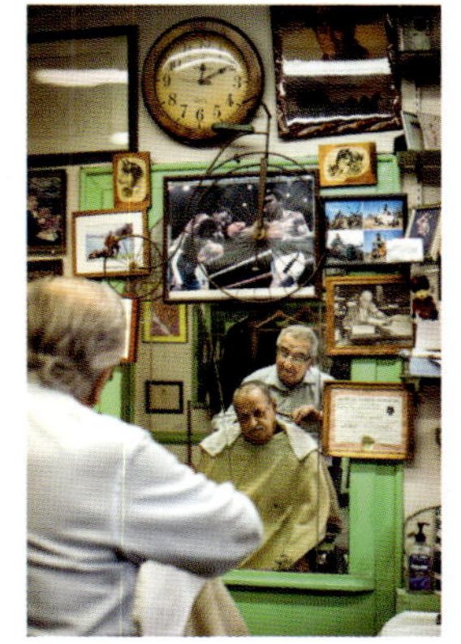
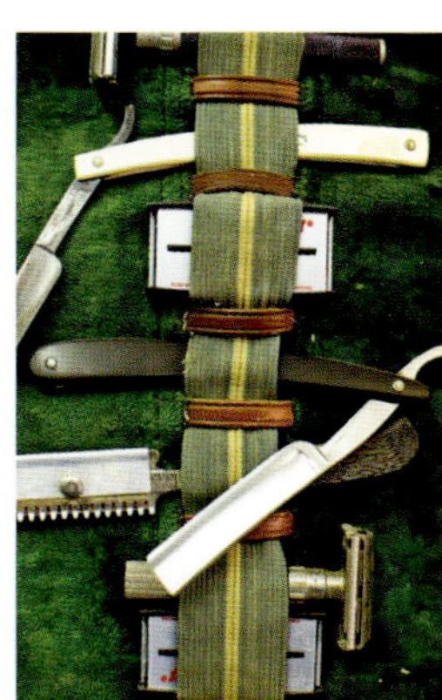

"Yup, I've been doing this 54 years.
Might make it another 54,
I don't know."

– Honest John Deitrich, Burlington, Kansas

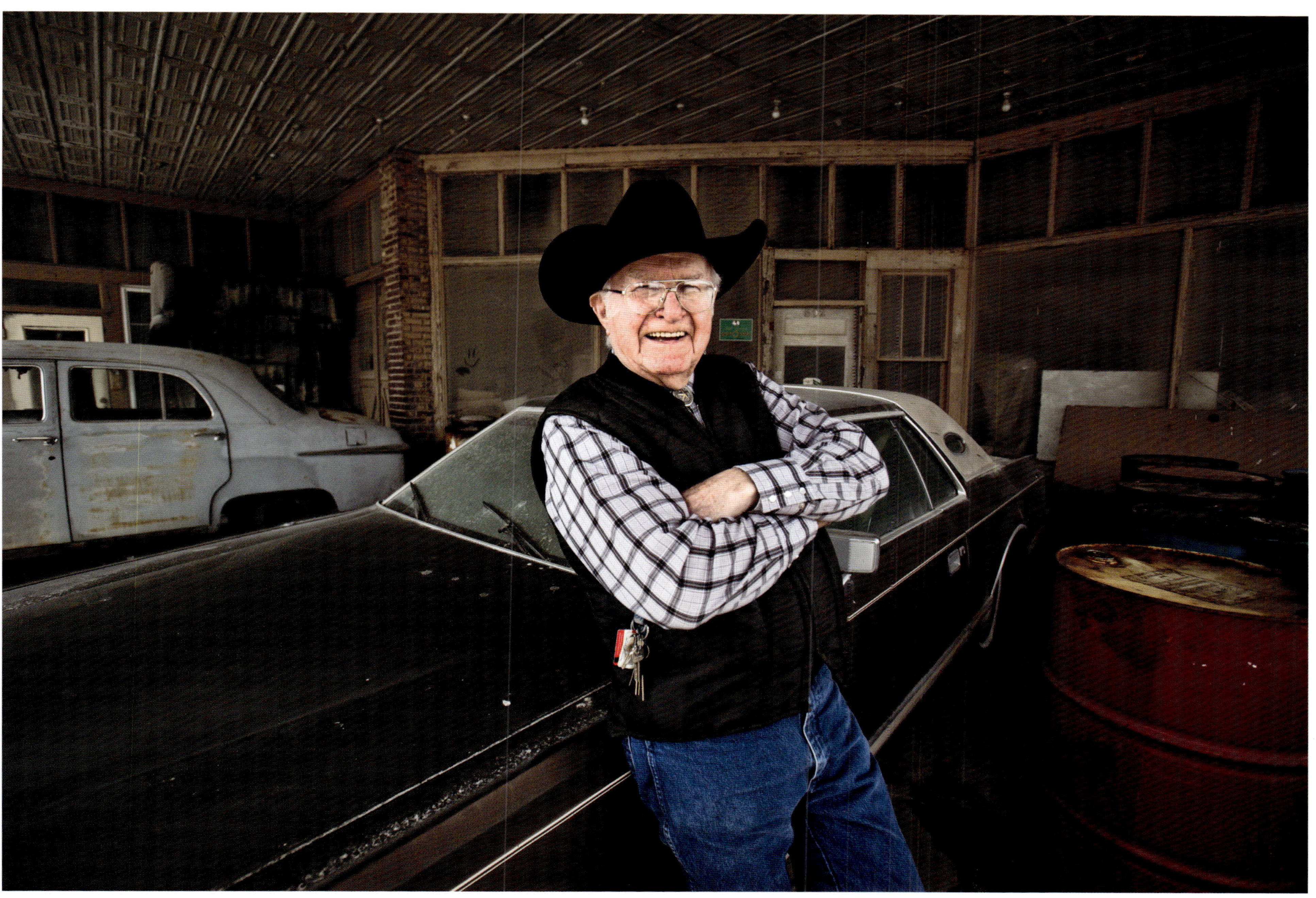

Honest John Deitrich, Burlington, Kansas

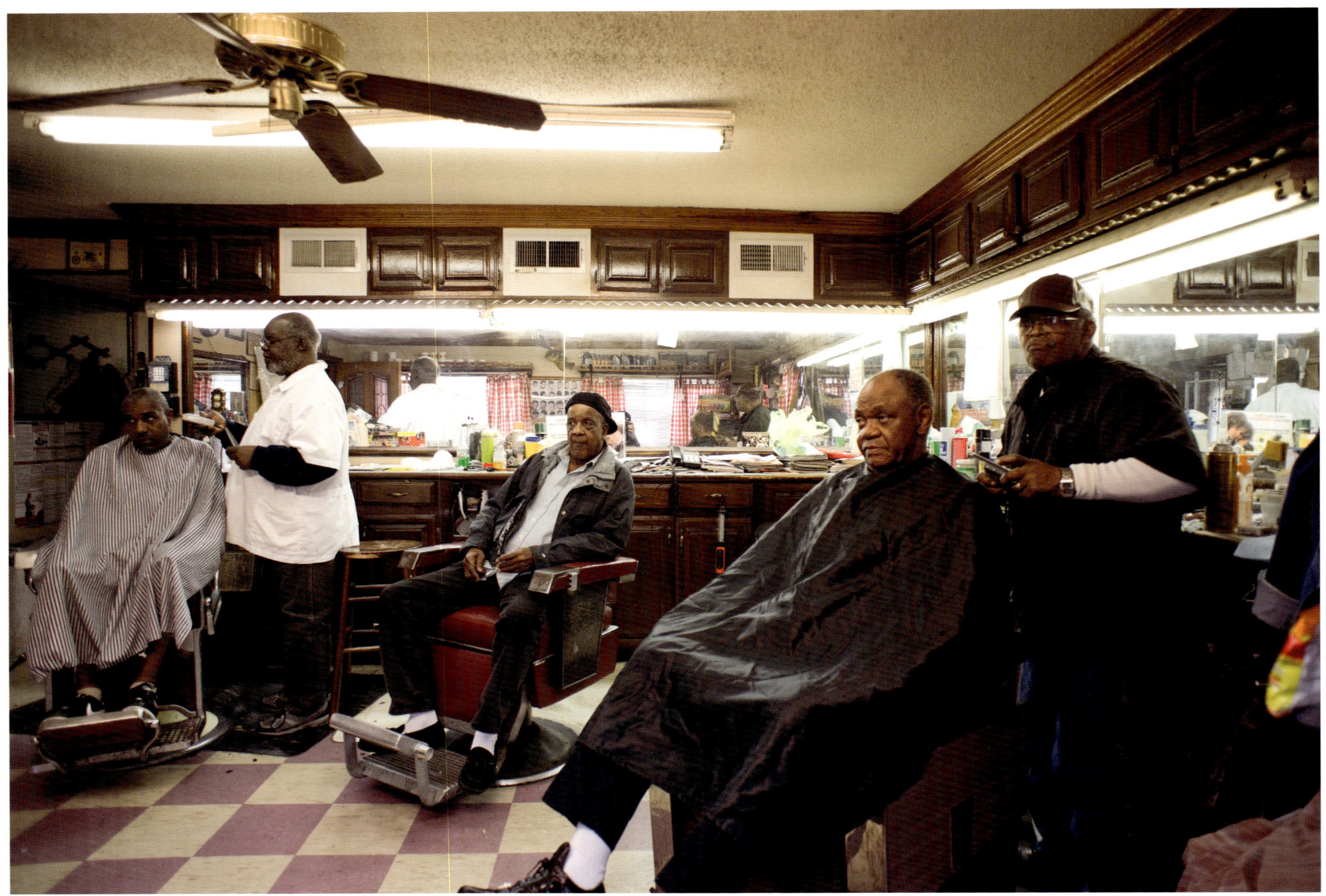

Harold's Barbershop and snack parlour, New Orleans, Louisiana

“Harold Young.
My last name is Herald.
I was young before I was Herald.”

– Herald Young, Harold’s Barber and Snack Parlor, New Orleans, Louisiana

ED
JACQUES
Ed's Barbershop
50 Years of GREAT HAIRCUTS
1958 - 2008
Barbershop will be closing at 4:00pm on Saturdays
TUES TO FRI
8 TO 530
SAT CLOSING
4:00
CLOSED MONDAY
Barbershop will be closing at 4:00pm on Saturdays

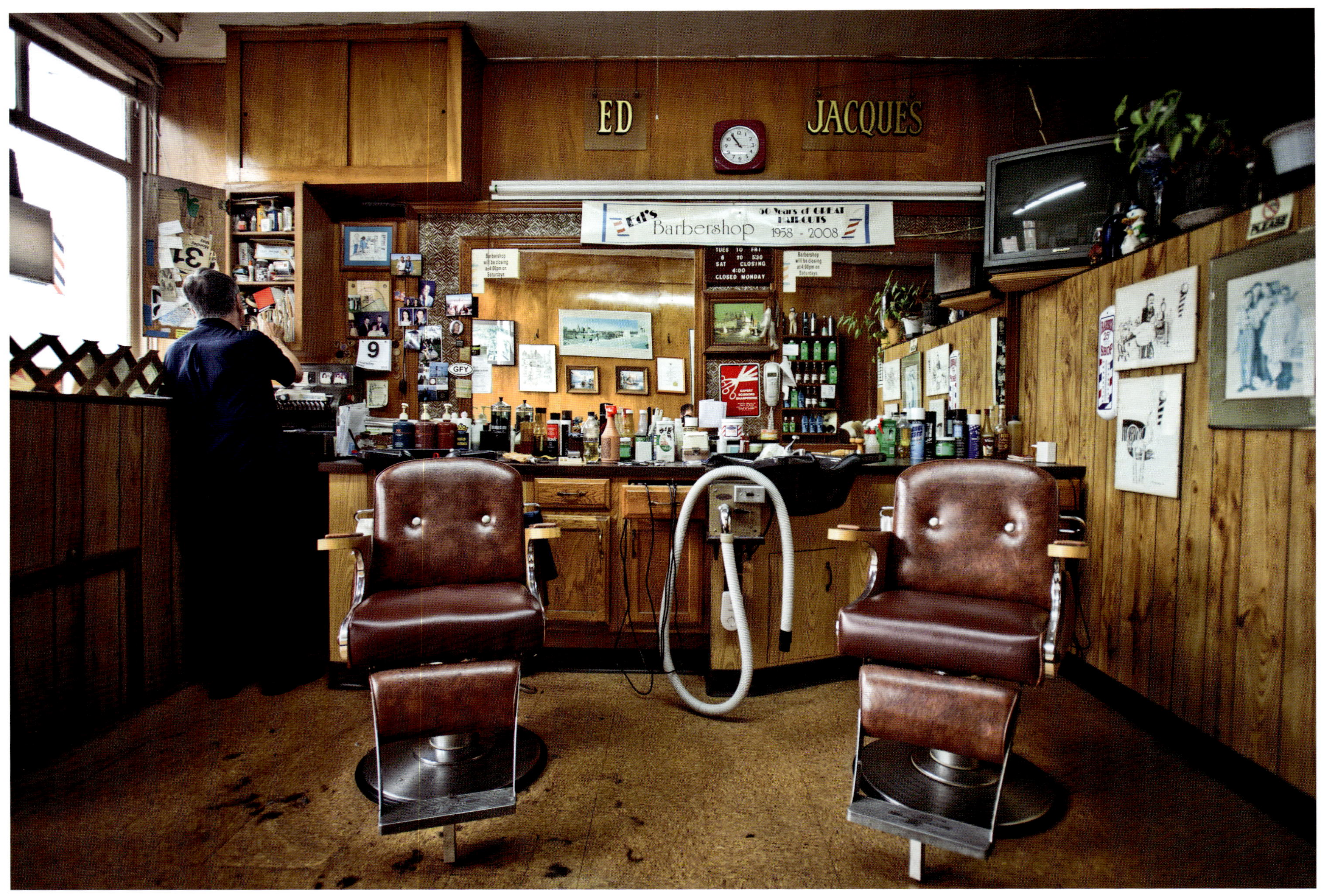

Ed's Barbershop, Providence, Rhode Island

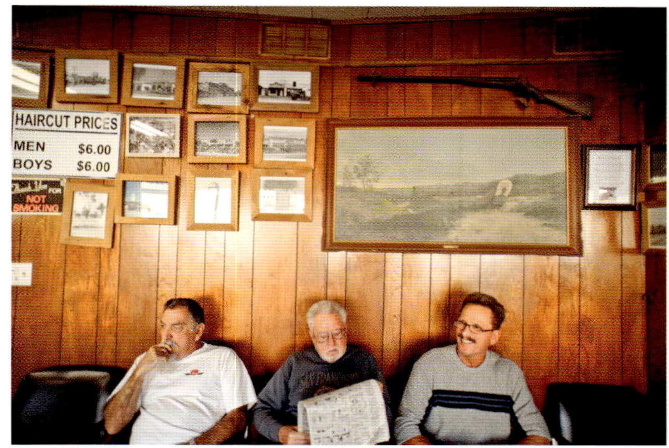
HAIRCUT PRICES
MEN $6.00
BOYS $6.00
NOT SMOKING

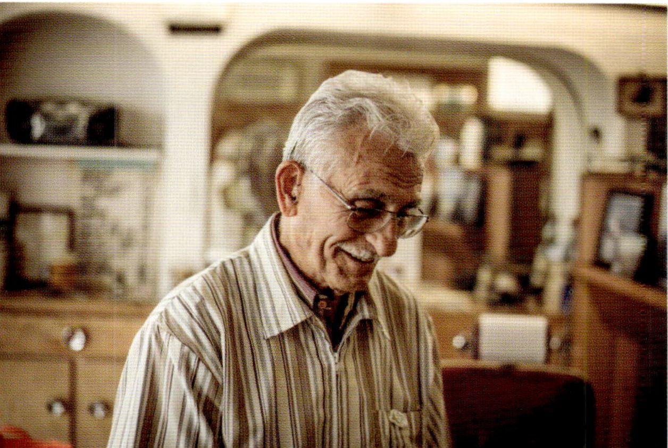

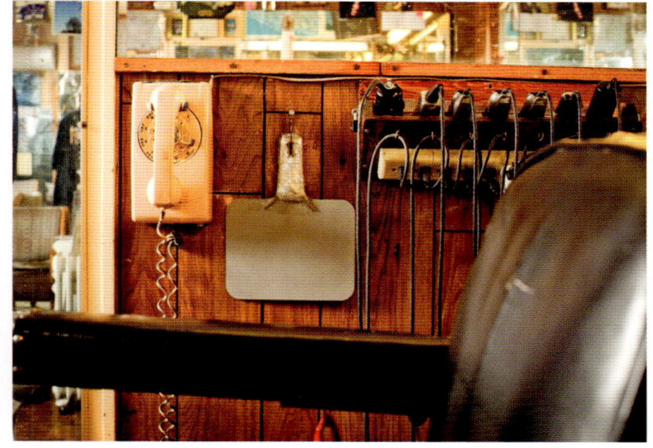

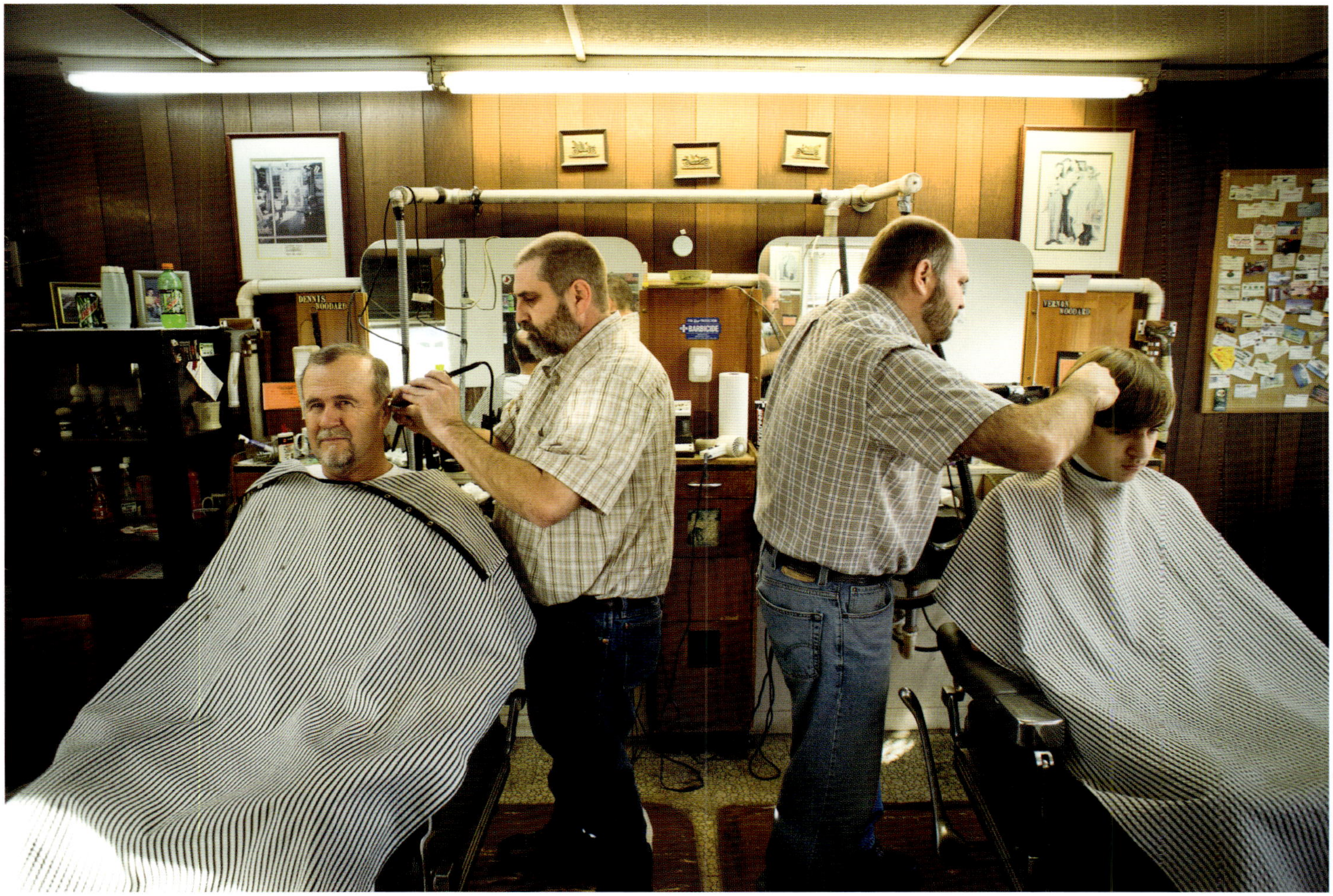

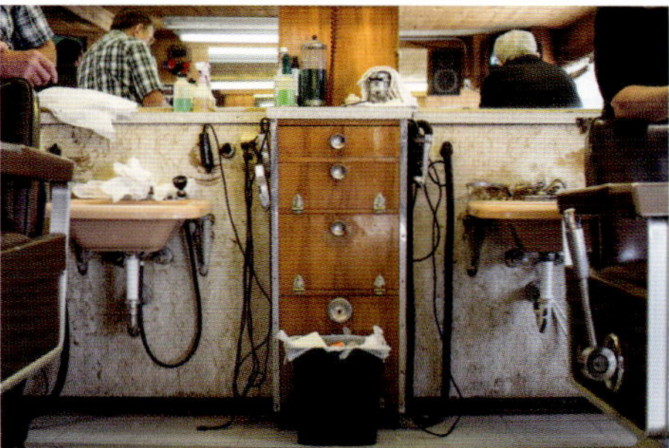

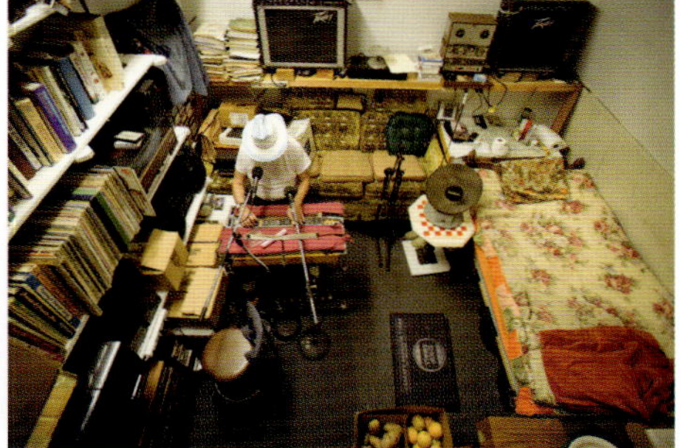

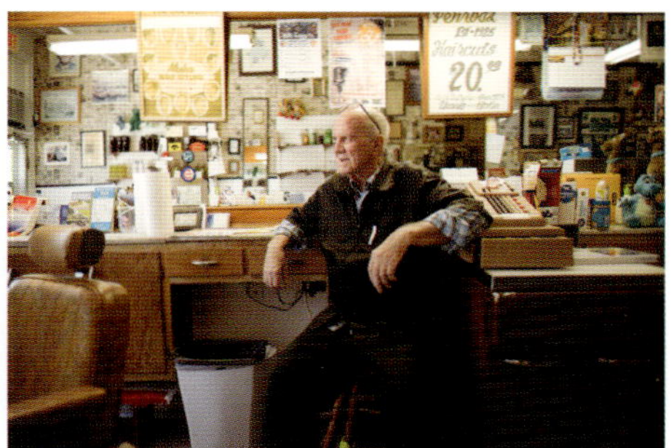

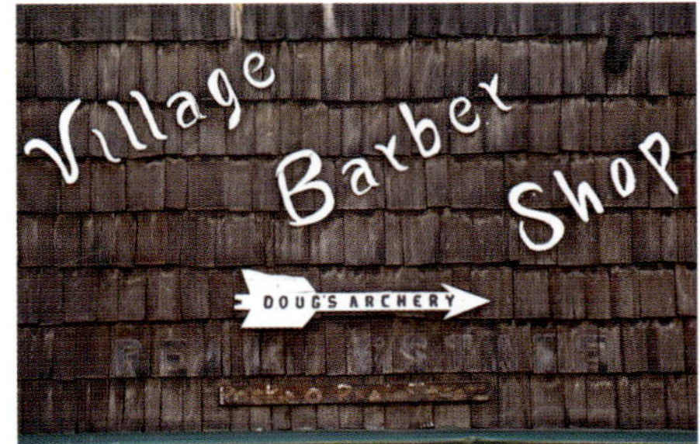
Village Barber Shop
DOUG'S ARCHERY

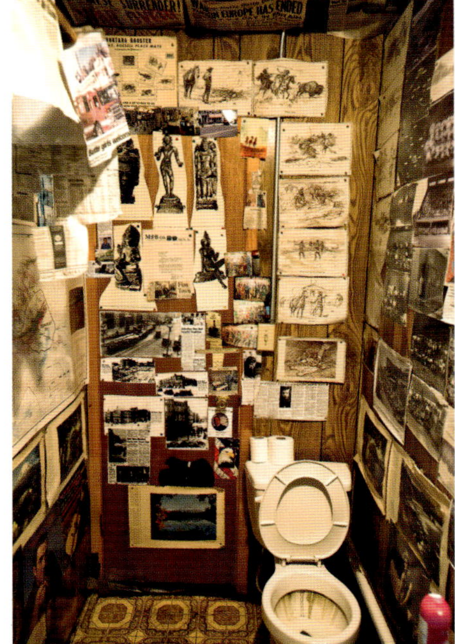

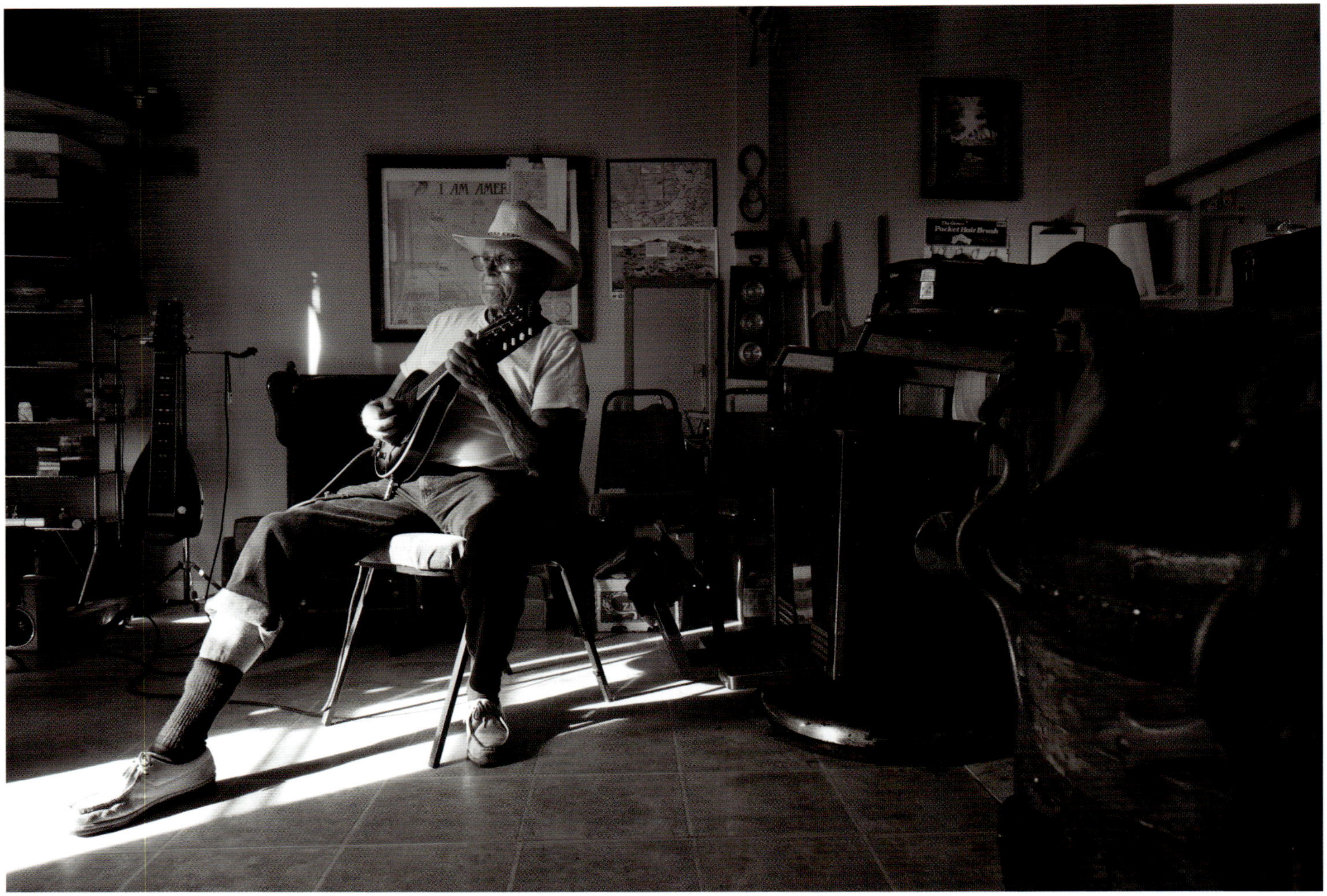

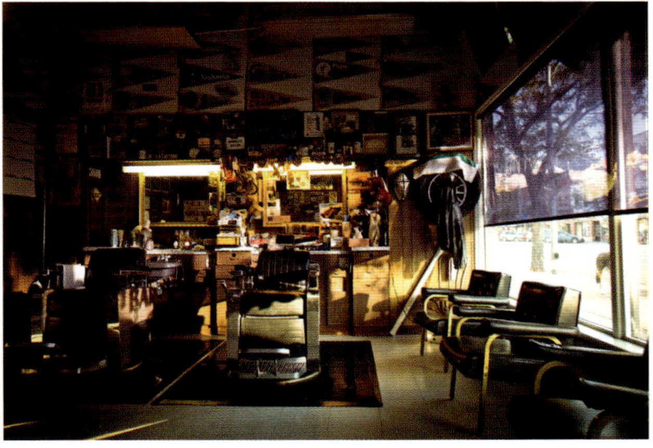

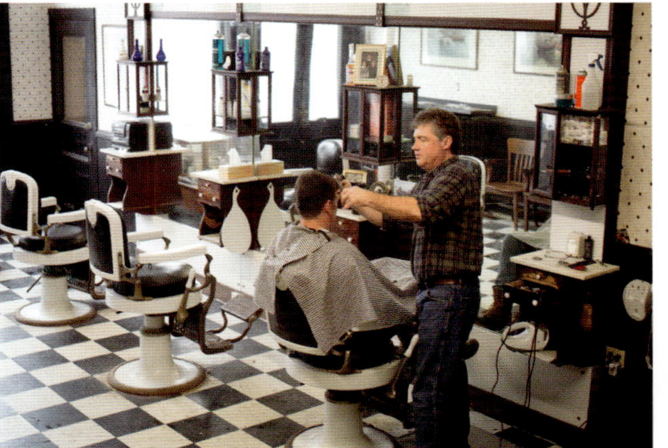

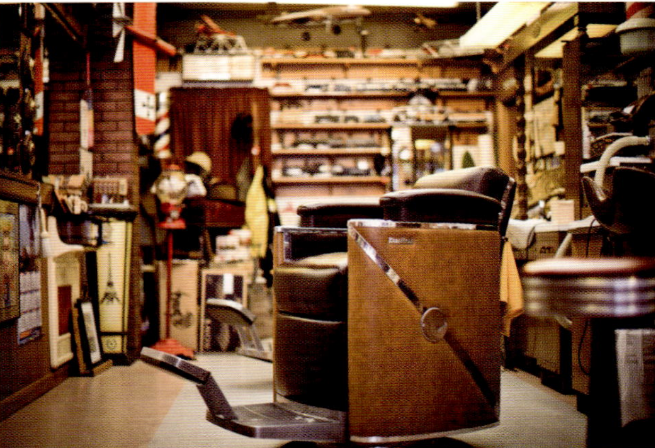

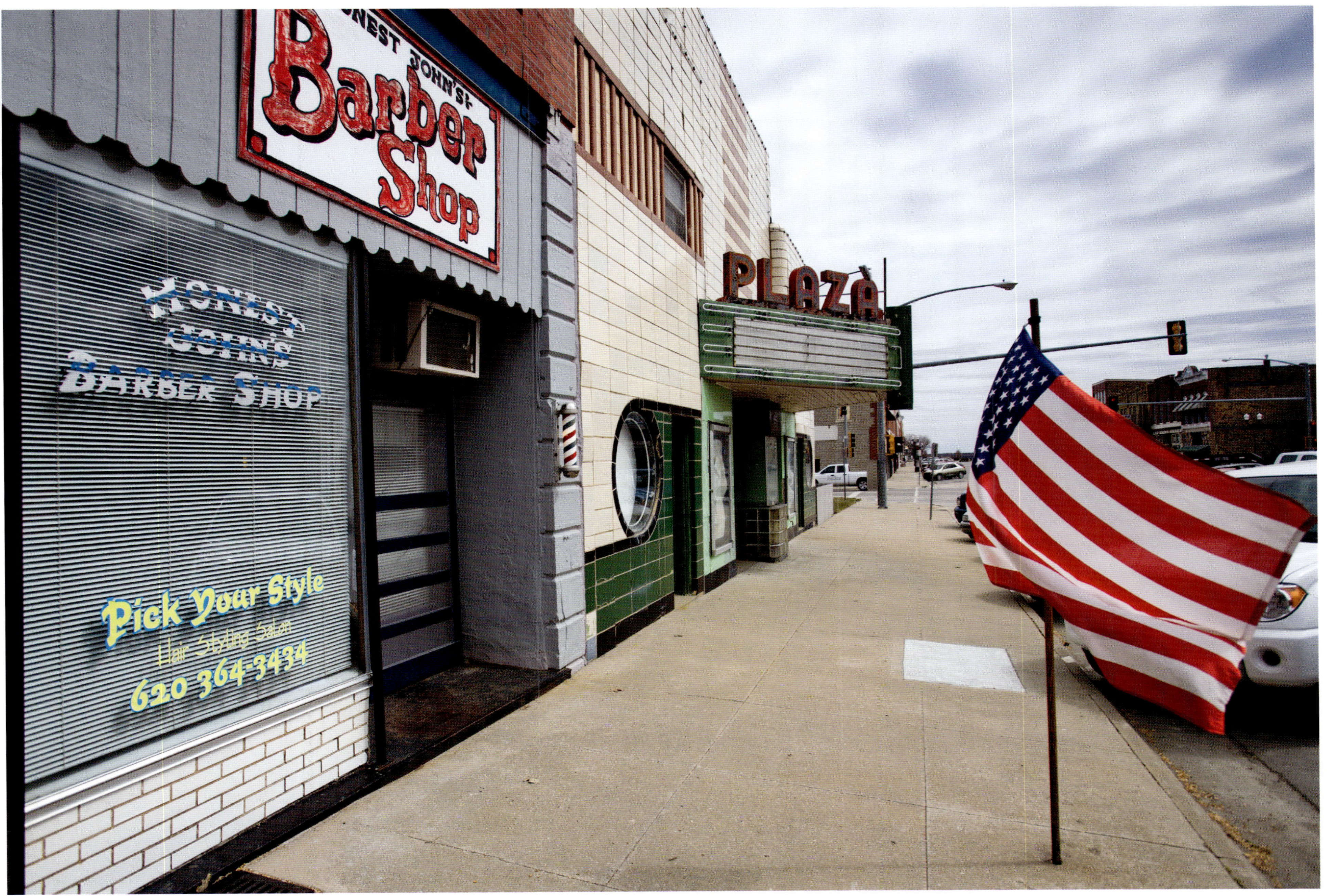

Honest John's Barbershop, Burlington, Kansas

"That old man that owned them hogs, he owned them so long, he looked just like 'em."

– Customer, Browning Barbershop, Sparks, Georgia

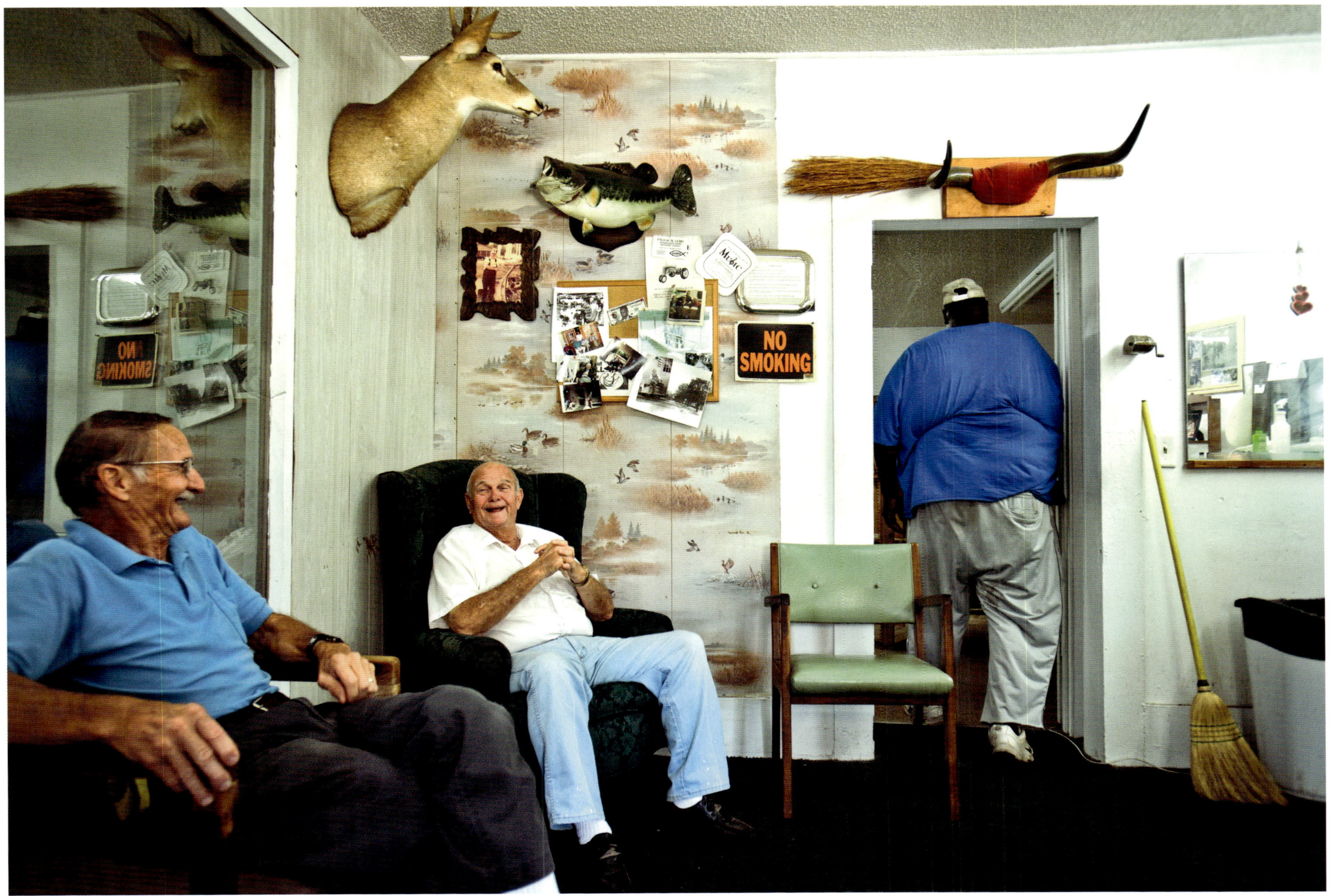

Browning Barbershop, Sparks, Georgia

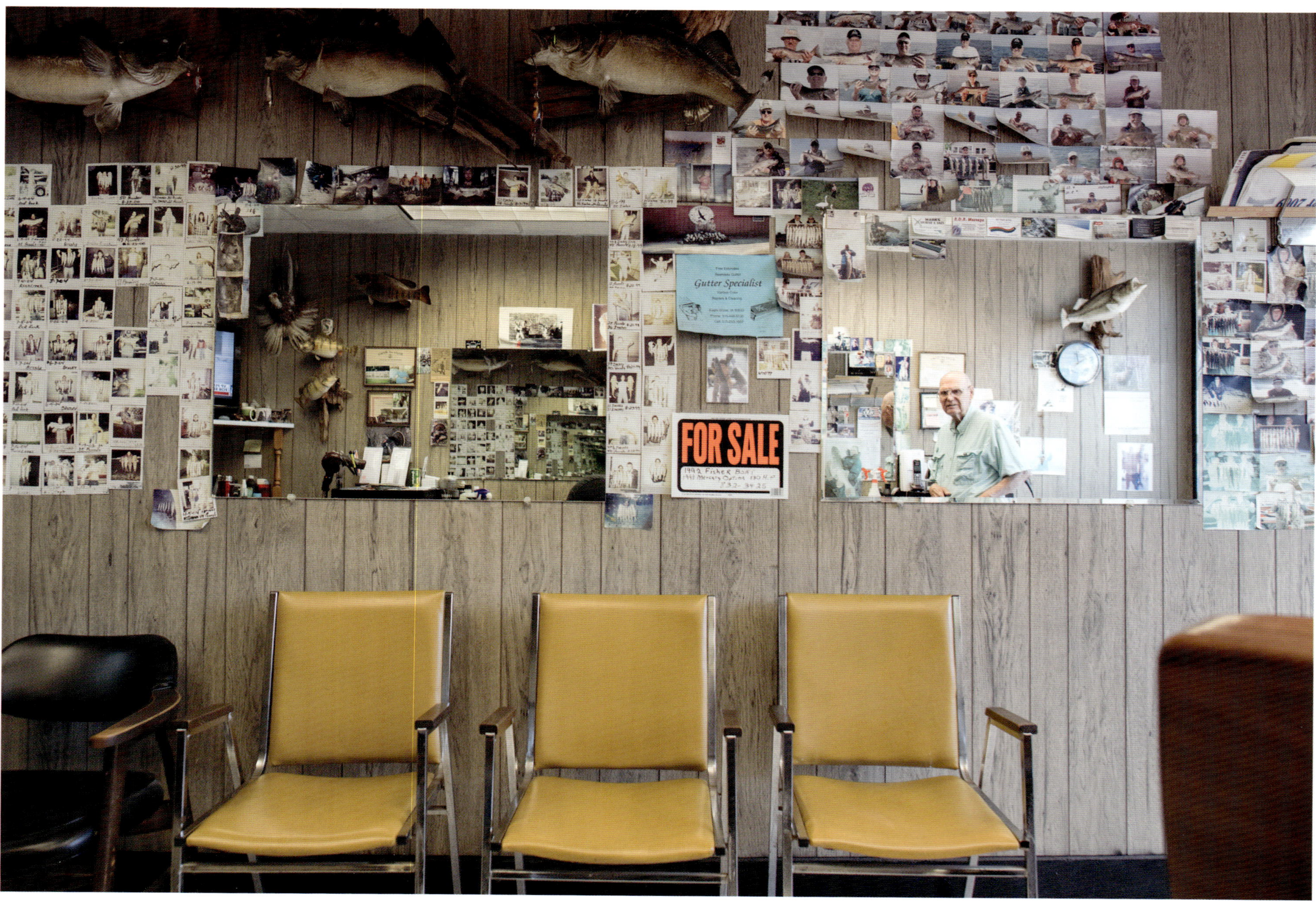

Al's Barbershop, Webster City, Iowa

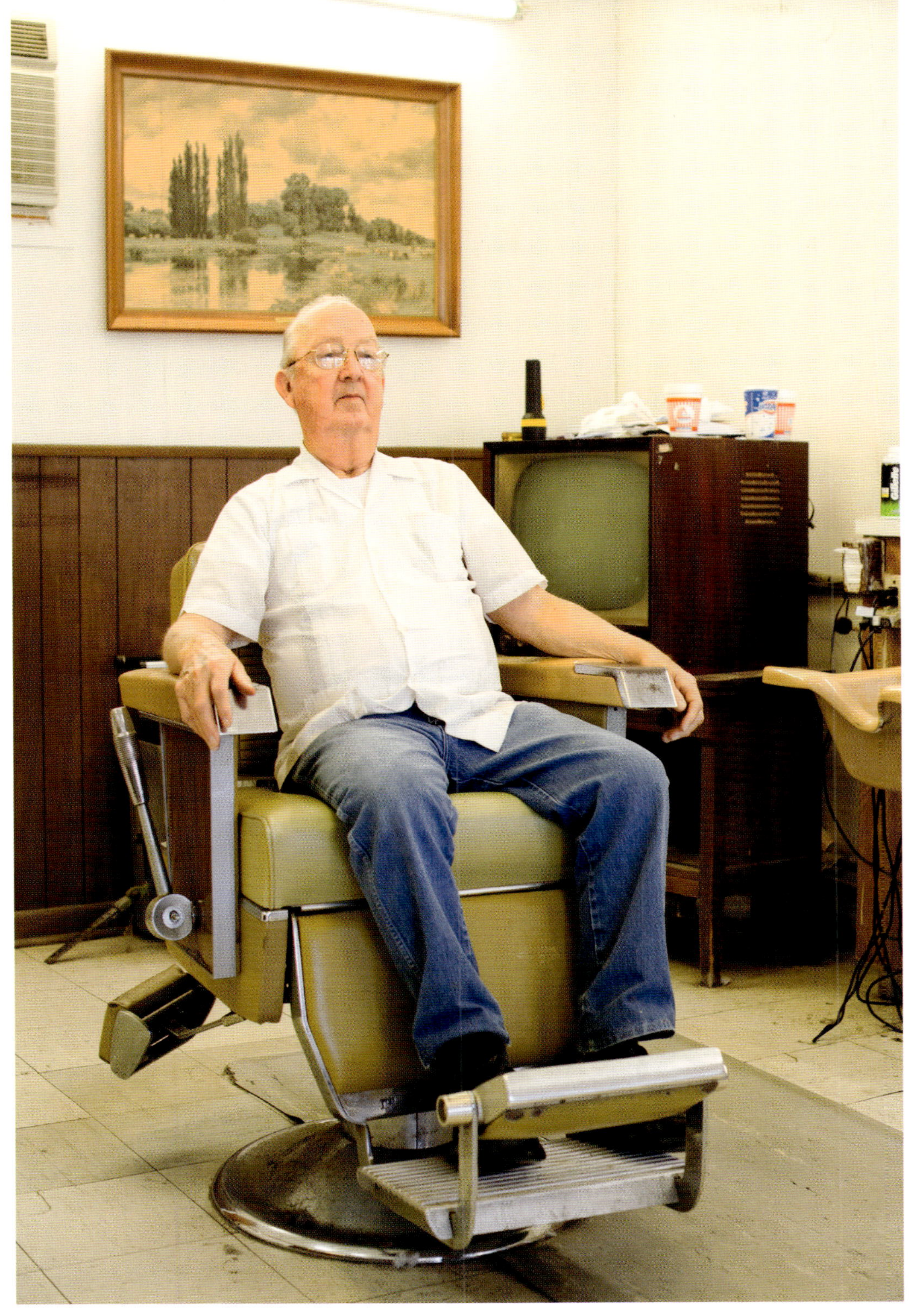

Cowey Barbershop, Gonzalez, Texas

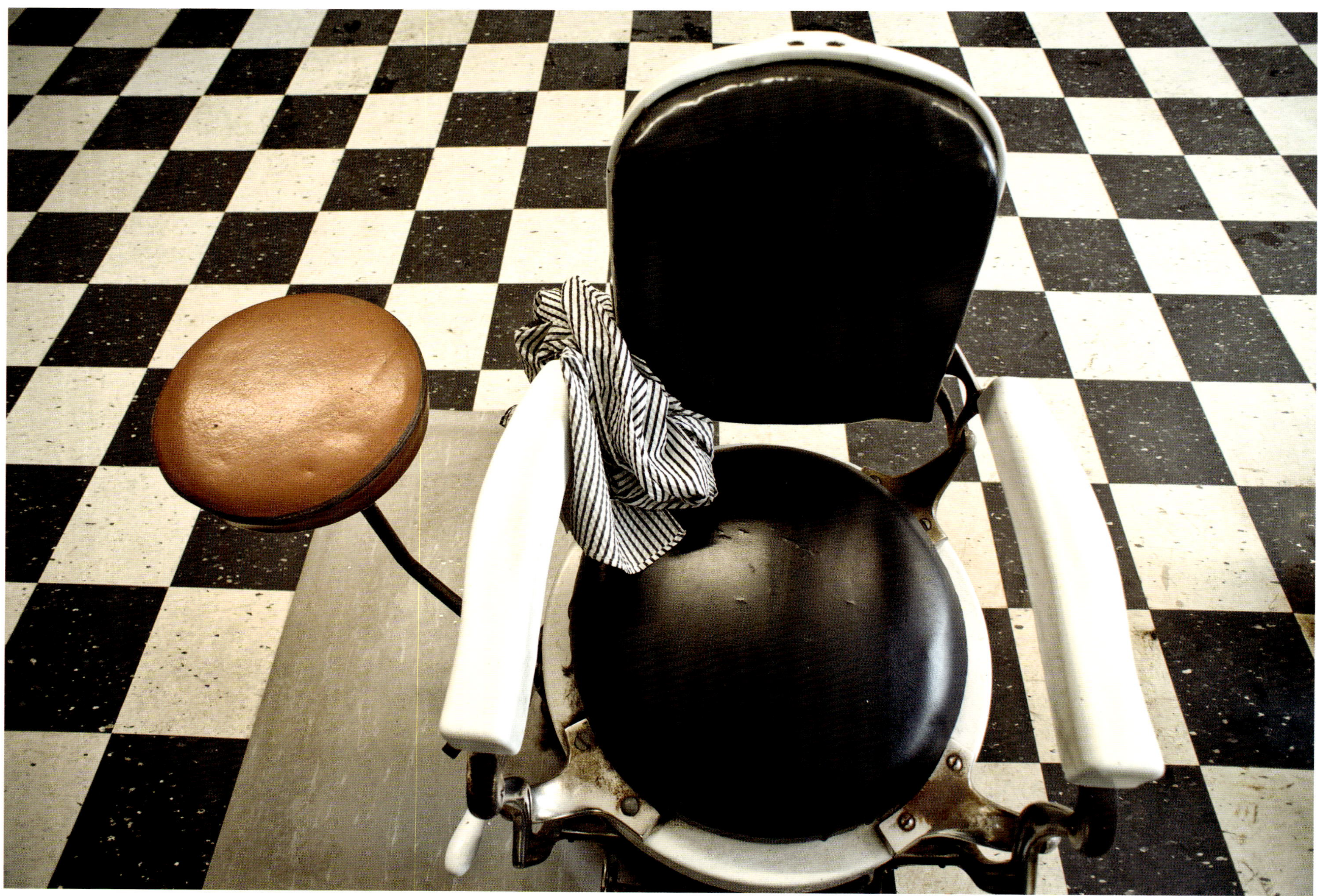

Jones Barbershop, Bennington, Vermont

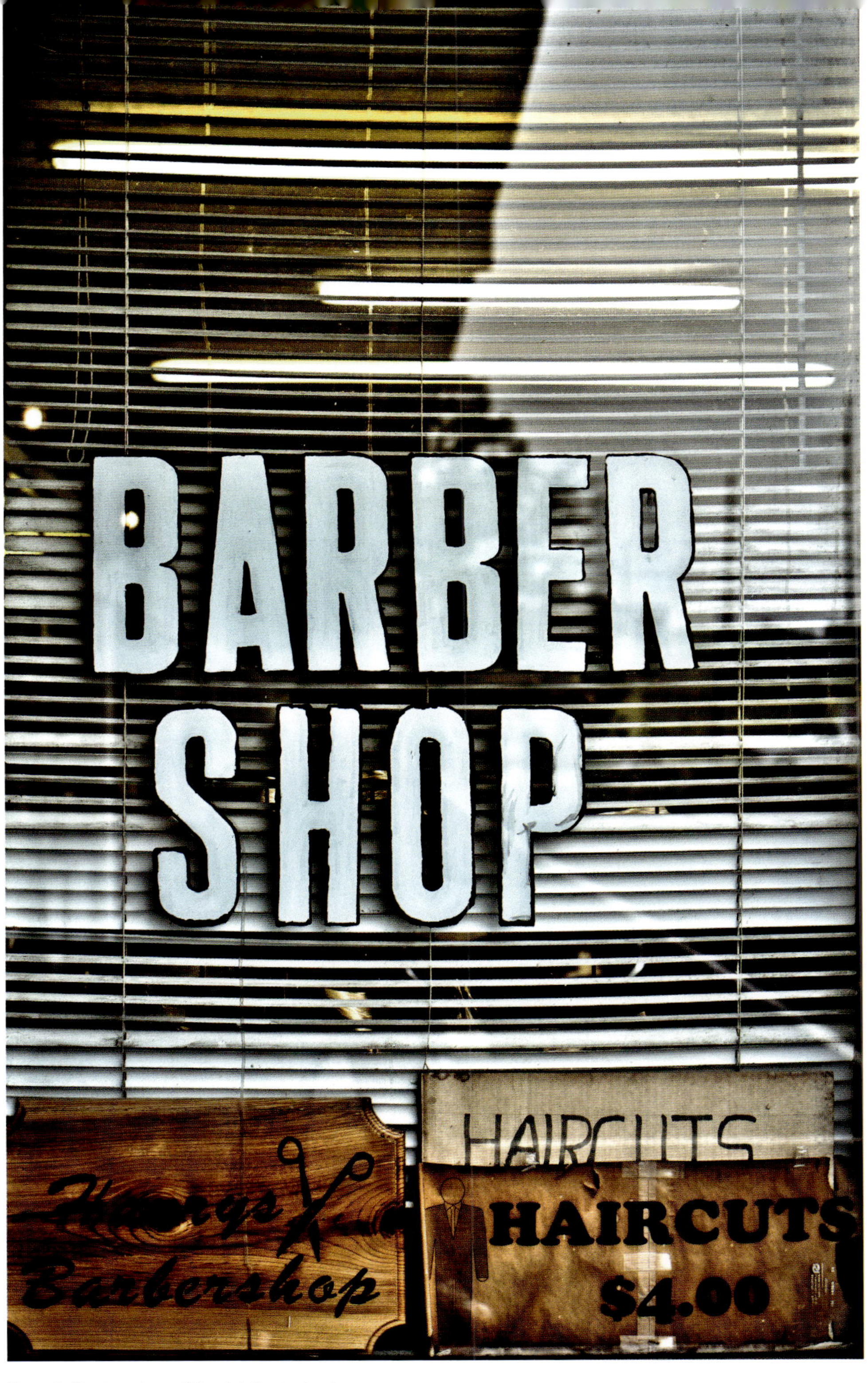

Harry's Barbershop, Biloxi, Mississippi

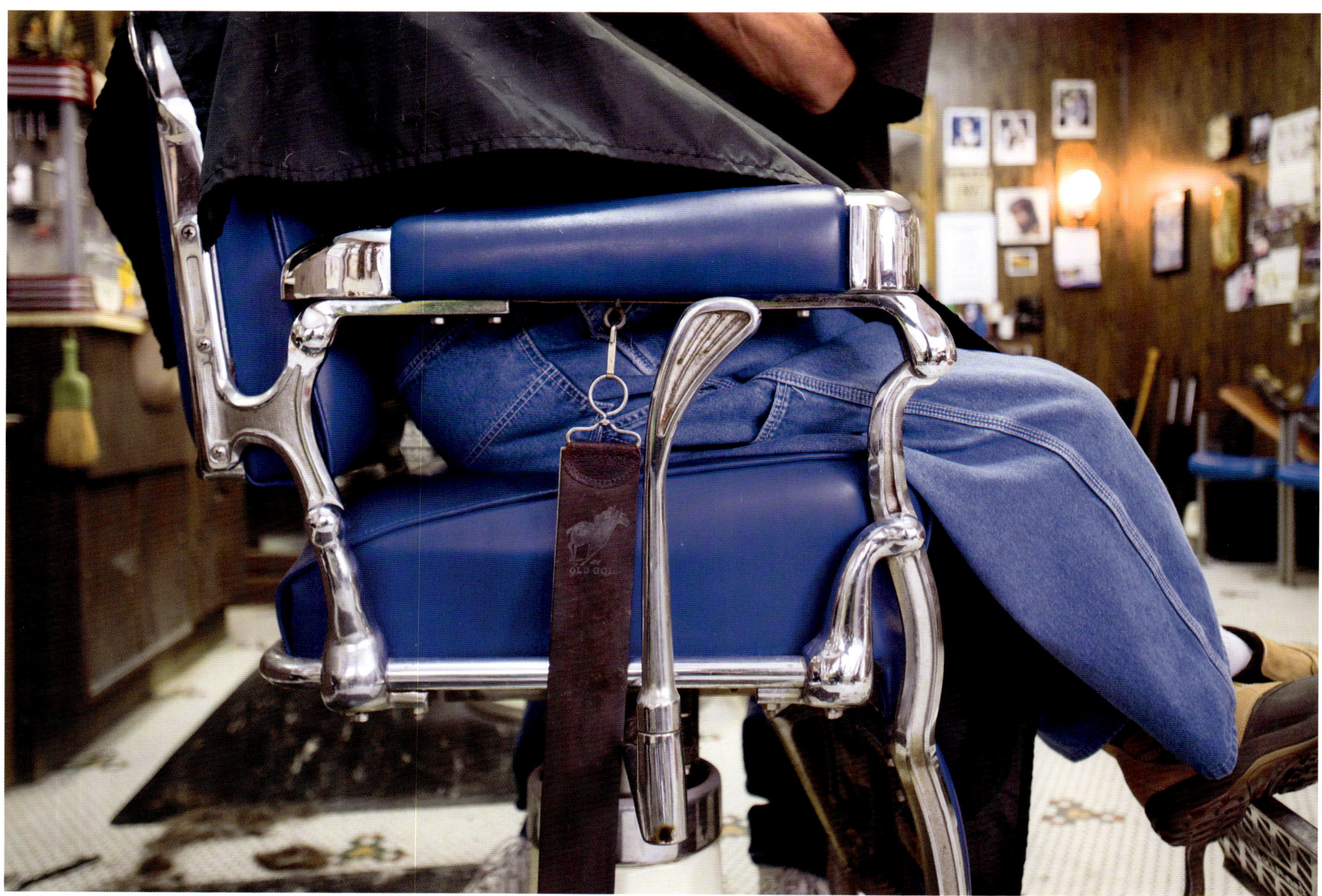

Smith's Barbershop, Excelsior Springs, Missouri

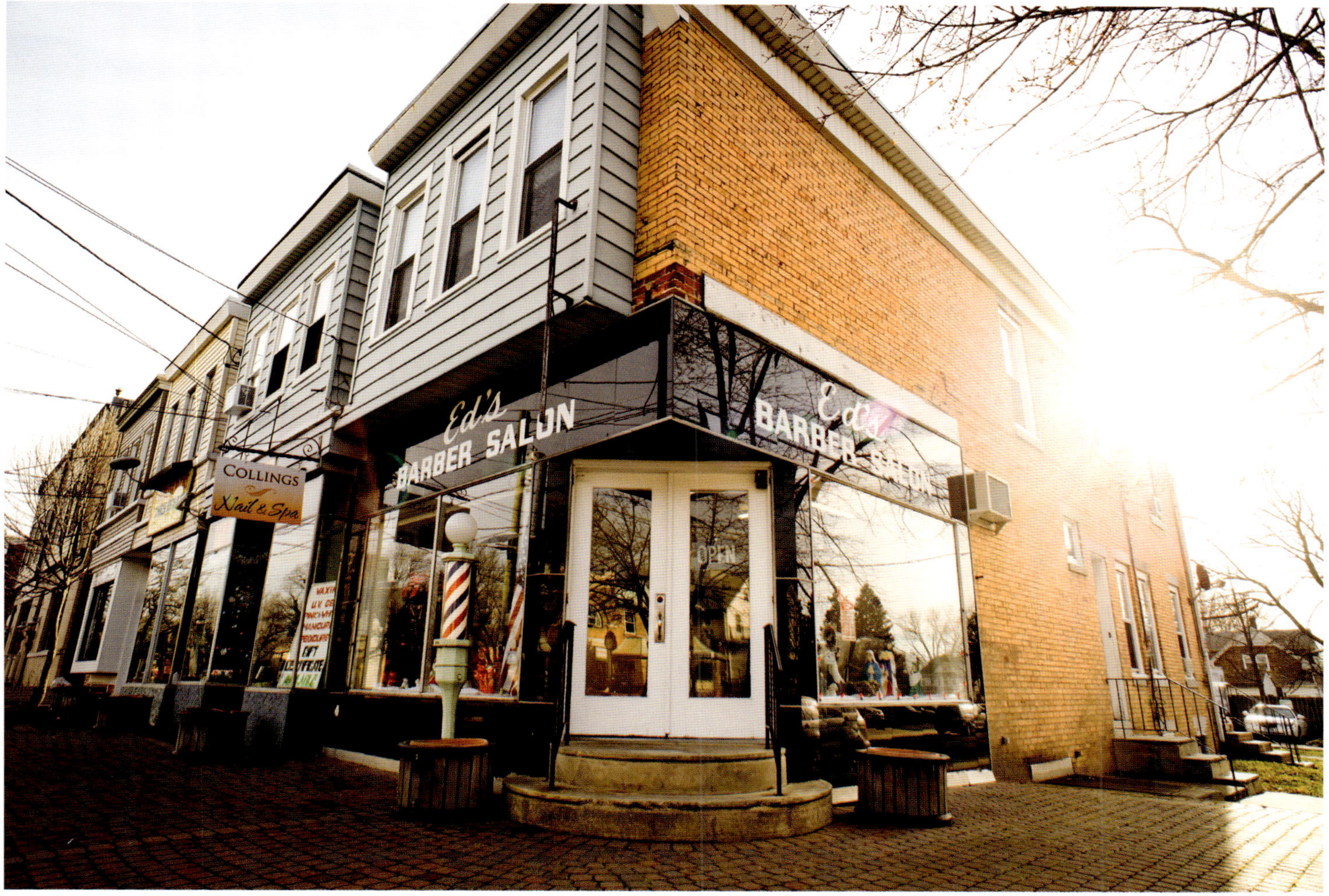

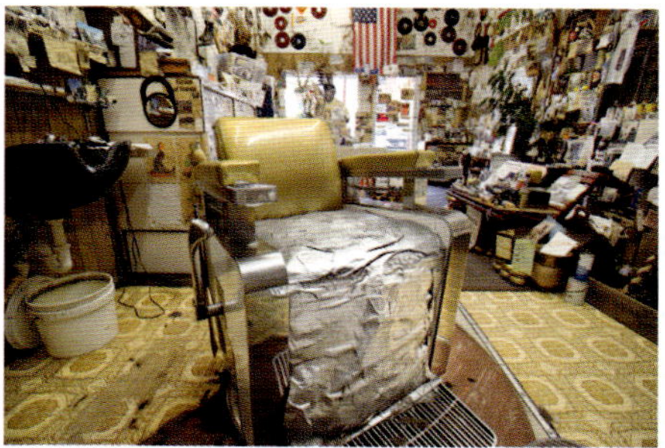

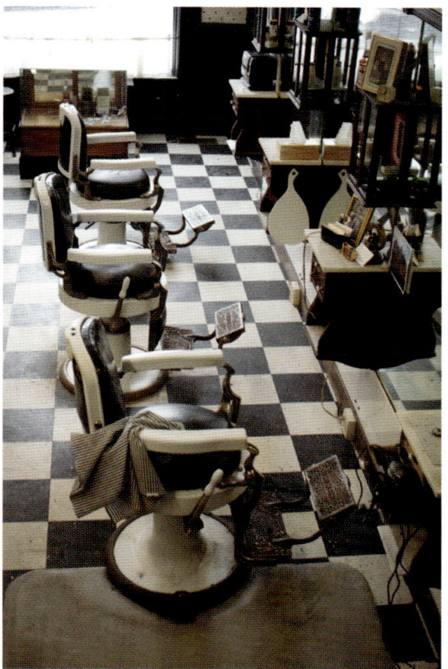

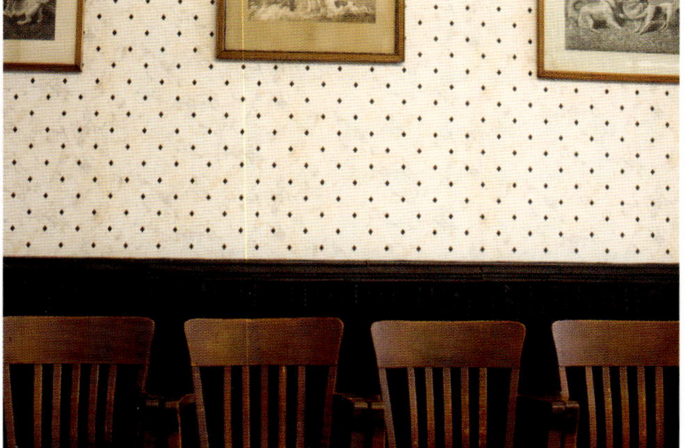

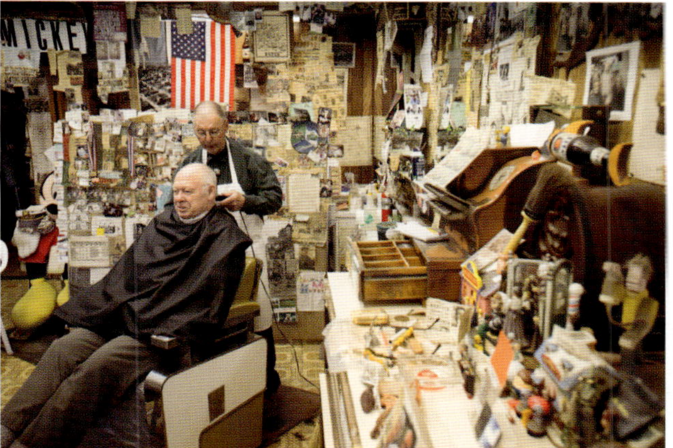

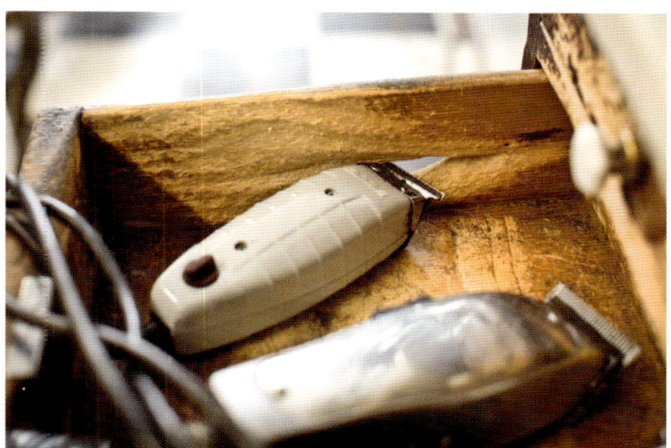

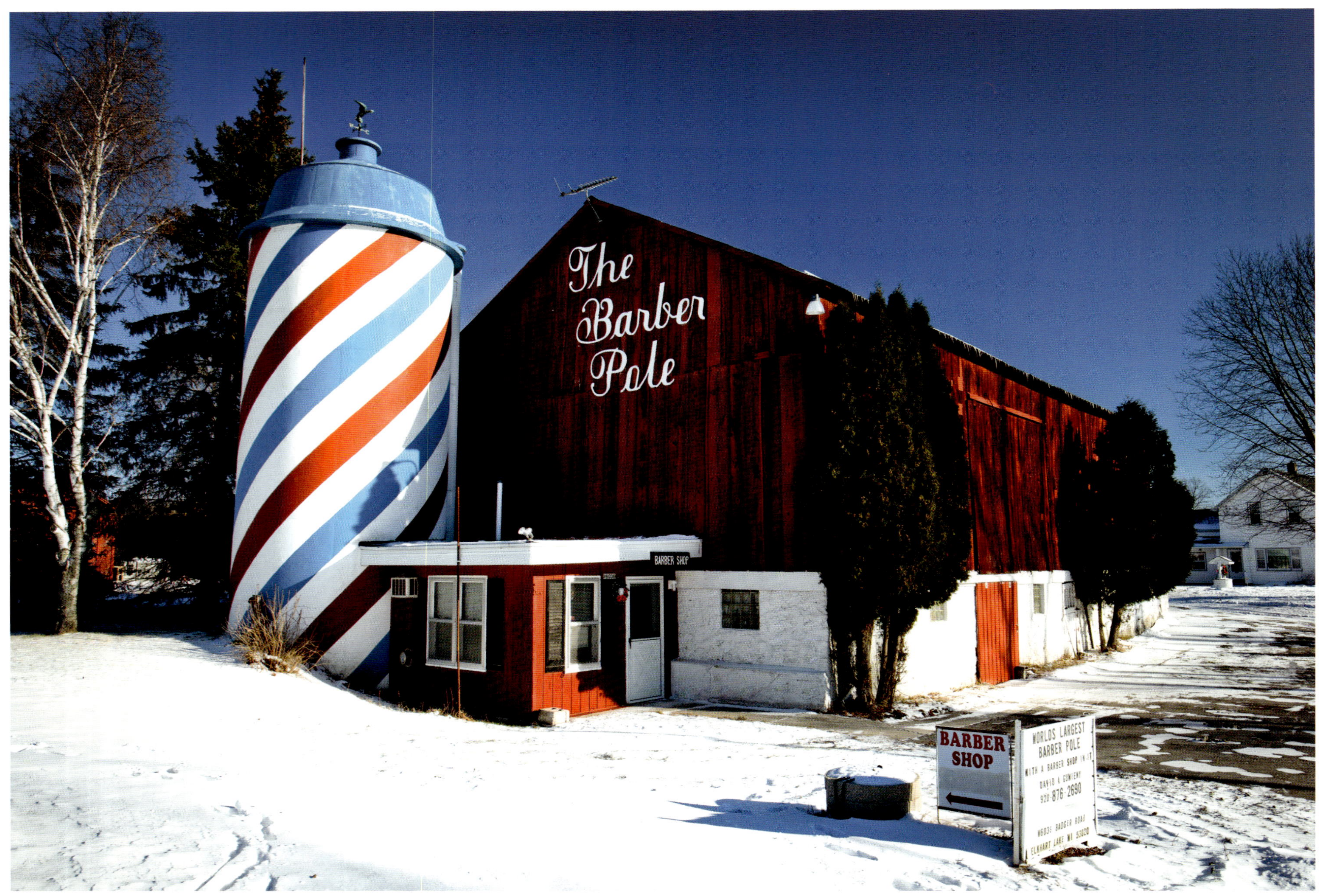

The Barber Pole, Elkhart Lake, Wisconsin

"Back in the day, the waiting room was the bar, and most people would go home without a haircut."

– David Gumieny, The Barber Pole, Elkhart Lake, Wisconsin

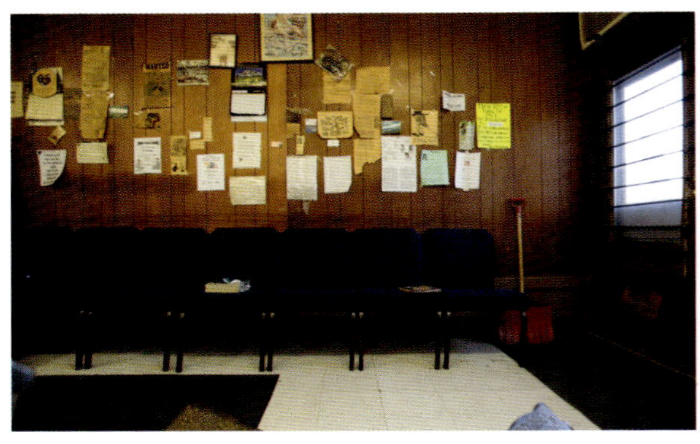
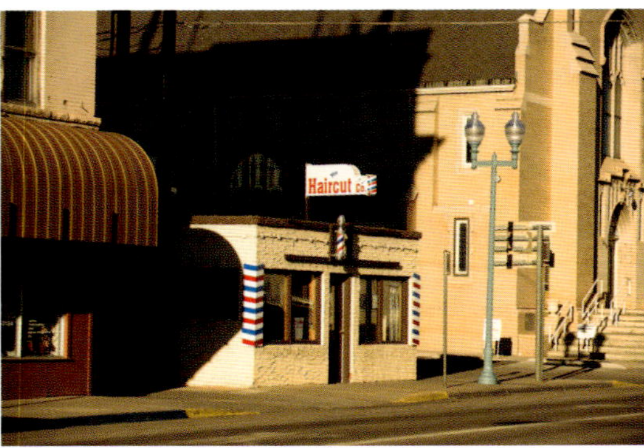
Haircut
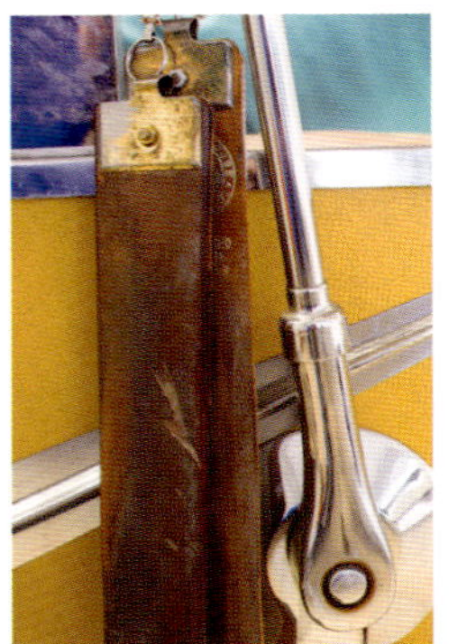
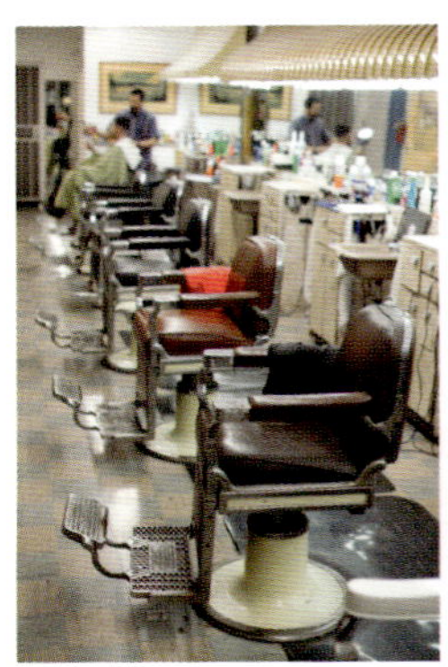
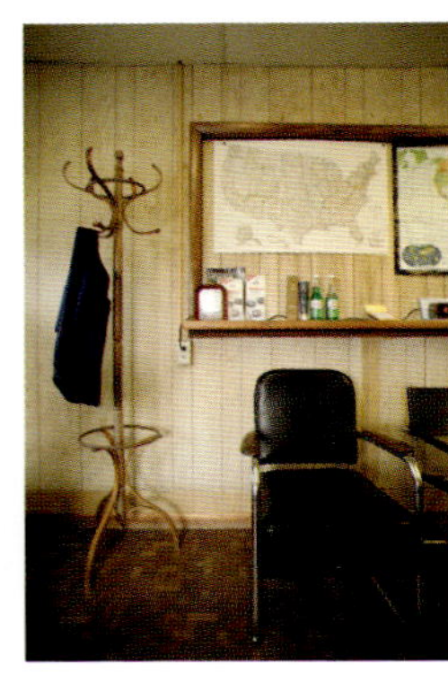
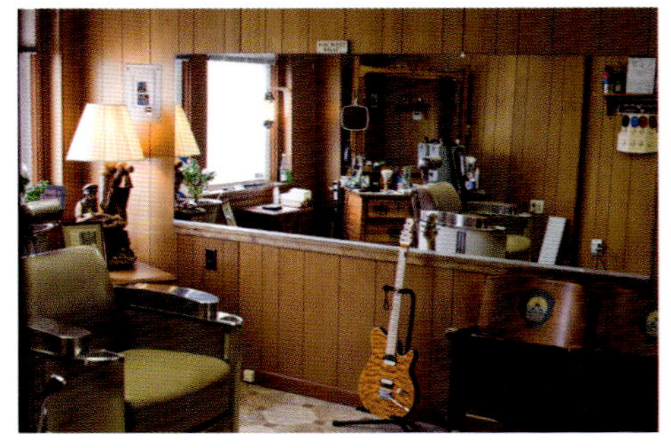
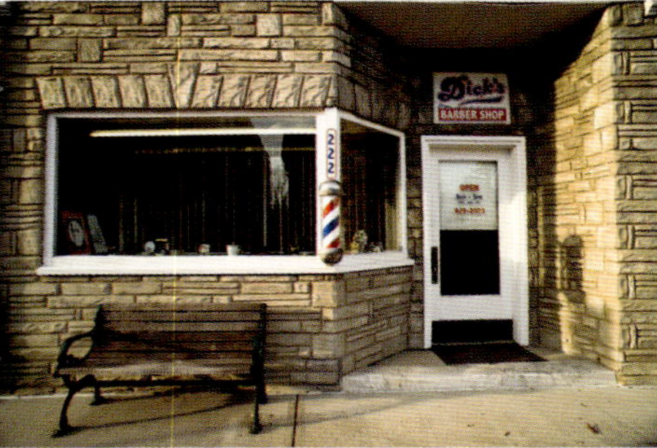
Dick's
BARBER SHOP
222
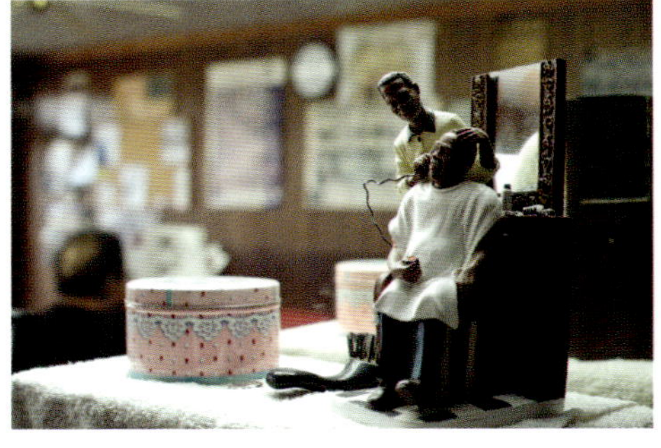
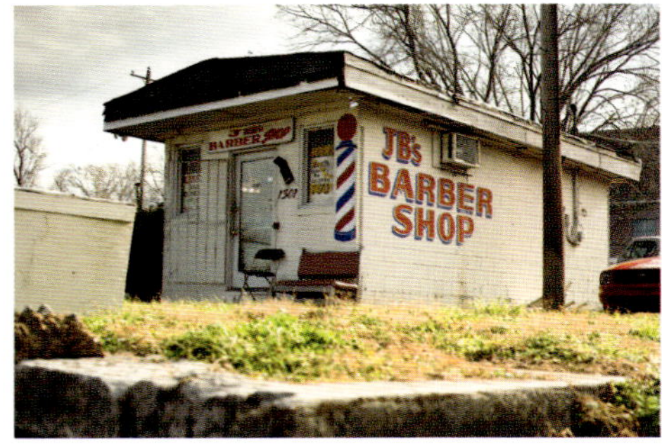
JB's
BARBER
SHOP
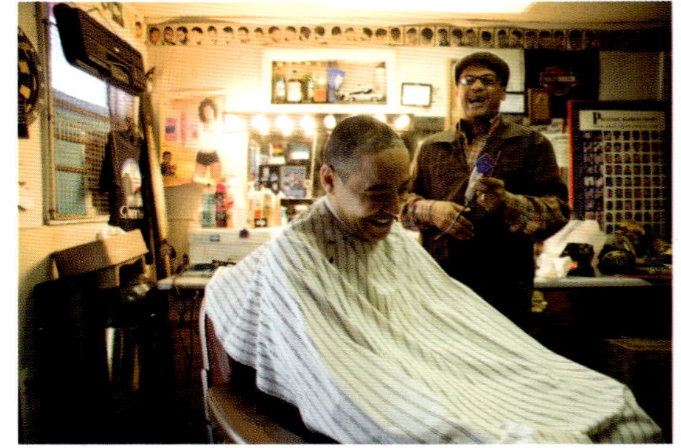
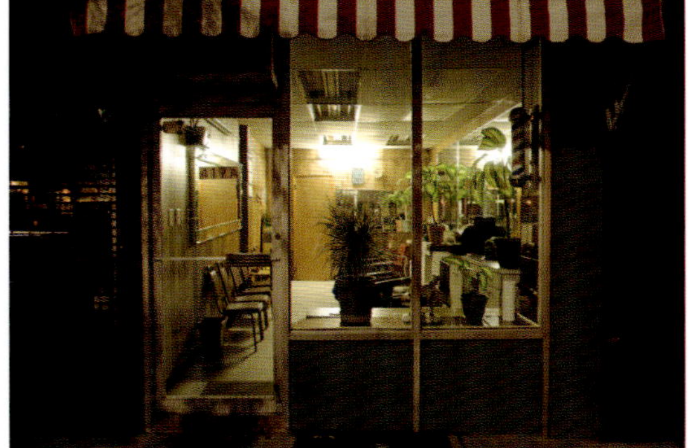
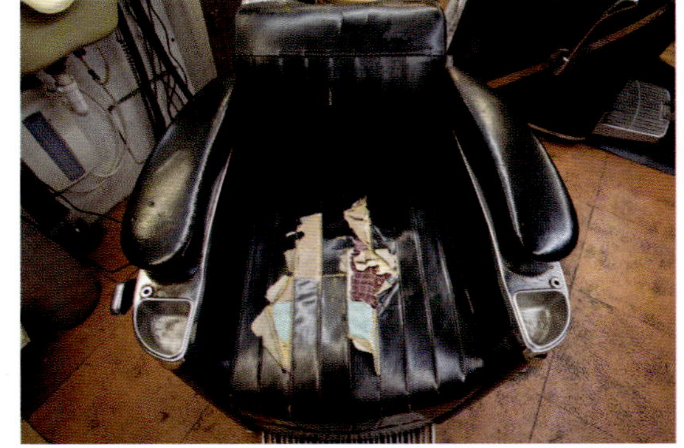
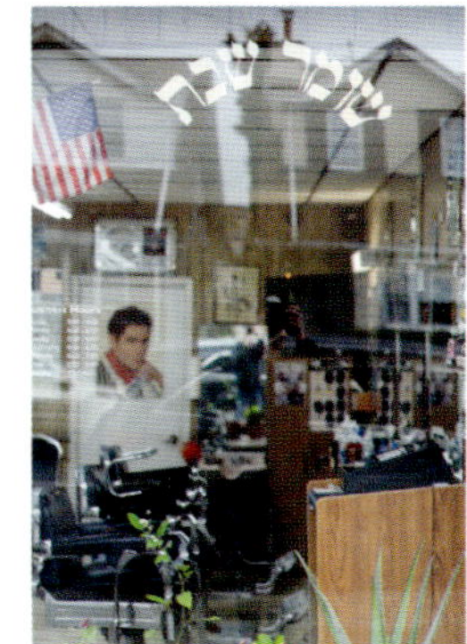
שומר שבת
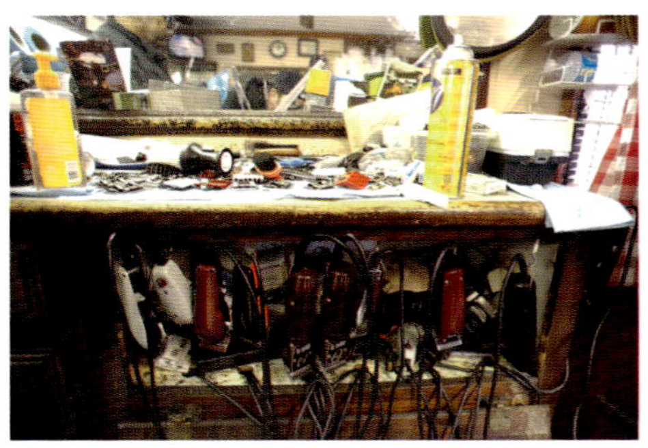
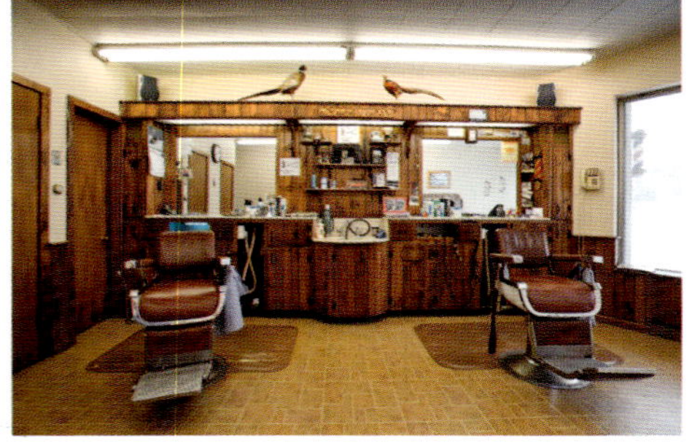
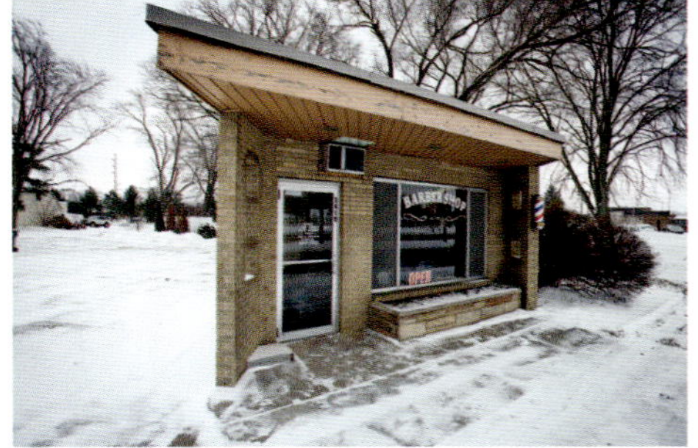
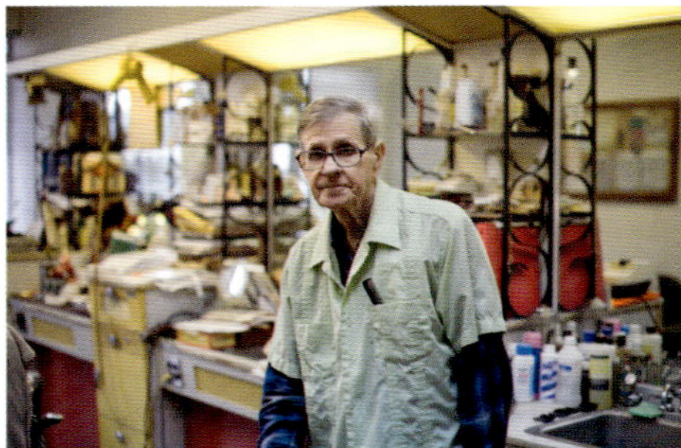

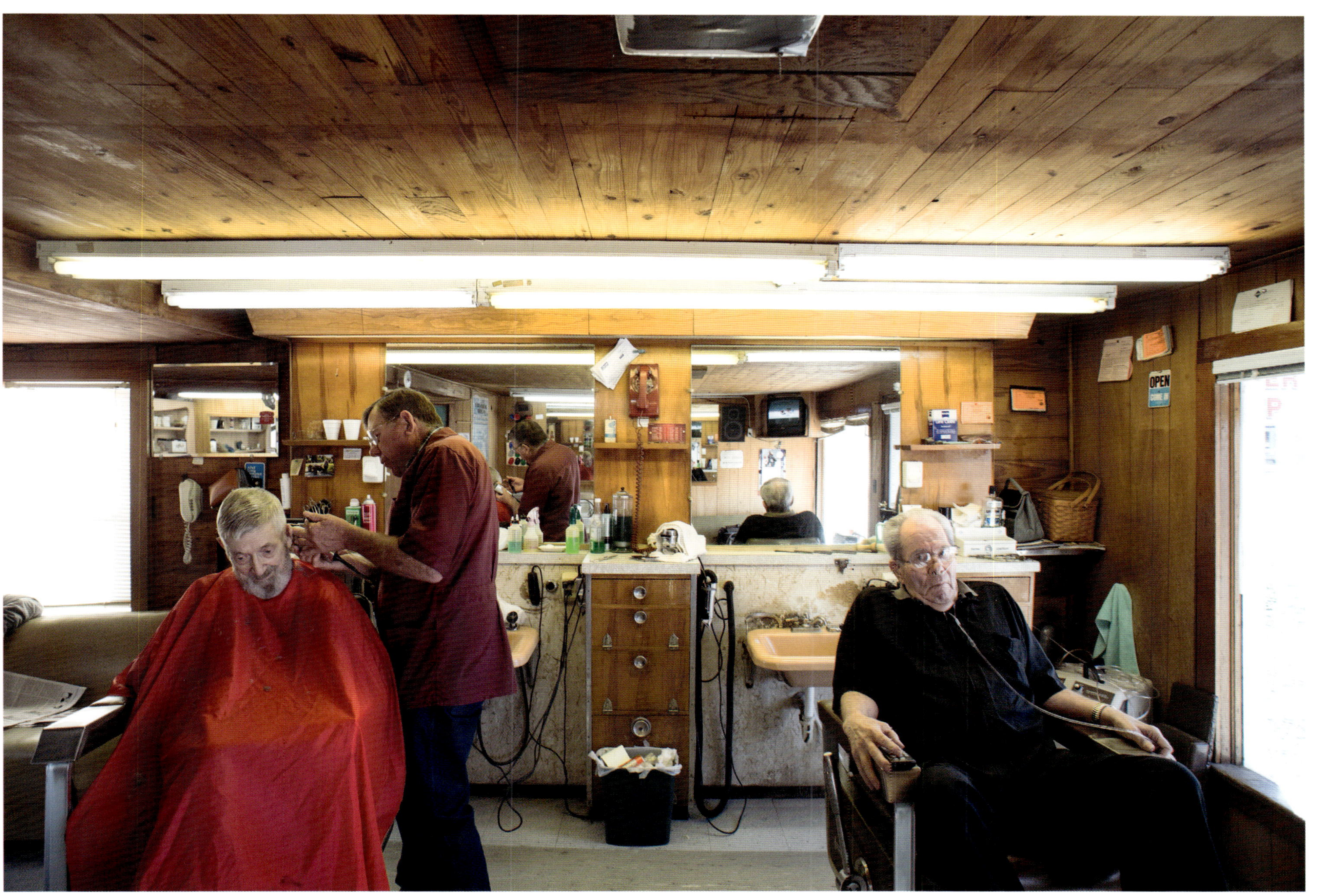

Don and John's Barbershop, Springdale, Arizona

“I’ve got a customer 103 years old. Drove in on his own too.”

– Stan McLean, McLean’s Barbershop, Hyannis, Massachusetts

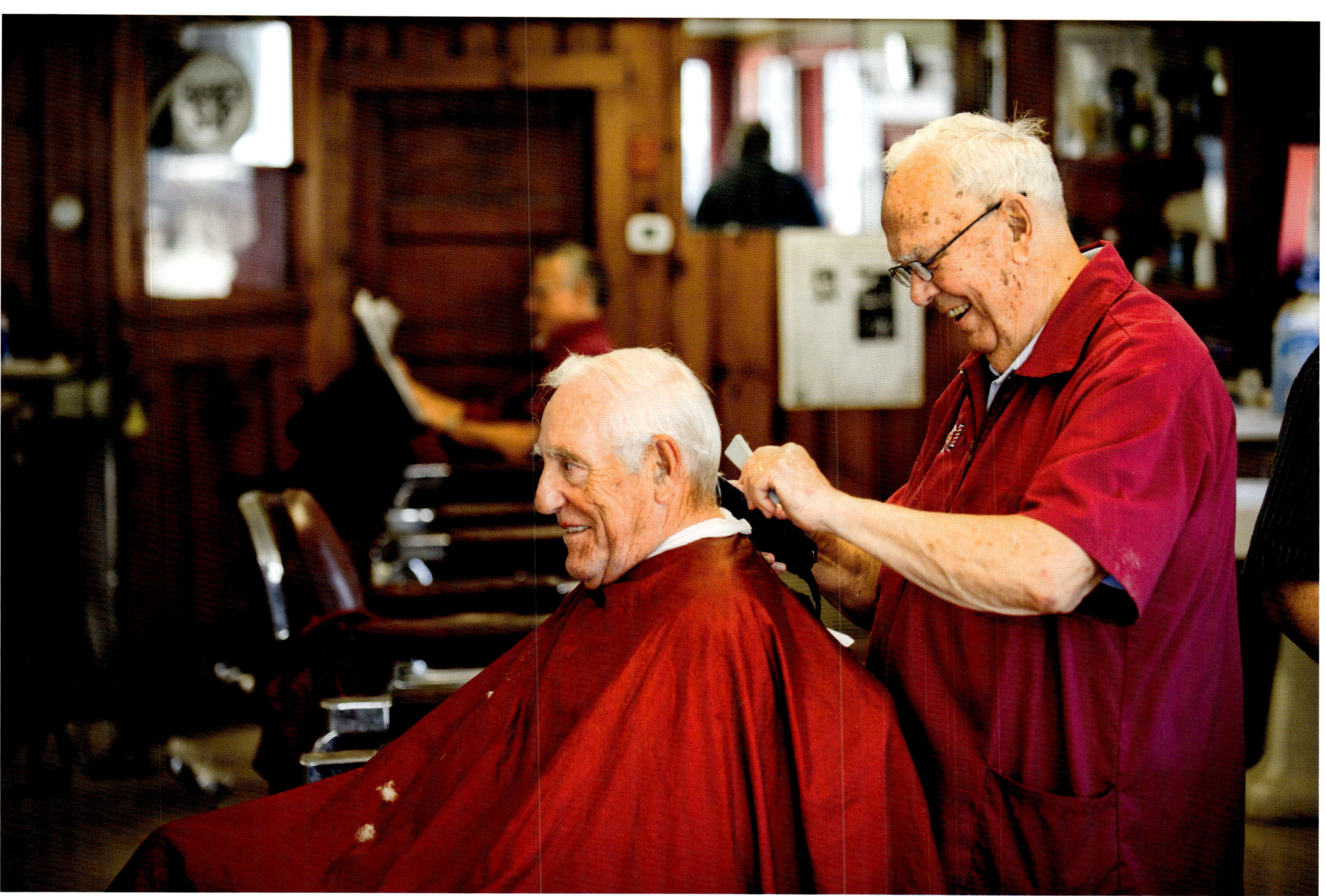

McLean's Barbershop, Hyannis, Massachusetts

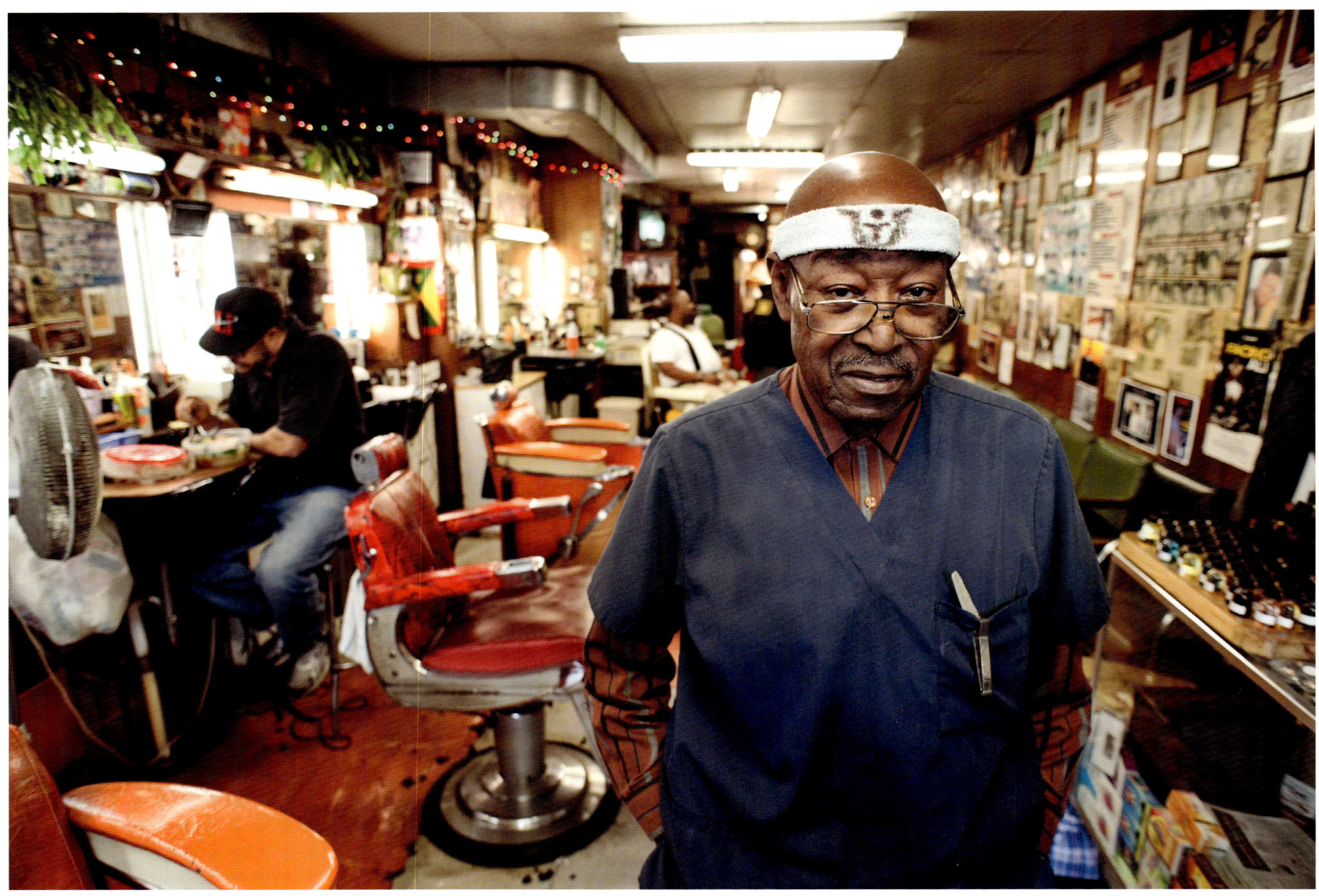

Stancil's Barbershop, Albany, New York

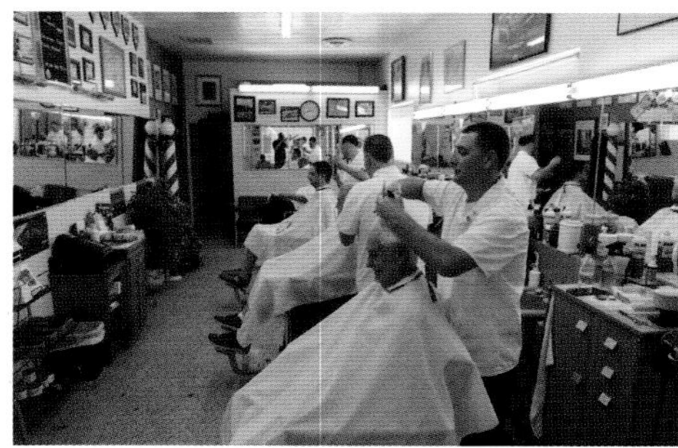

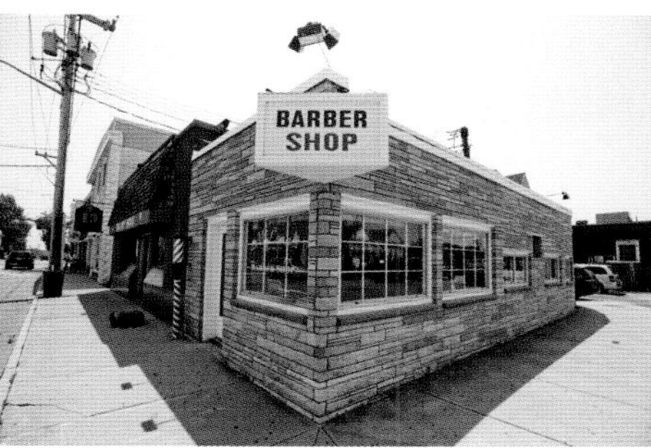

BARBER
SHOP

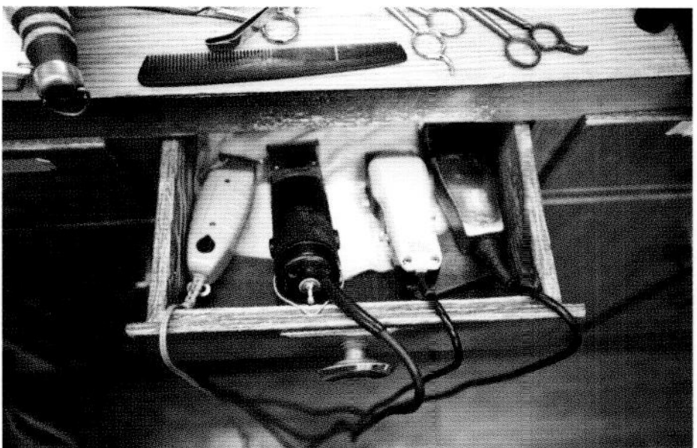

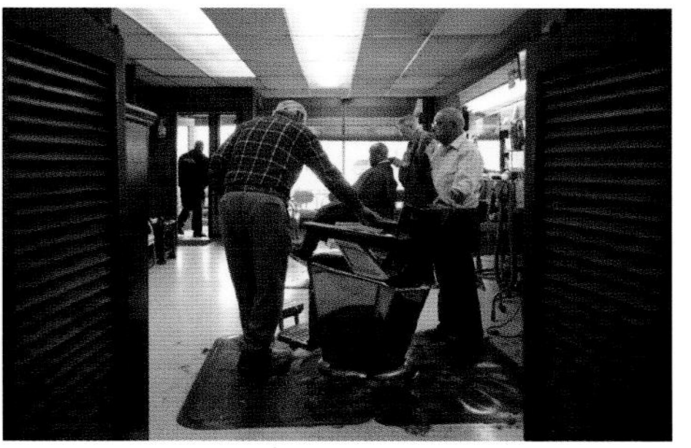

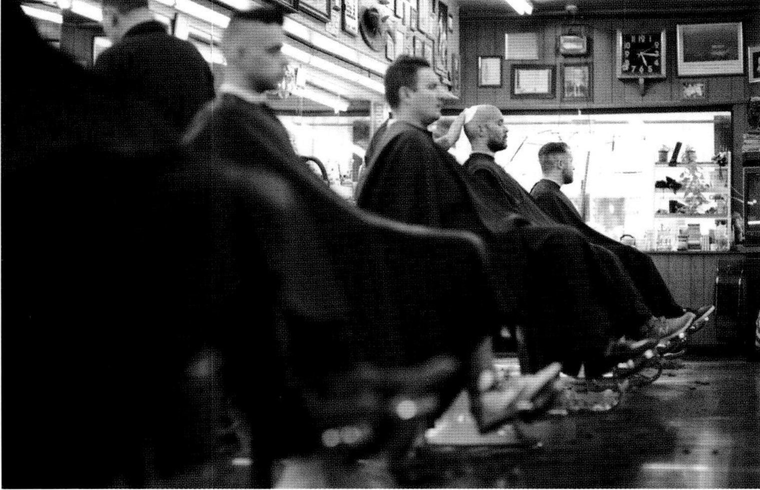

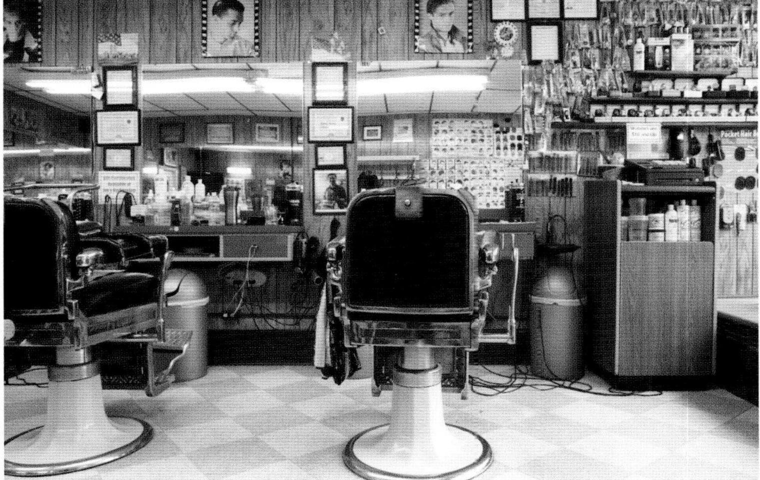

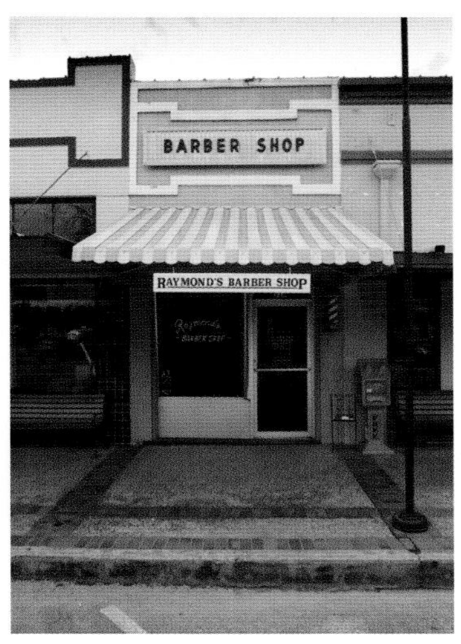

BARBER SHOP
RAYMOND'S BARBER SHOP

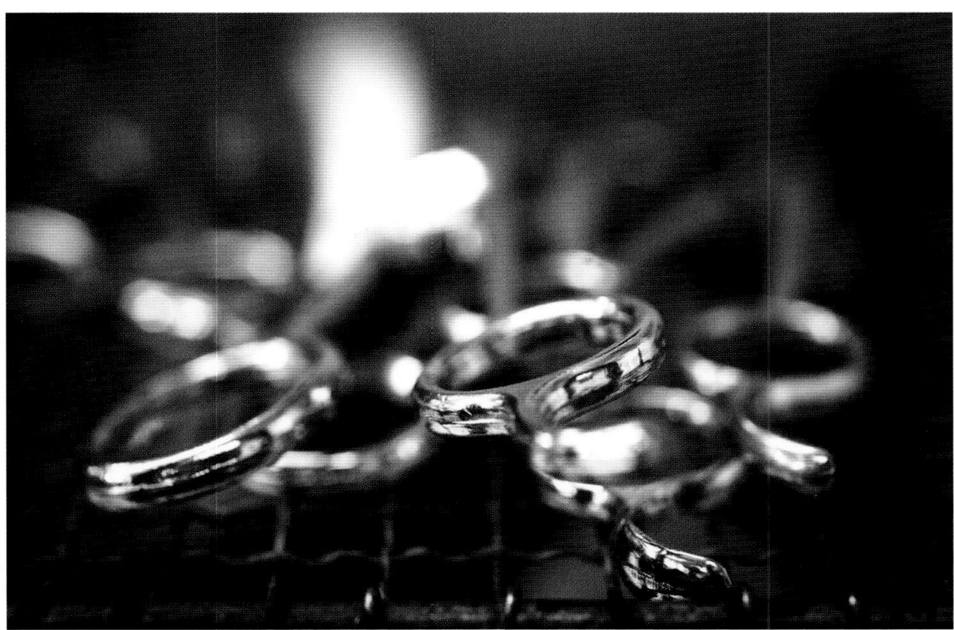

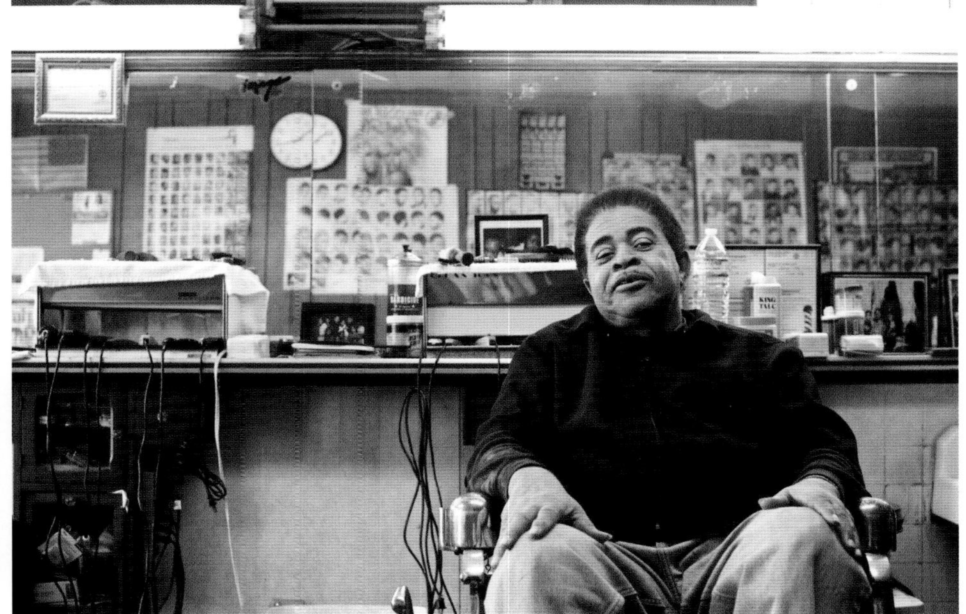

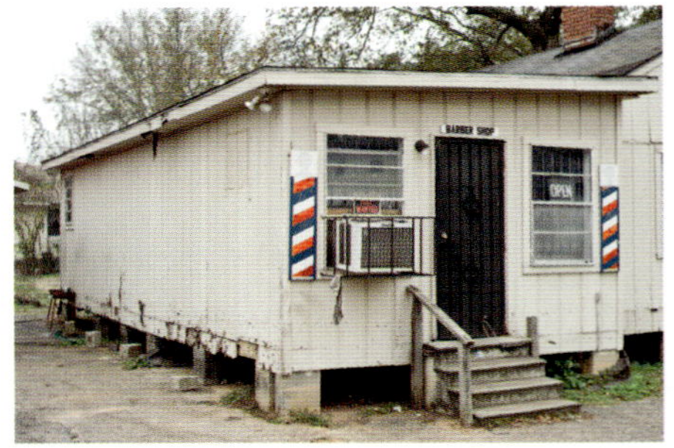
BARBER SHOP

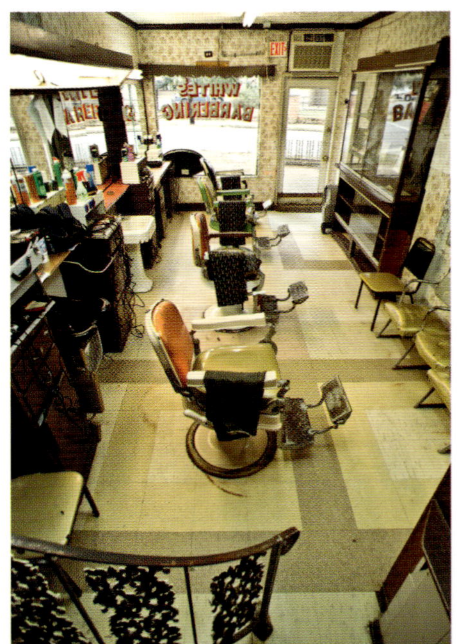

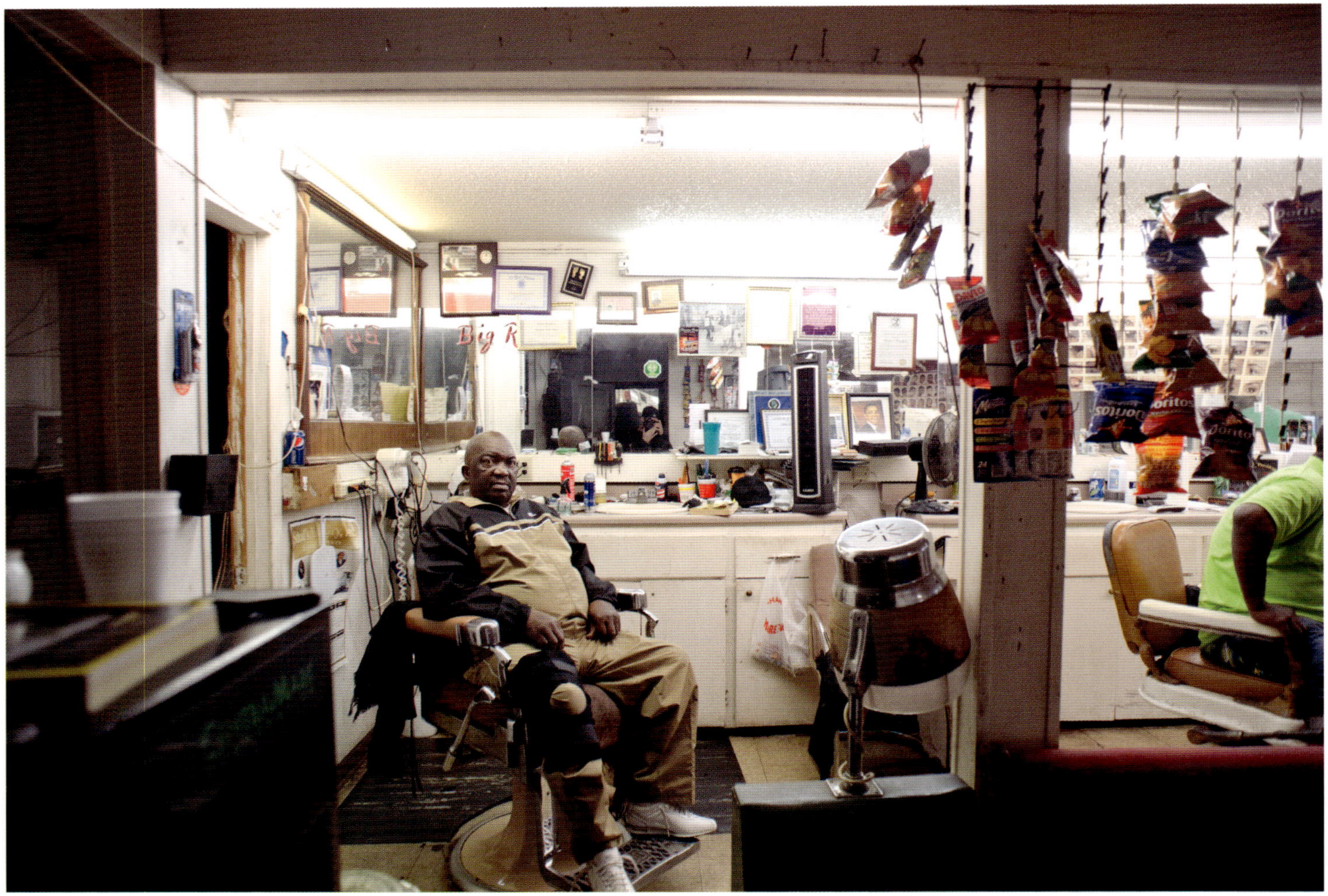

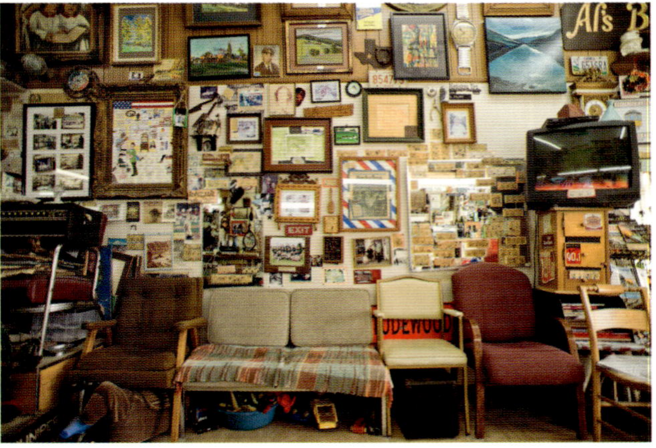

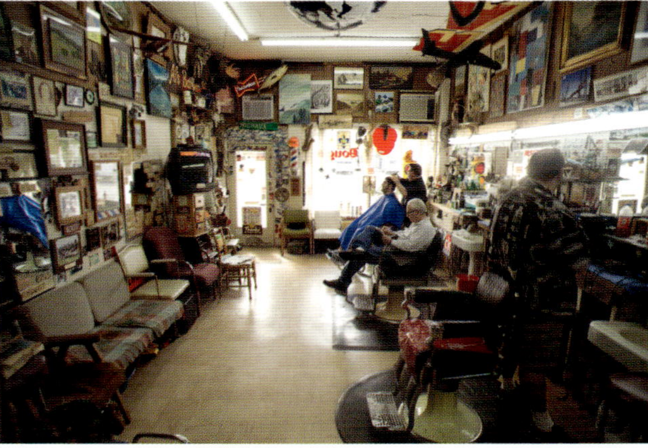

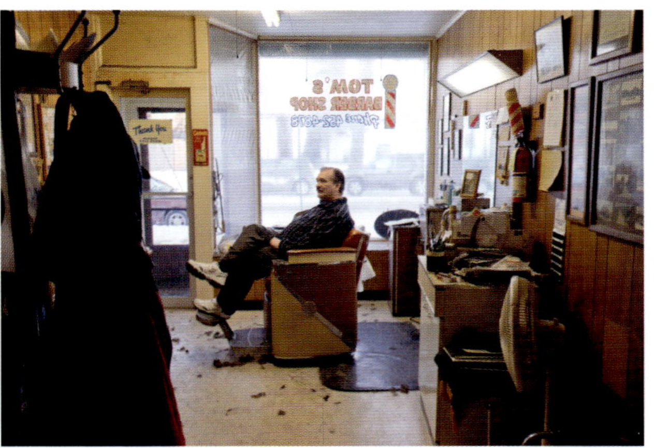

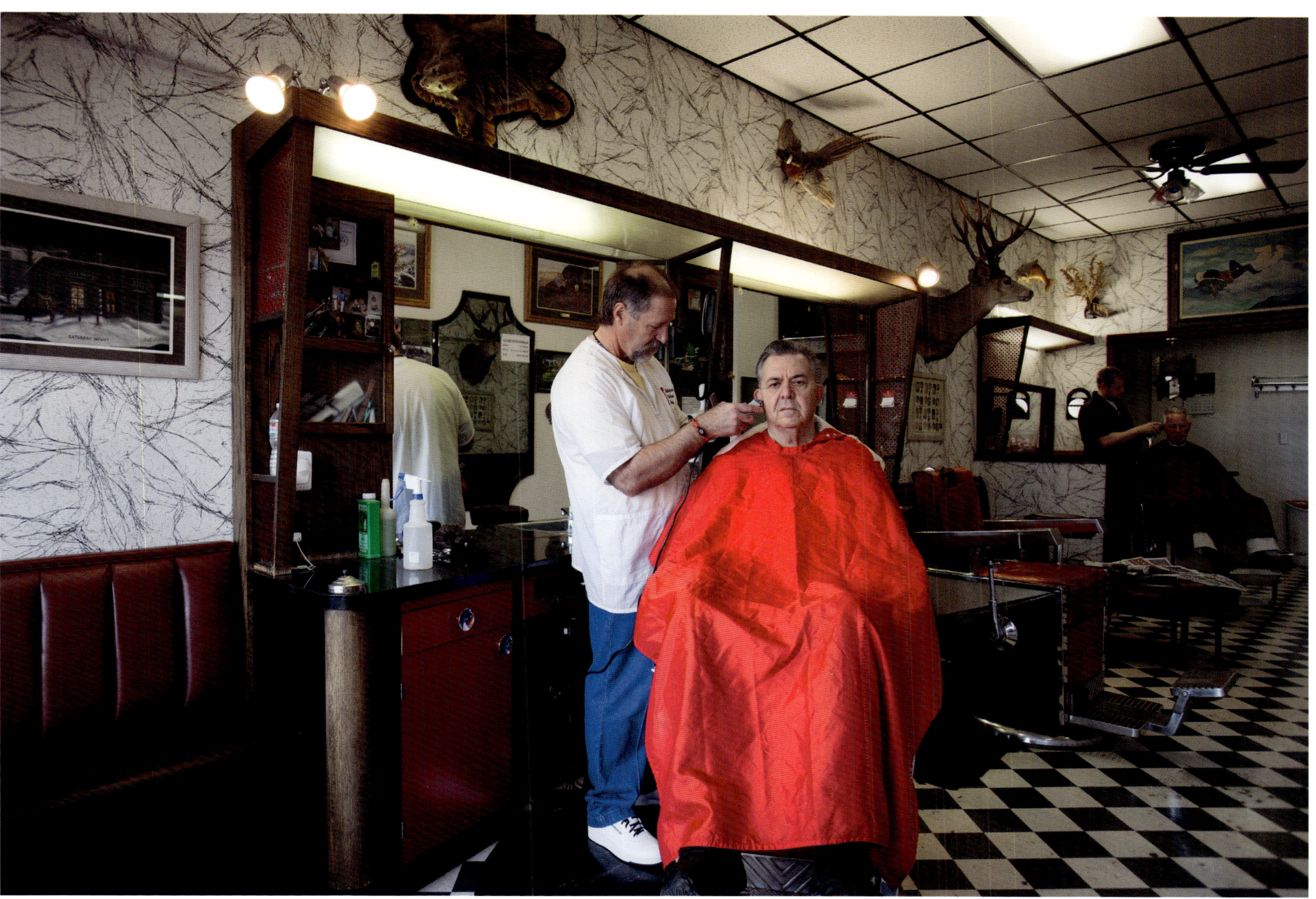

Holmes Barbershop, Cedar City, Utah

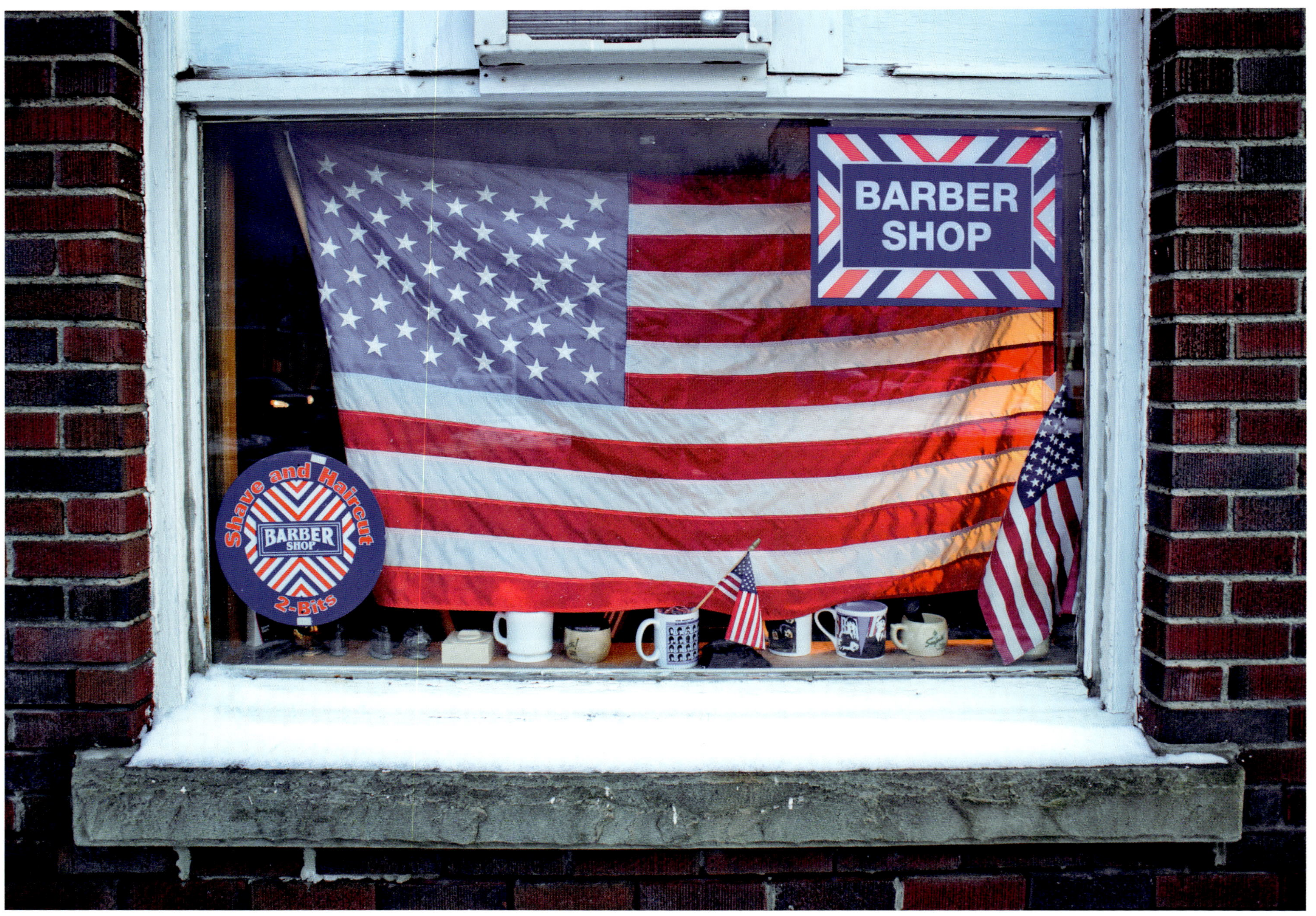

Unknown, Pennsylvania

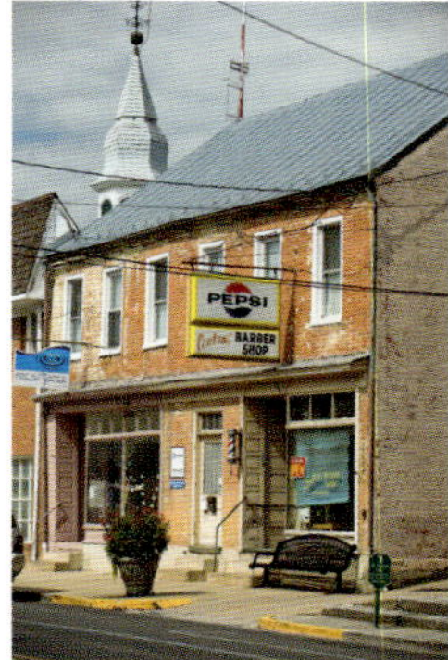
PEPSI
BARBER SHOP

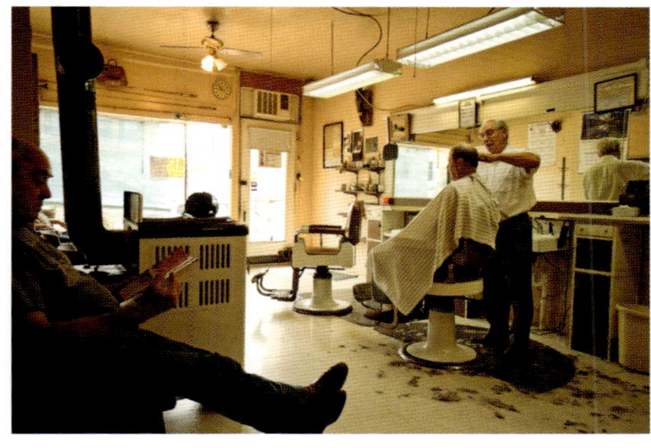

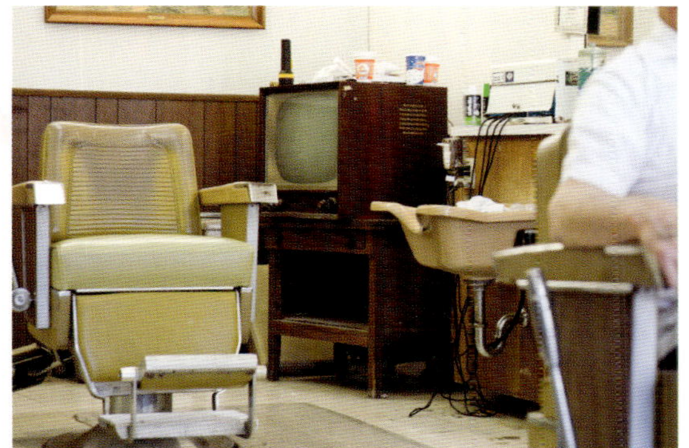

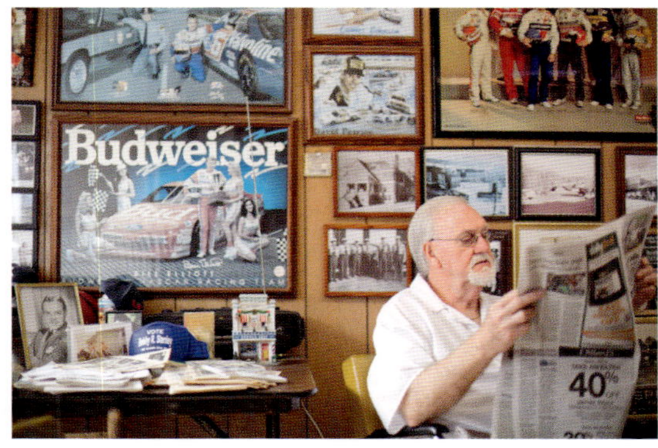
Budweiser

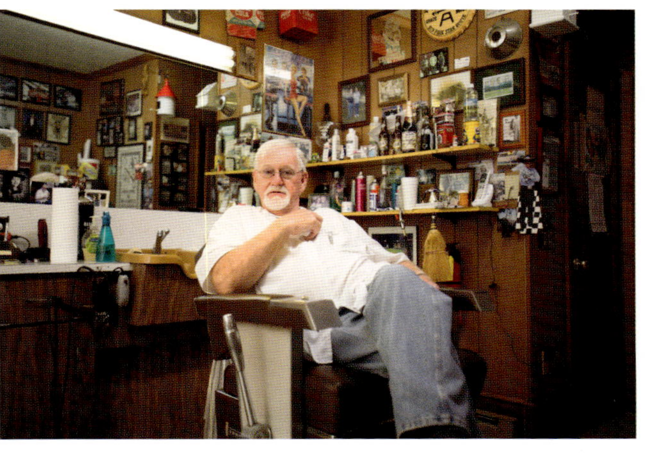

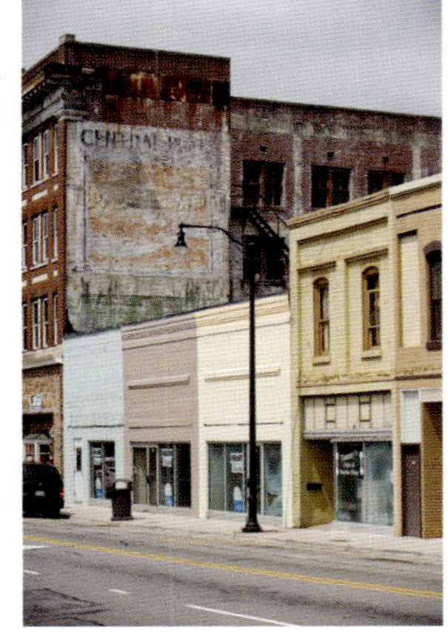

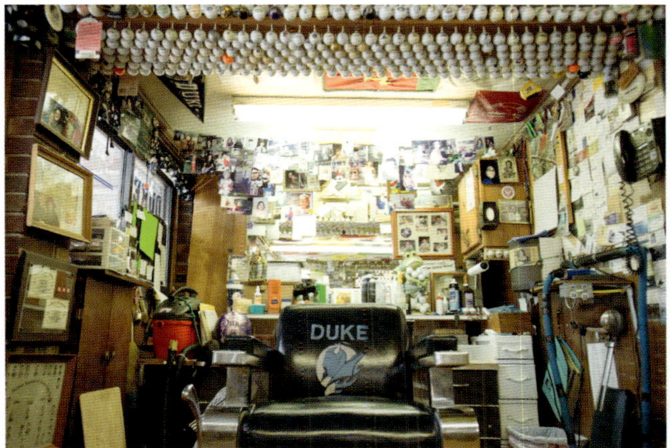
DUKE

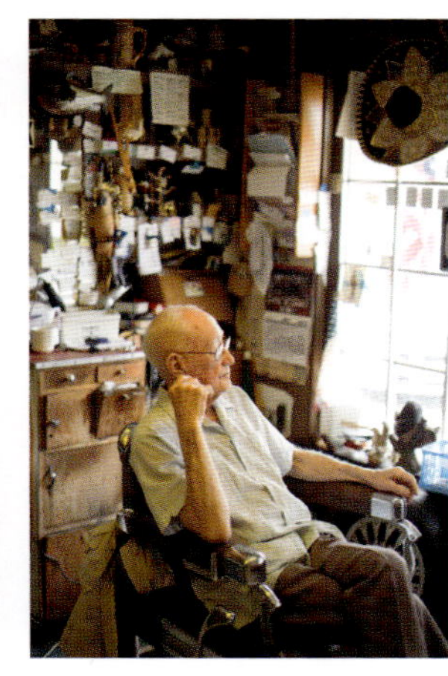

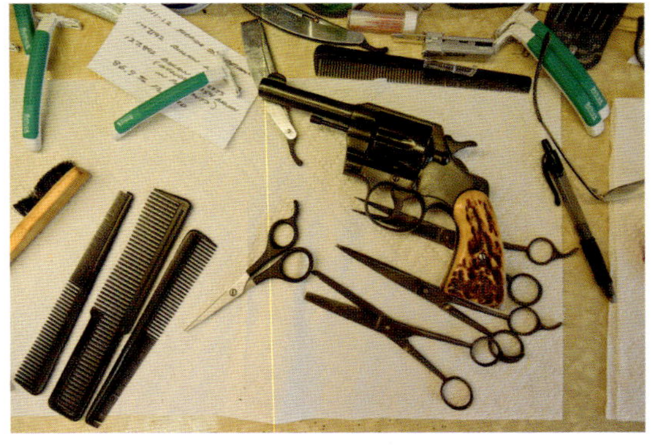

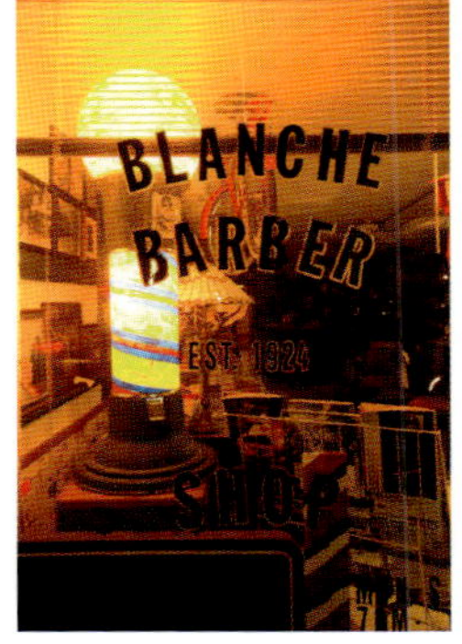
BLANCHE
BARBER
EST. 1924

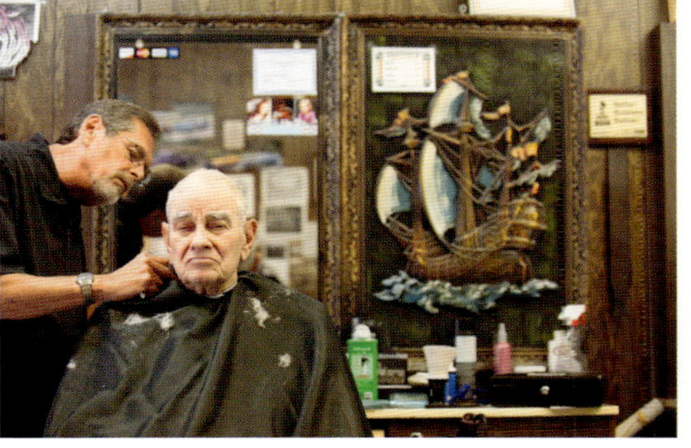

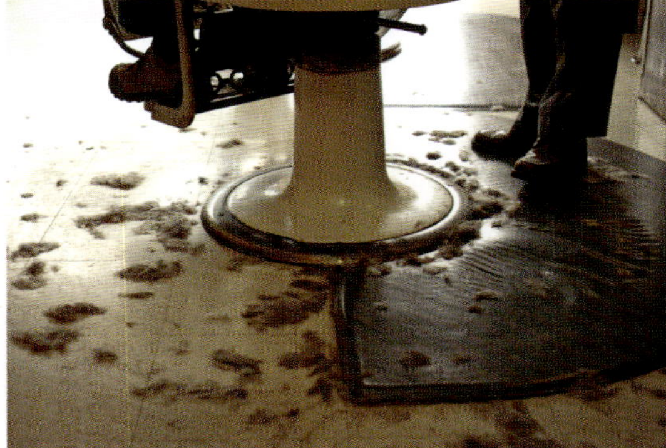

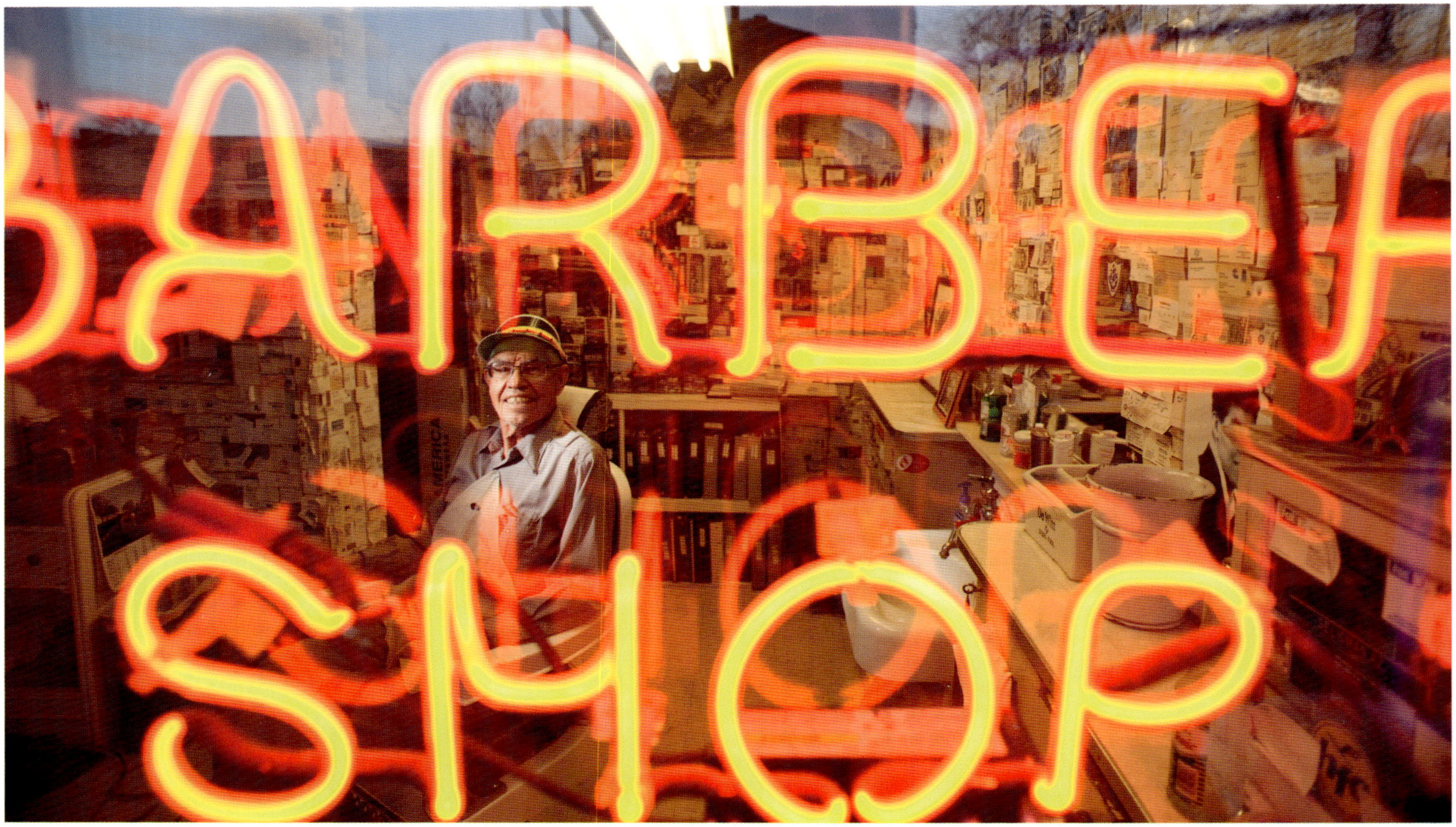

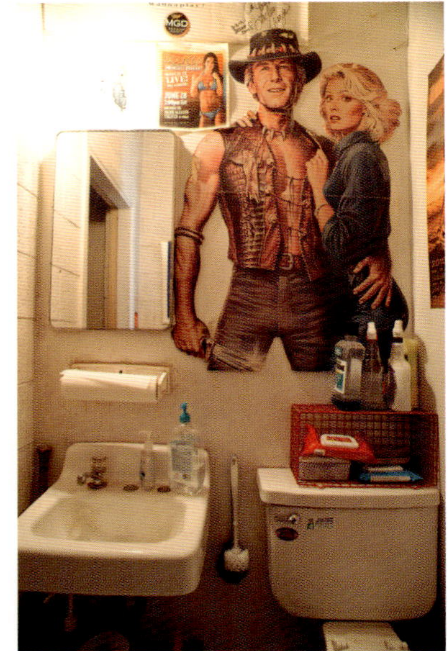

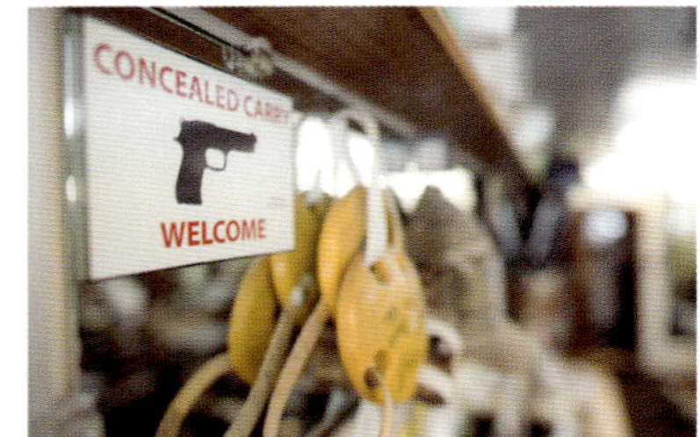
CONCEALED CARR
WELCOME

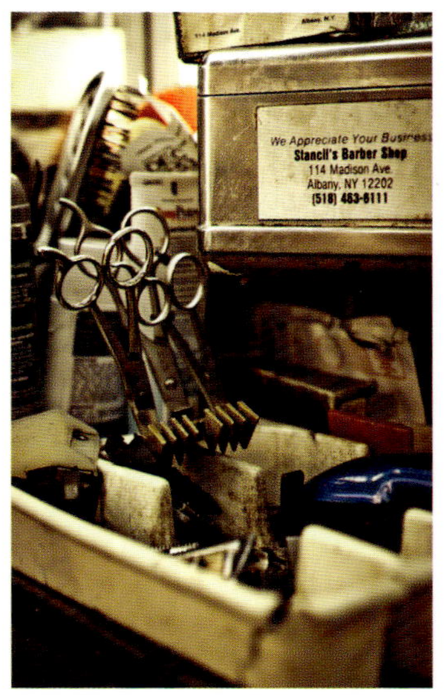
We Appreciate Your Business
Stancil's Barber Shop
114 Madison Ave.
Albany, NY 12202
(518) 463-6111

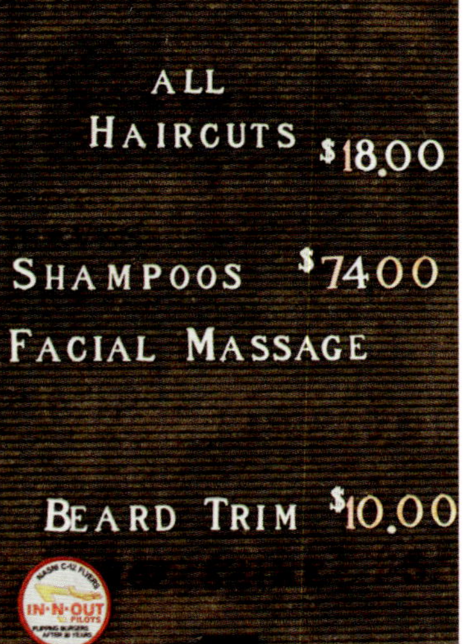
ALL
HAIRCUTS $18.00
SHAMPOOS $7.00
FACIAL MASSAGE
BEARD TRIM $10.00
IN-N-OUT

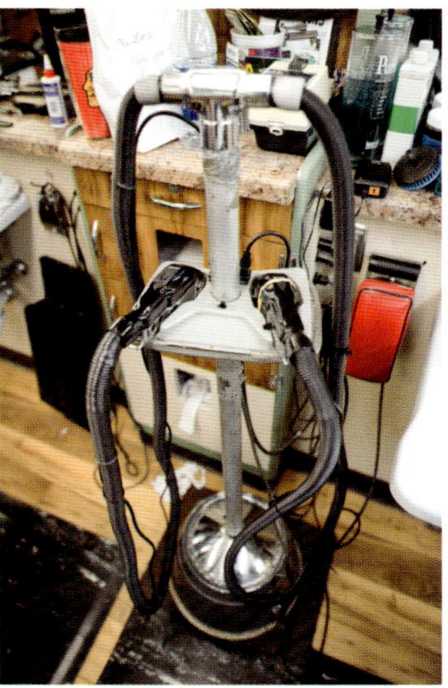

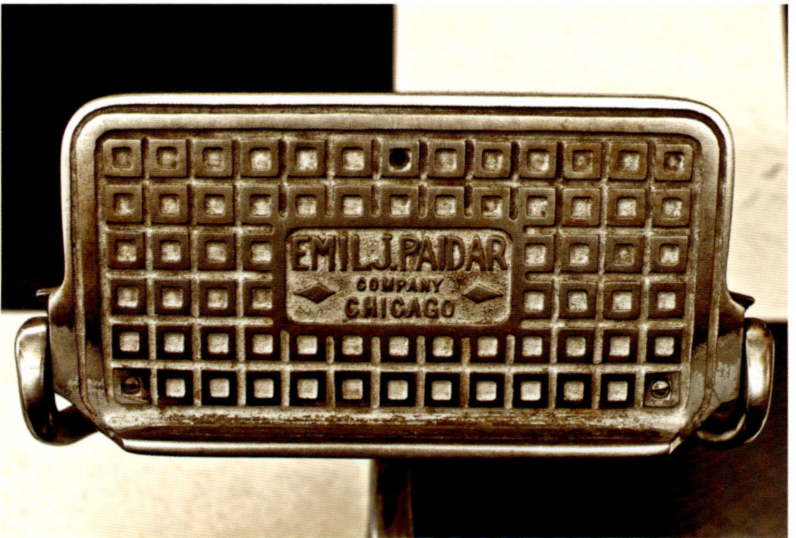
EMIL J. PAIDAR
COMPANY
CHICAGO

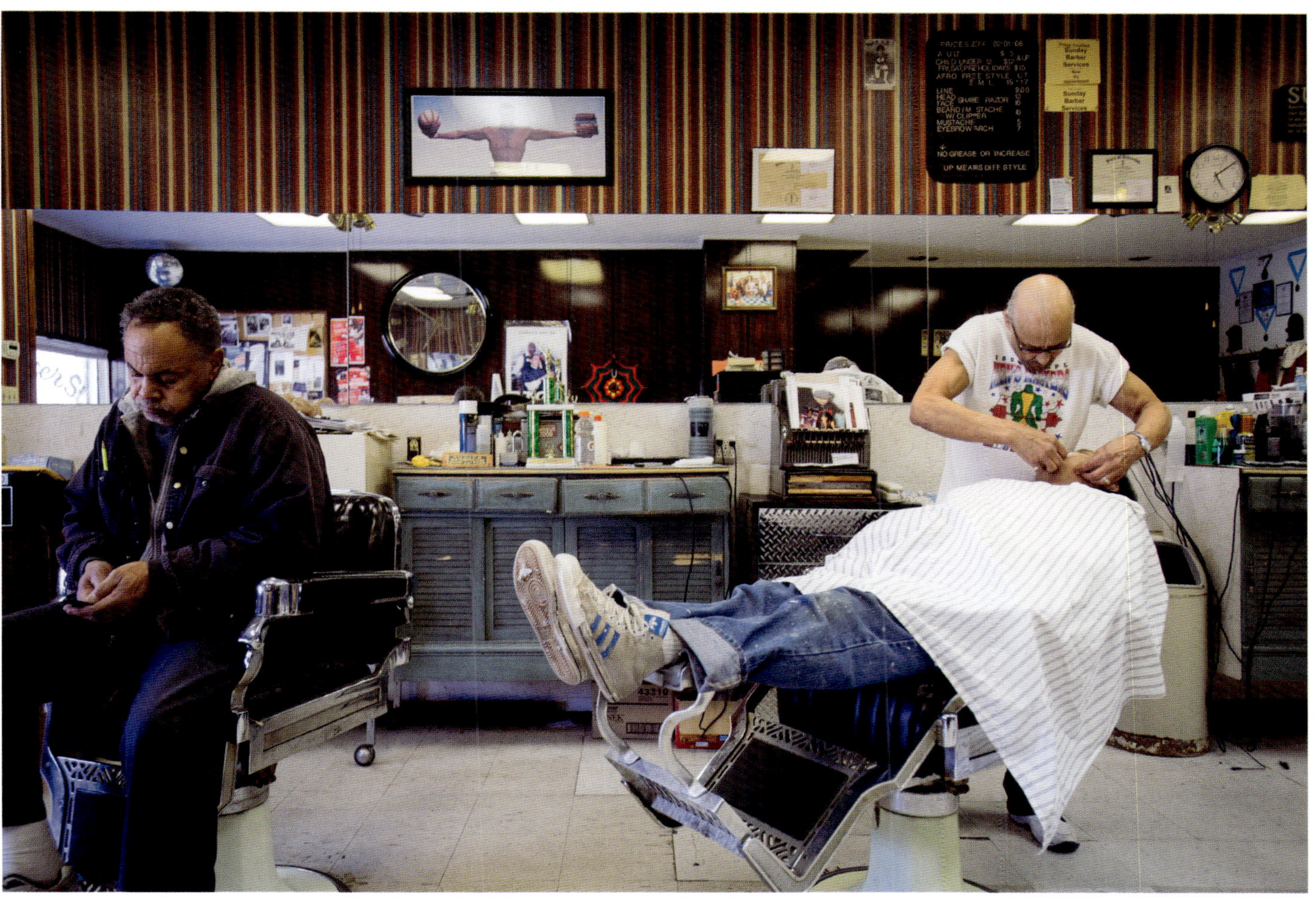

Goodwin's Spencer St. Barbershop, Omaha, Nebraska

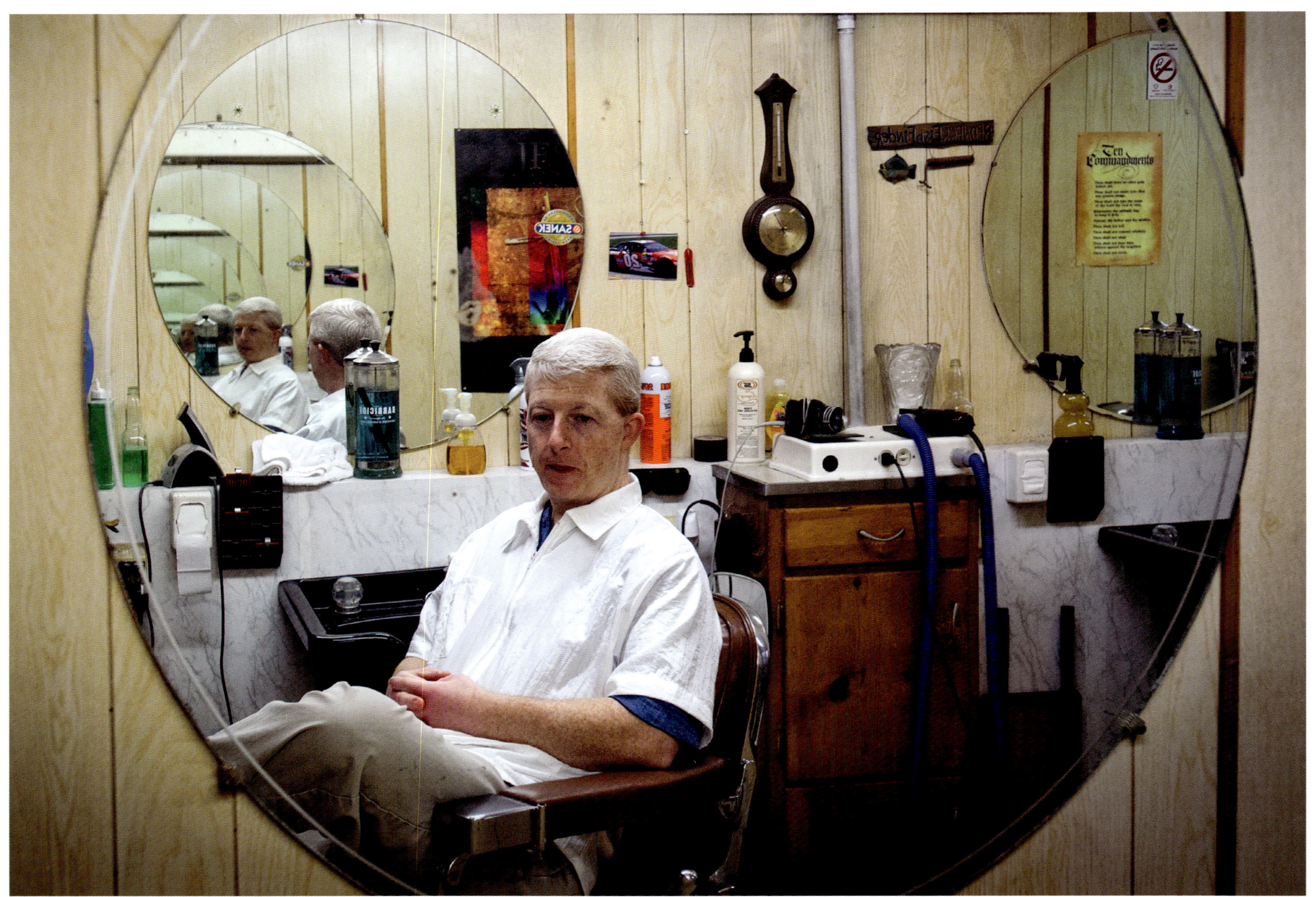

Neely's Barbershop, Winchester, Kentucky

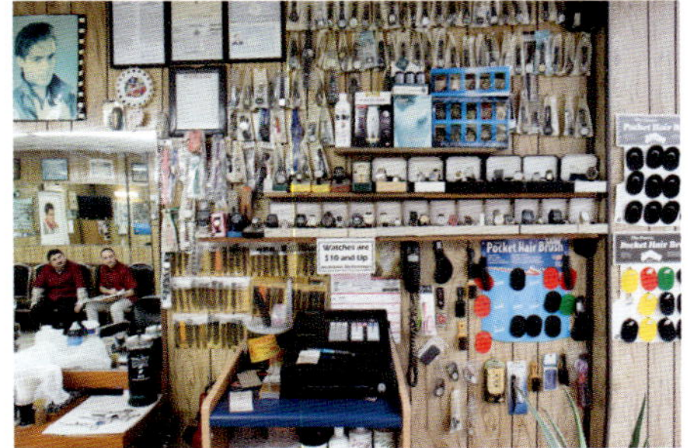

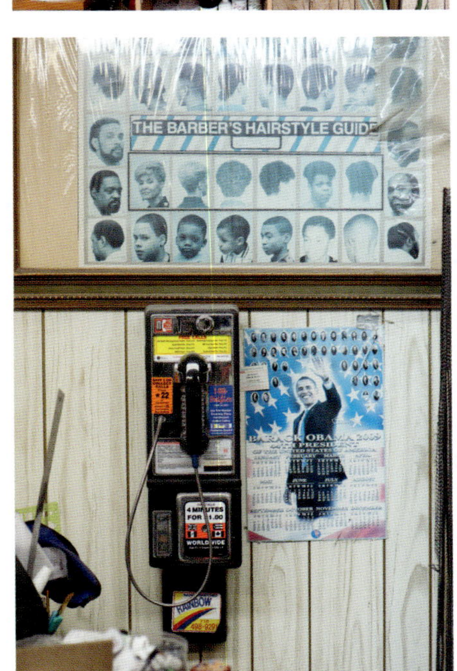
THE BARBER'S HAIRSTYLE GUIDE

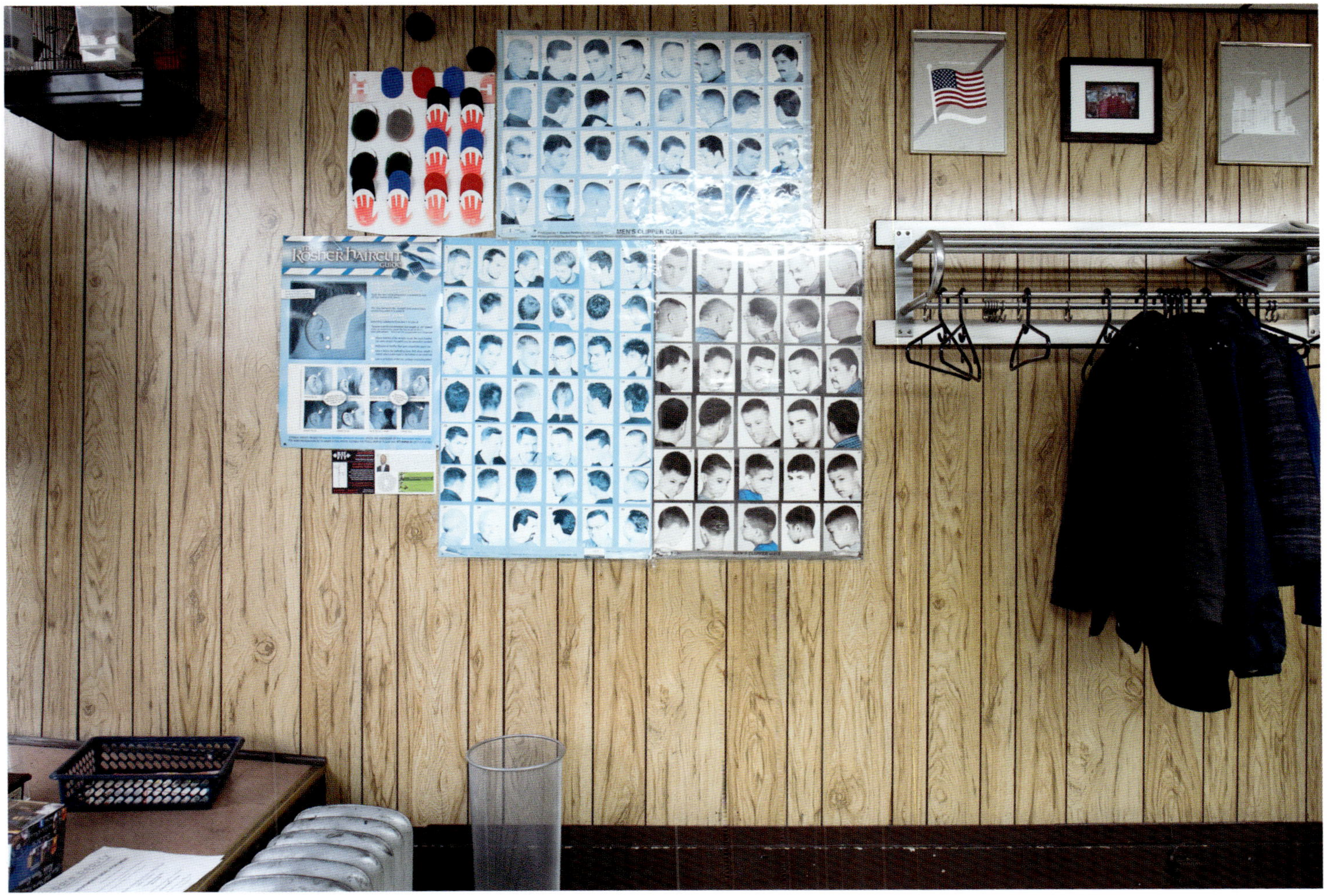

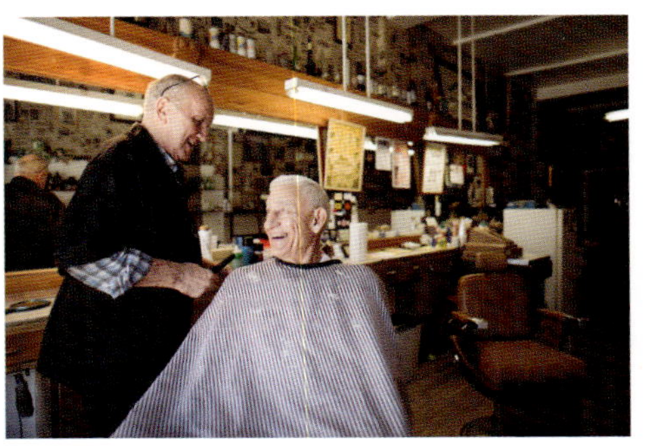

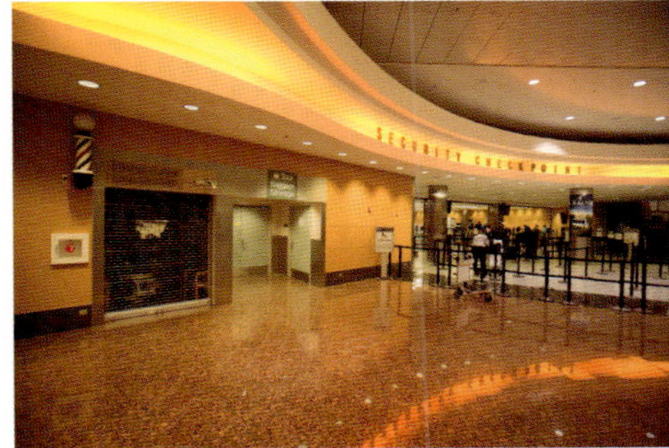

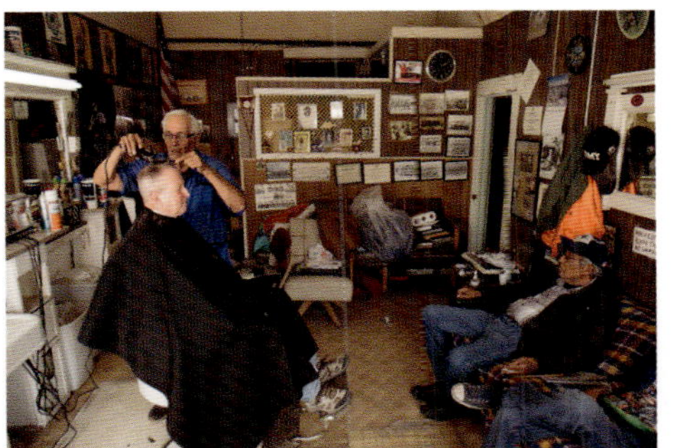

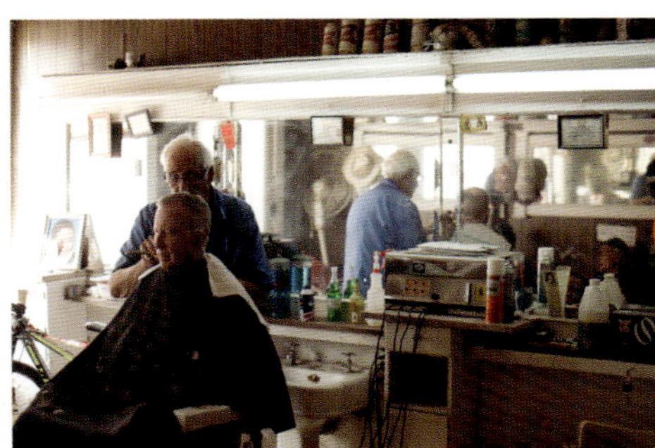

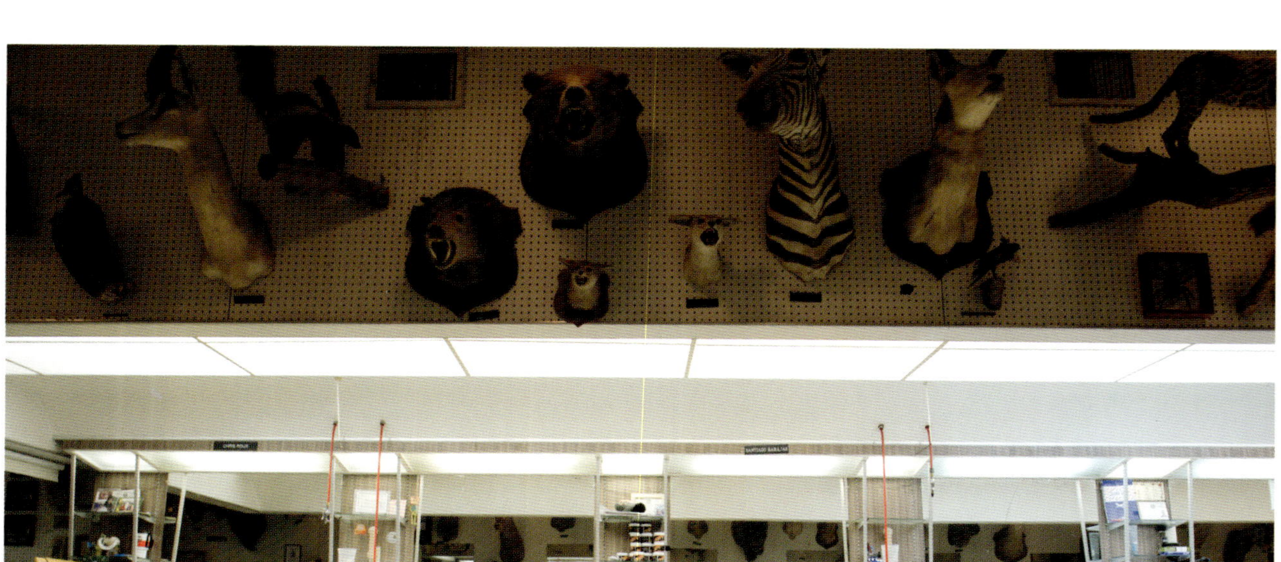

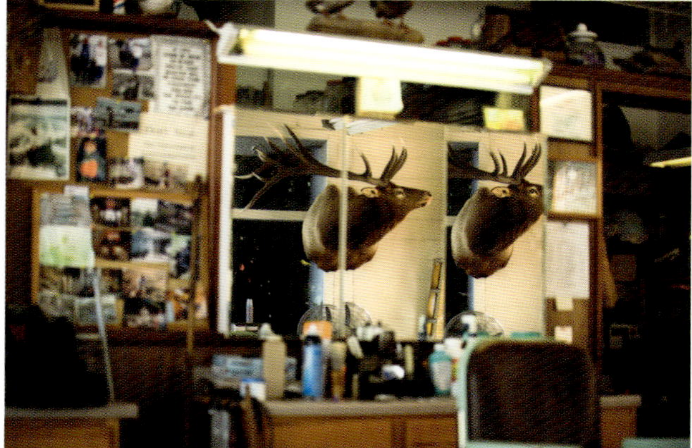

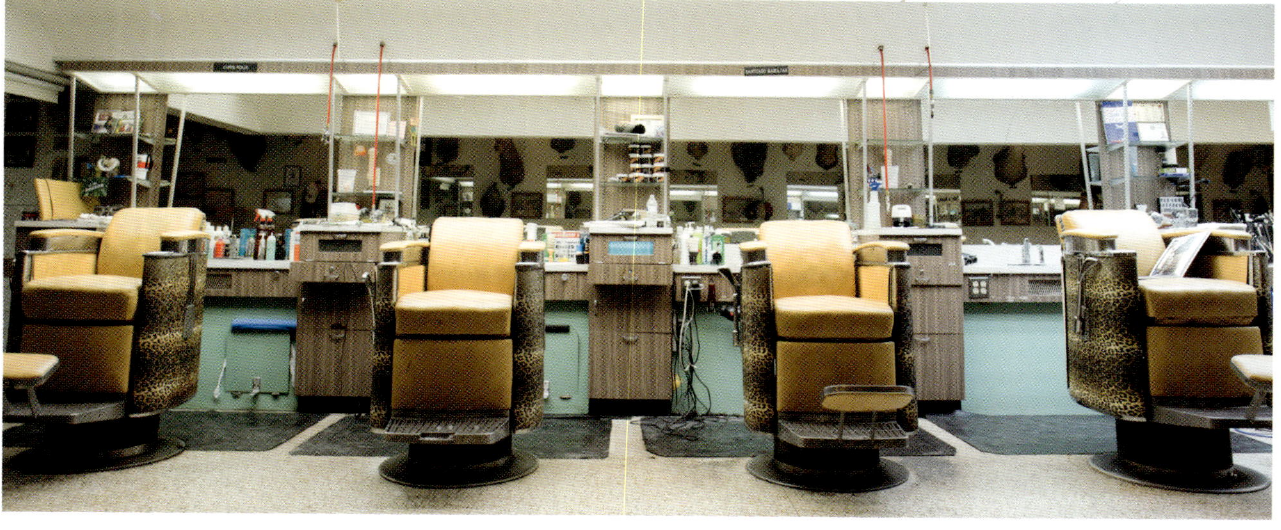

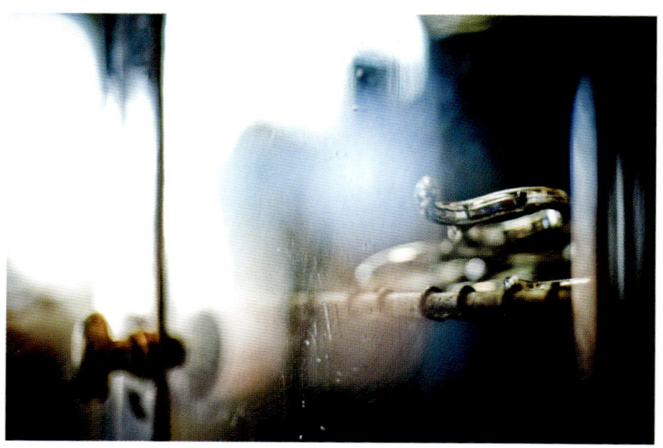

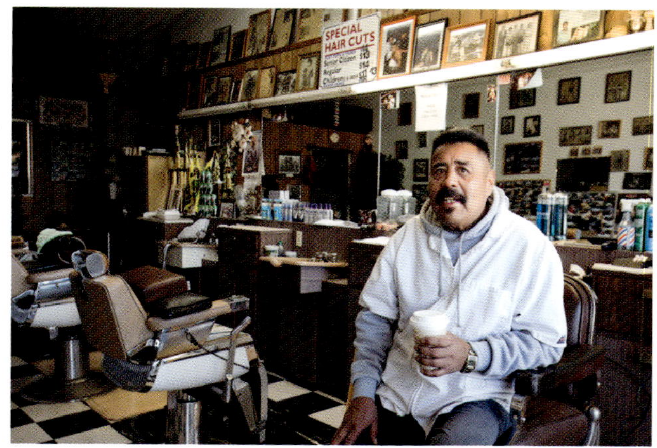
SPECIAL
HAIR CUTS

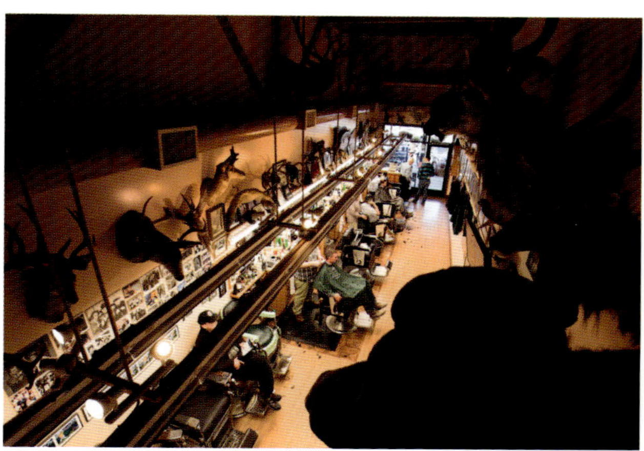

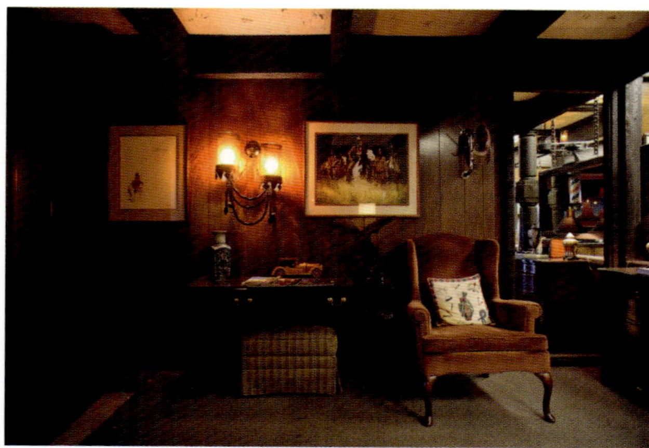

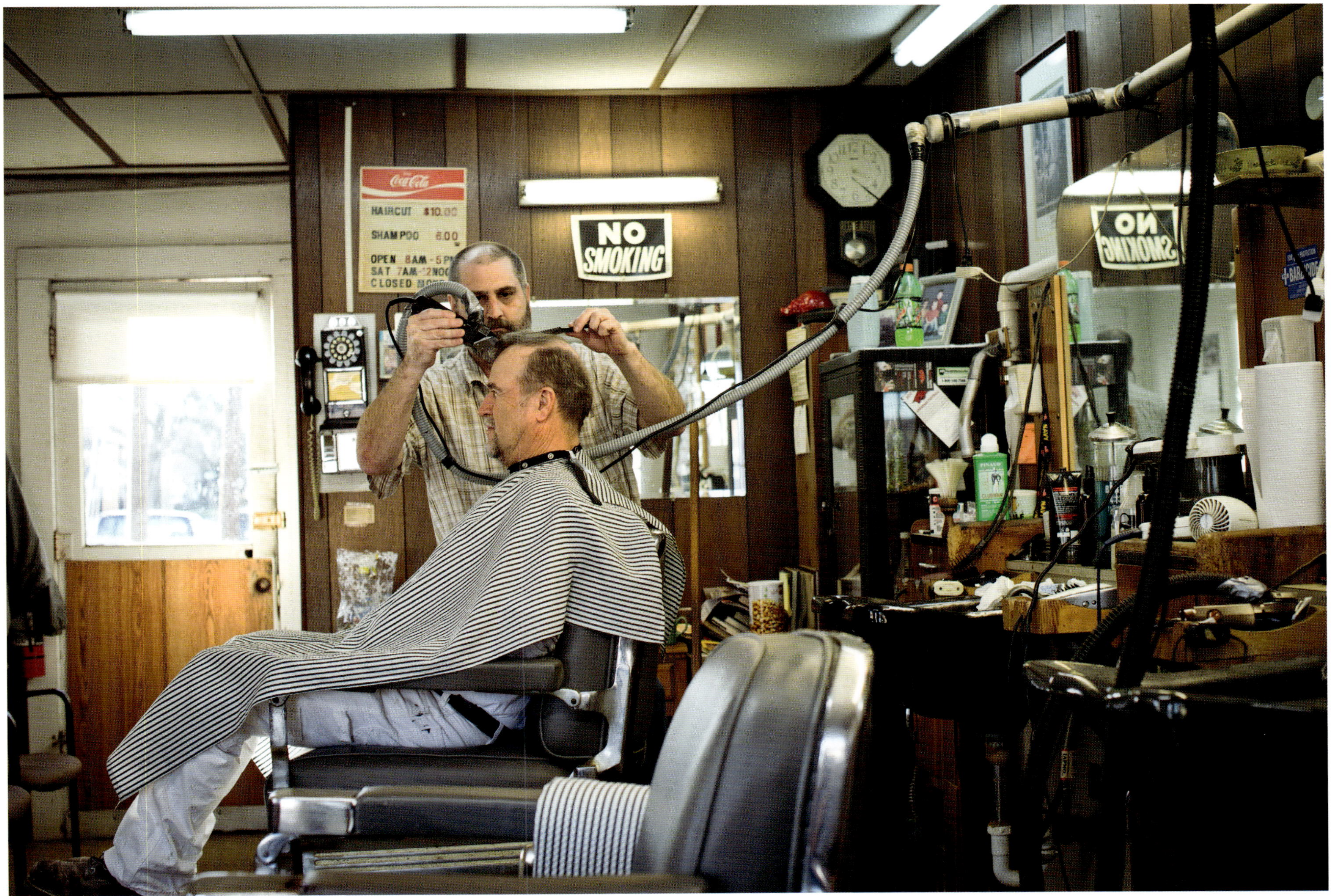

Woodard's Barbershop, Springdale, Arizona

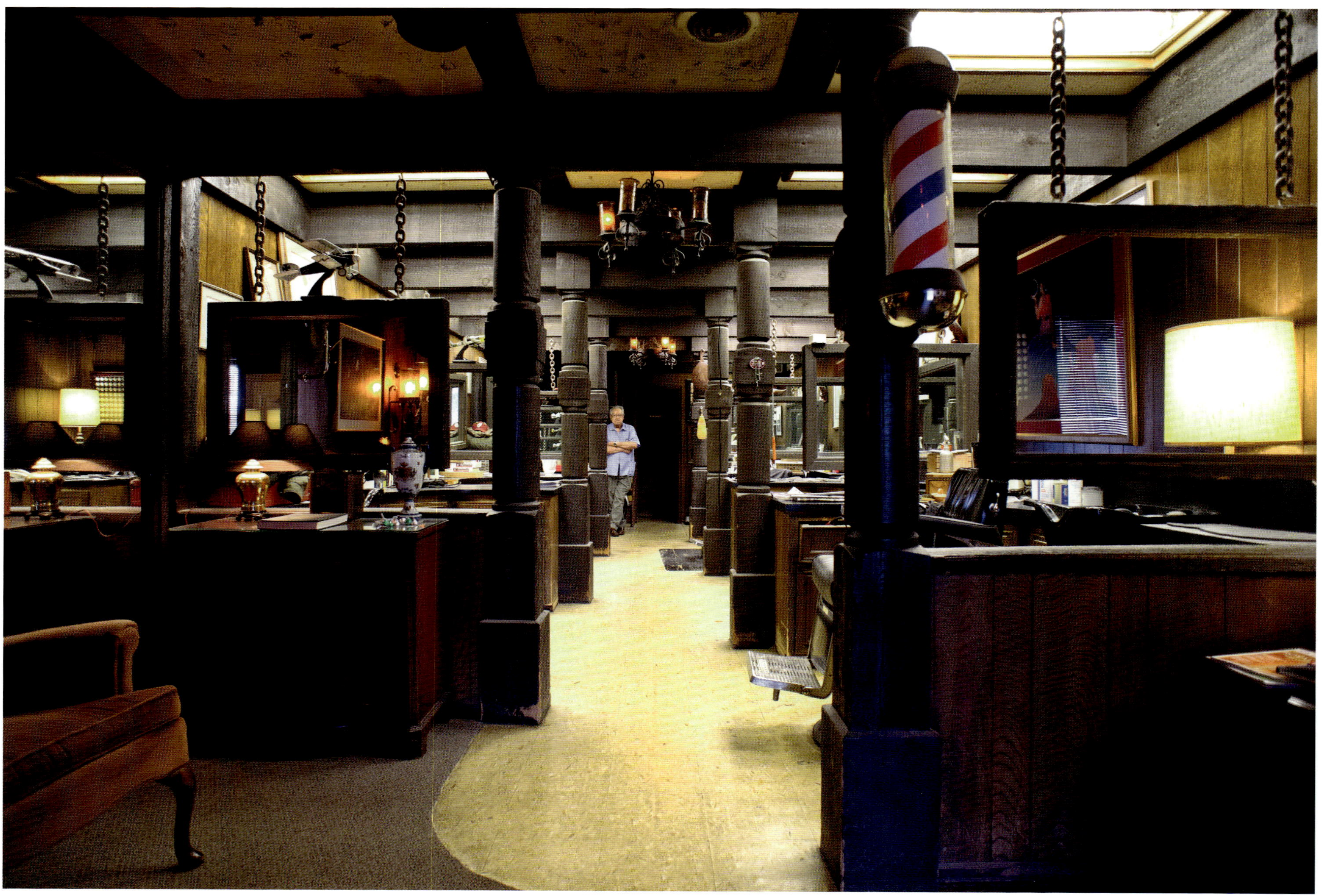

Continental Barbershop, Tulsa, Oklahoma

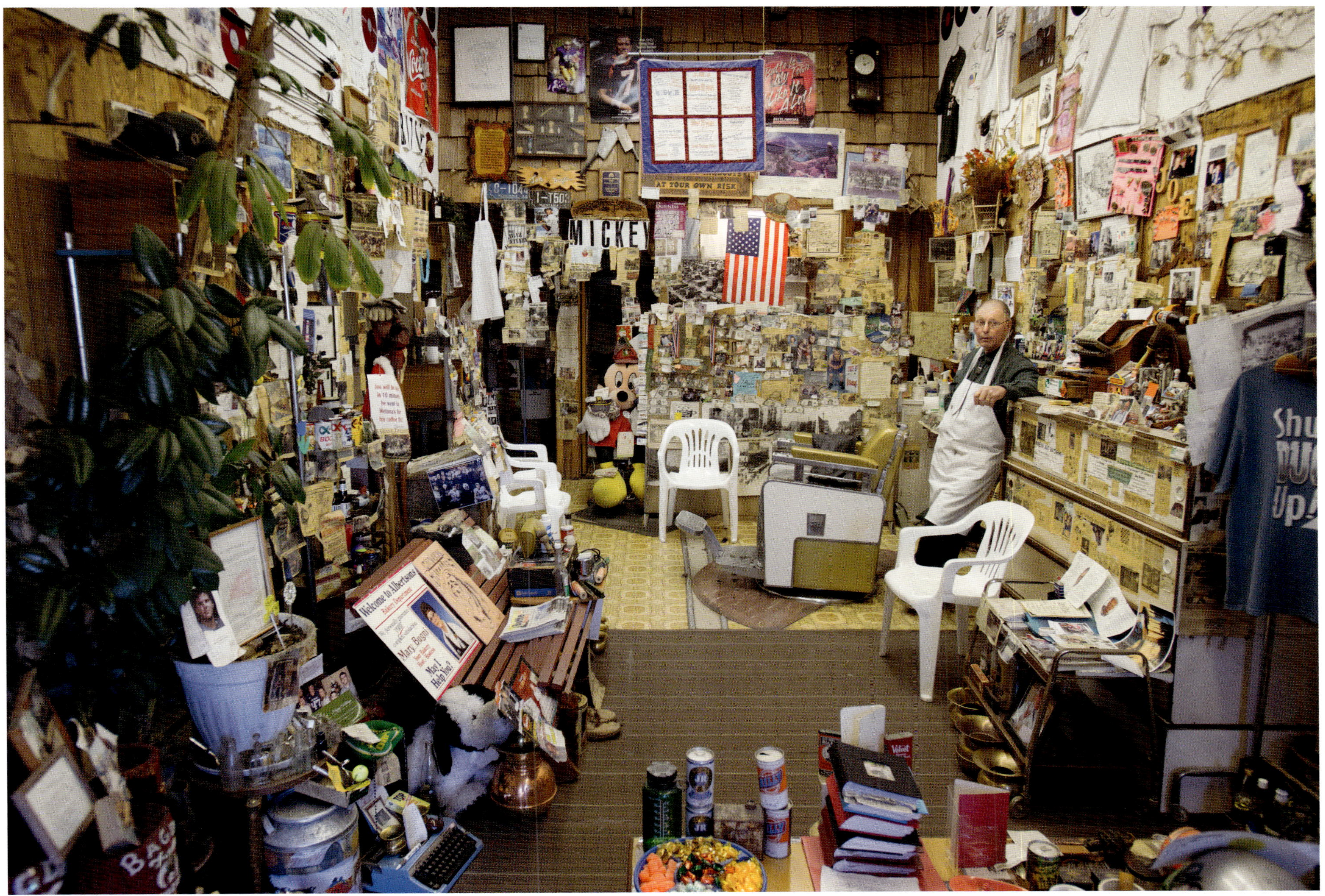

Amherst Ave. Barbershop, Butte, Montana

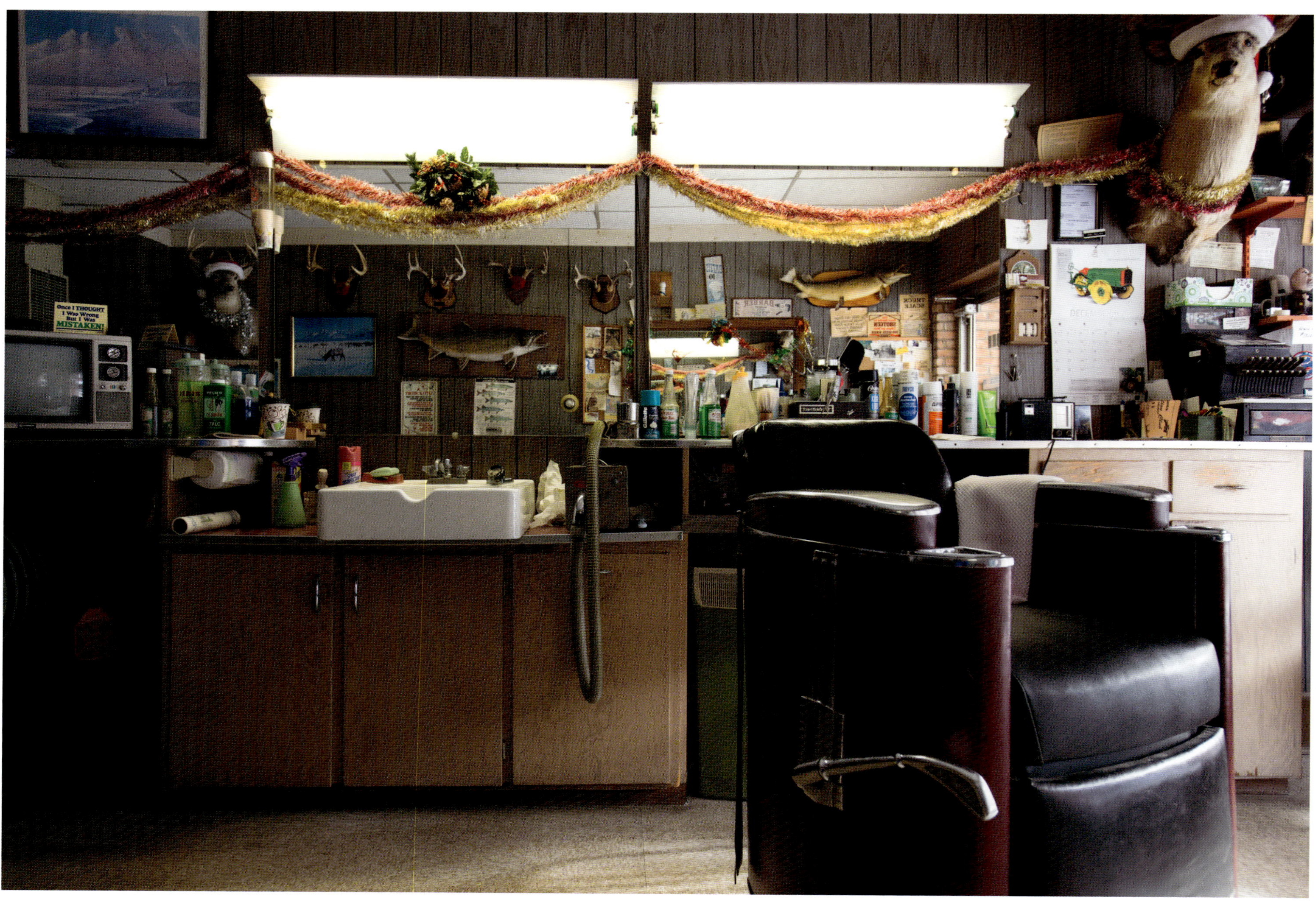

Tony's Barbershop, Sauk Center, Minnesota

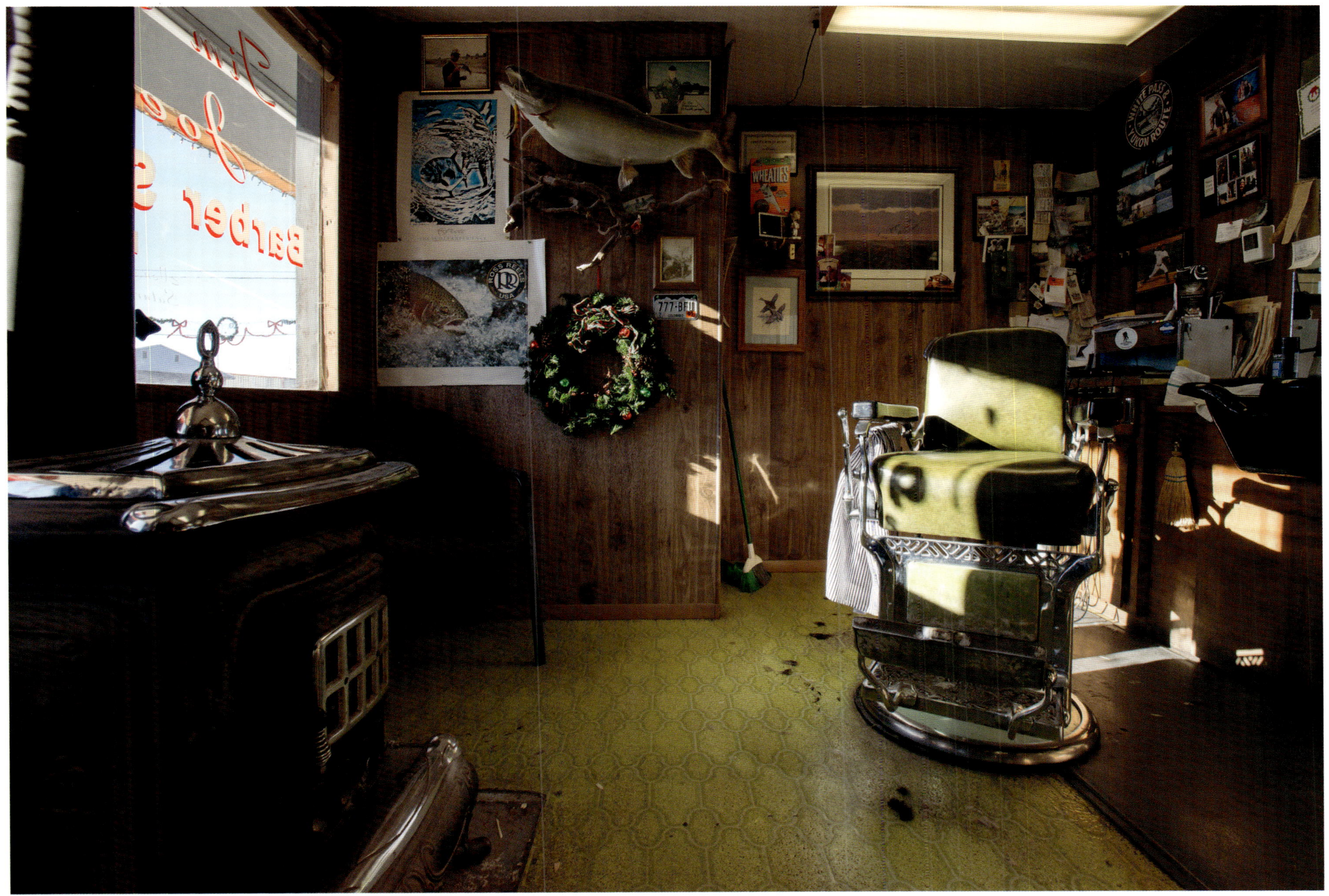

Tim's Barbershop, Montrose, Colorado

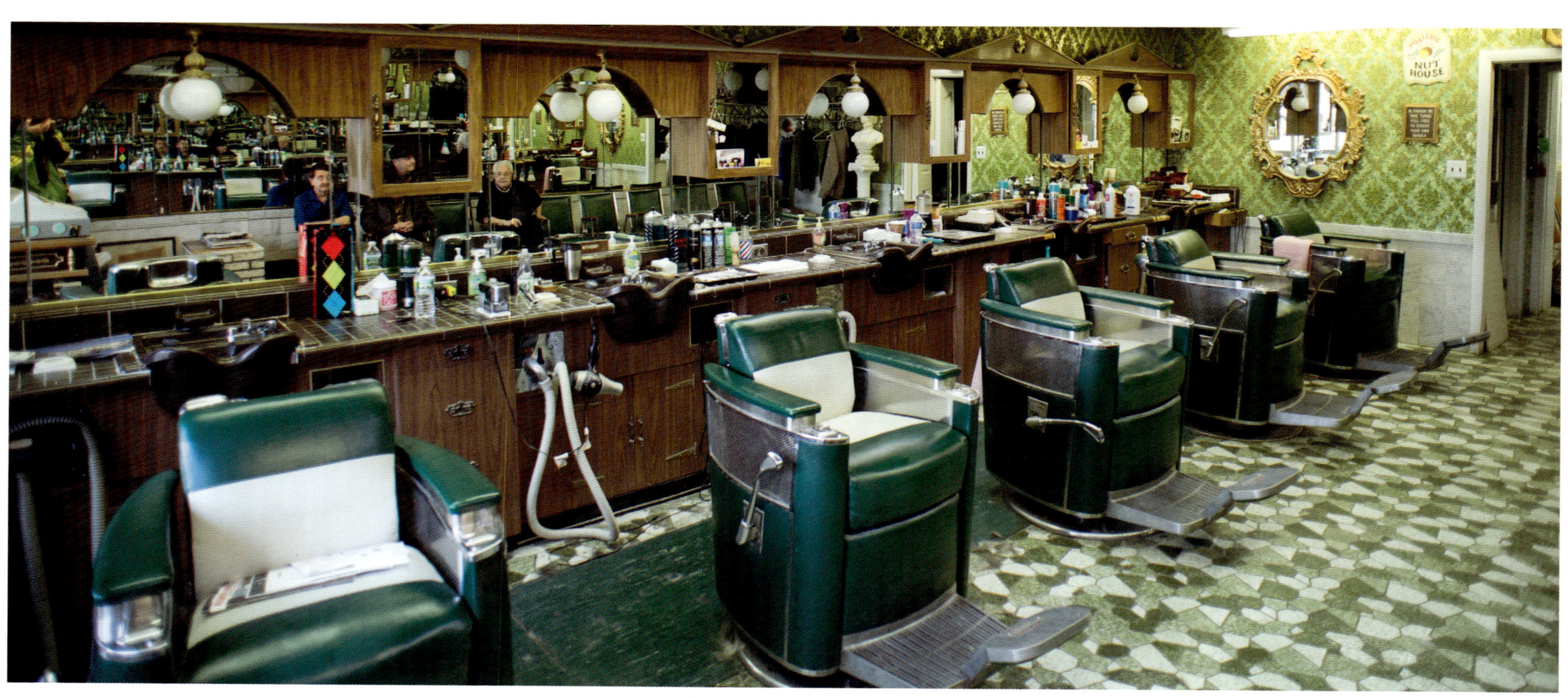

Unique Barbershop, Cherry Hill, New Jersey

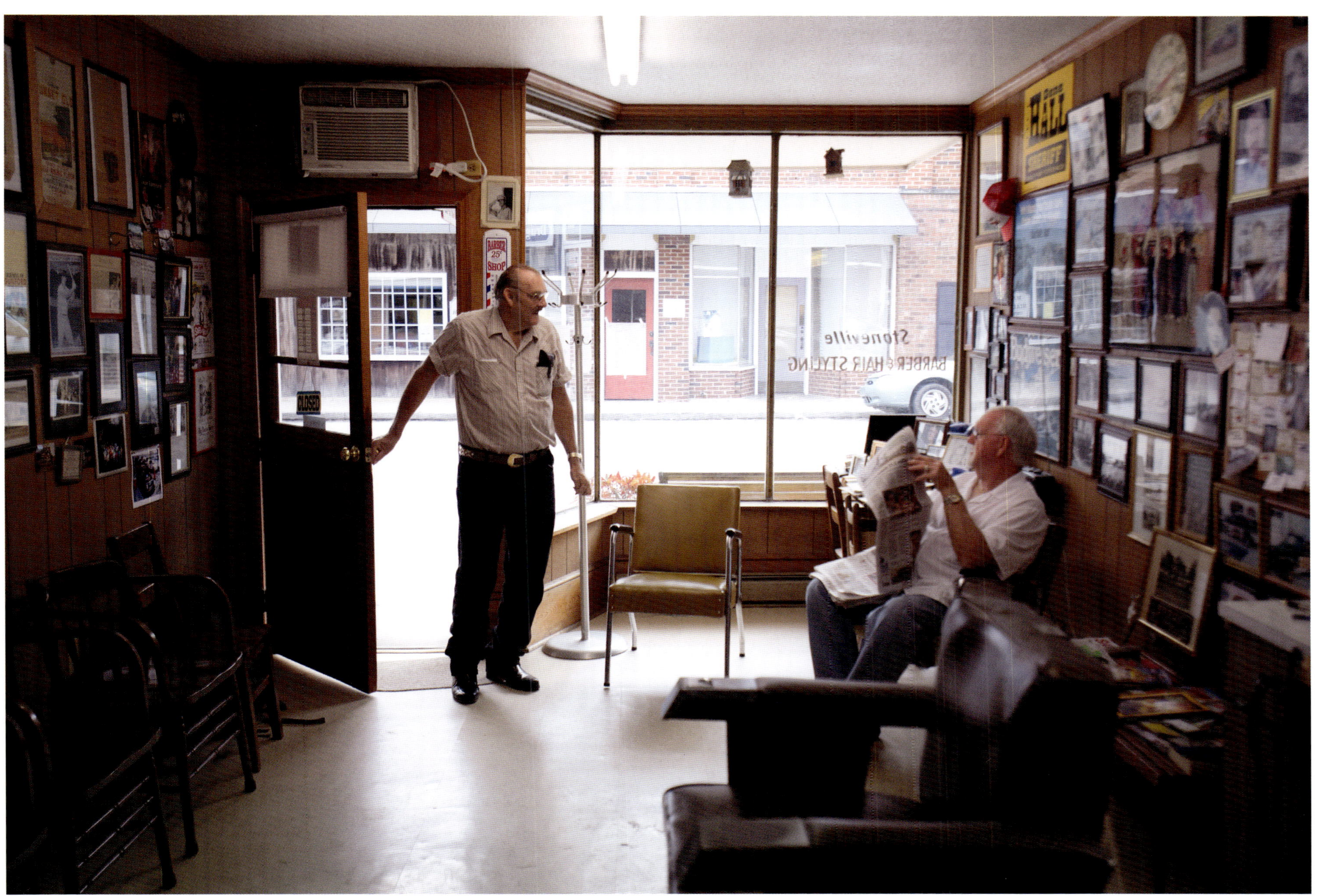

Stoneville Barbershop, Stoneville, North Carolina

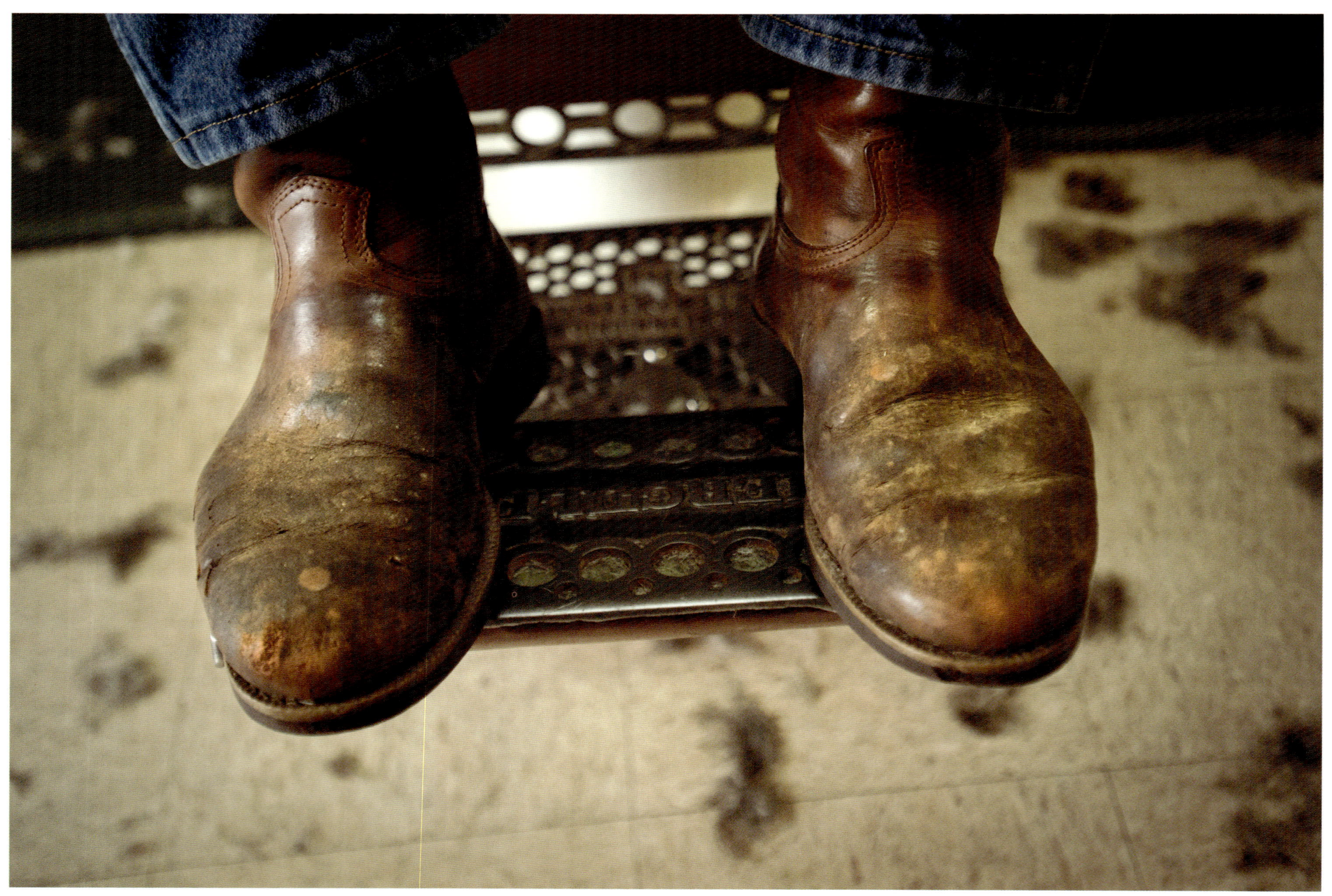

Central Barbershop, Woodstock, Virginia

"If it moves, we hunt it."

– Customer, Central Barbershop, Woodstock, Virginia

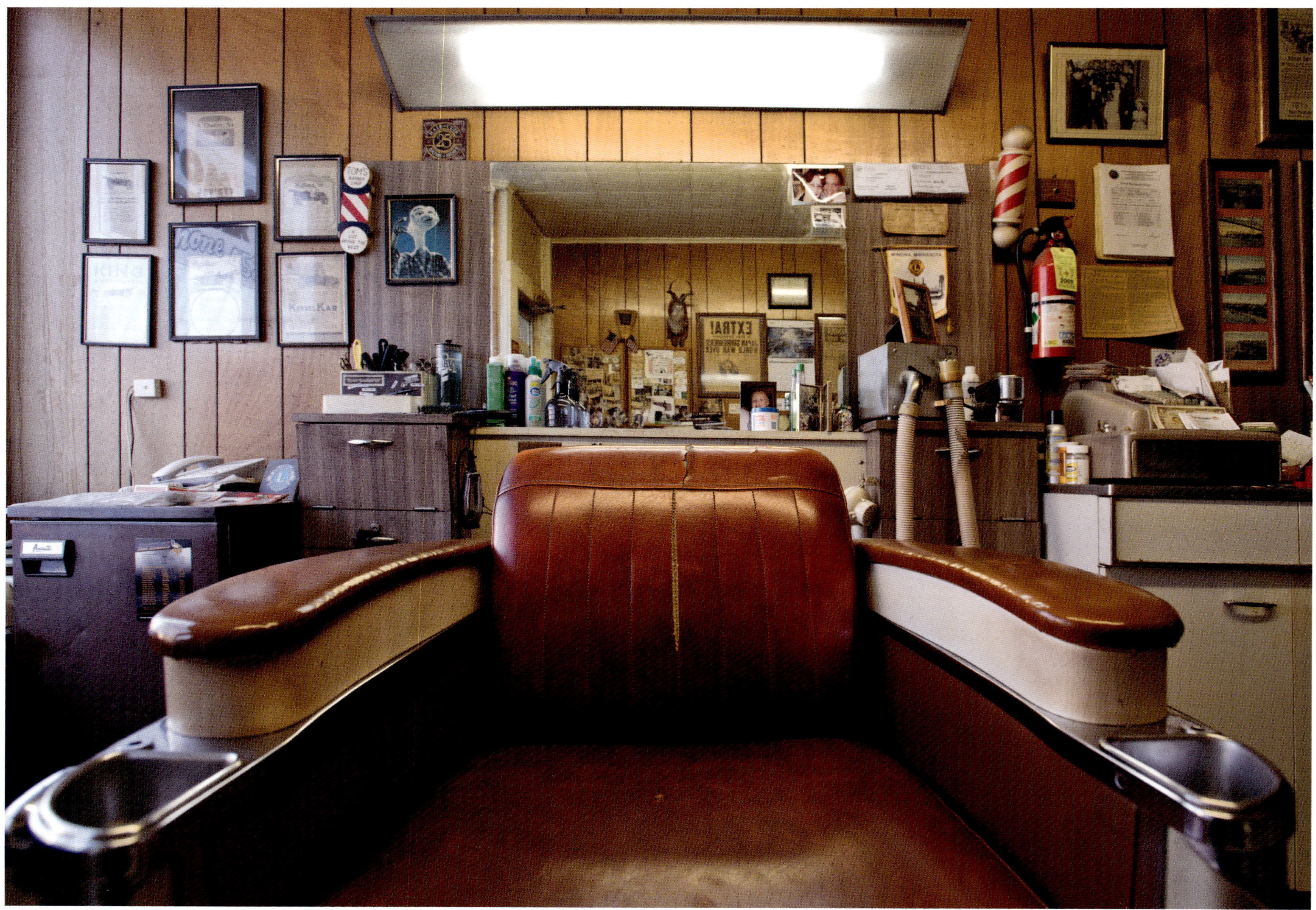

Tom's Barbershop, Winona, Minnesota

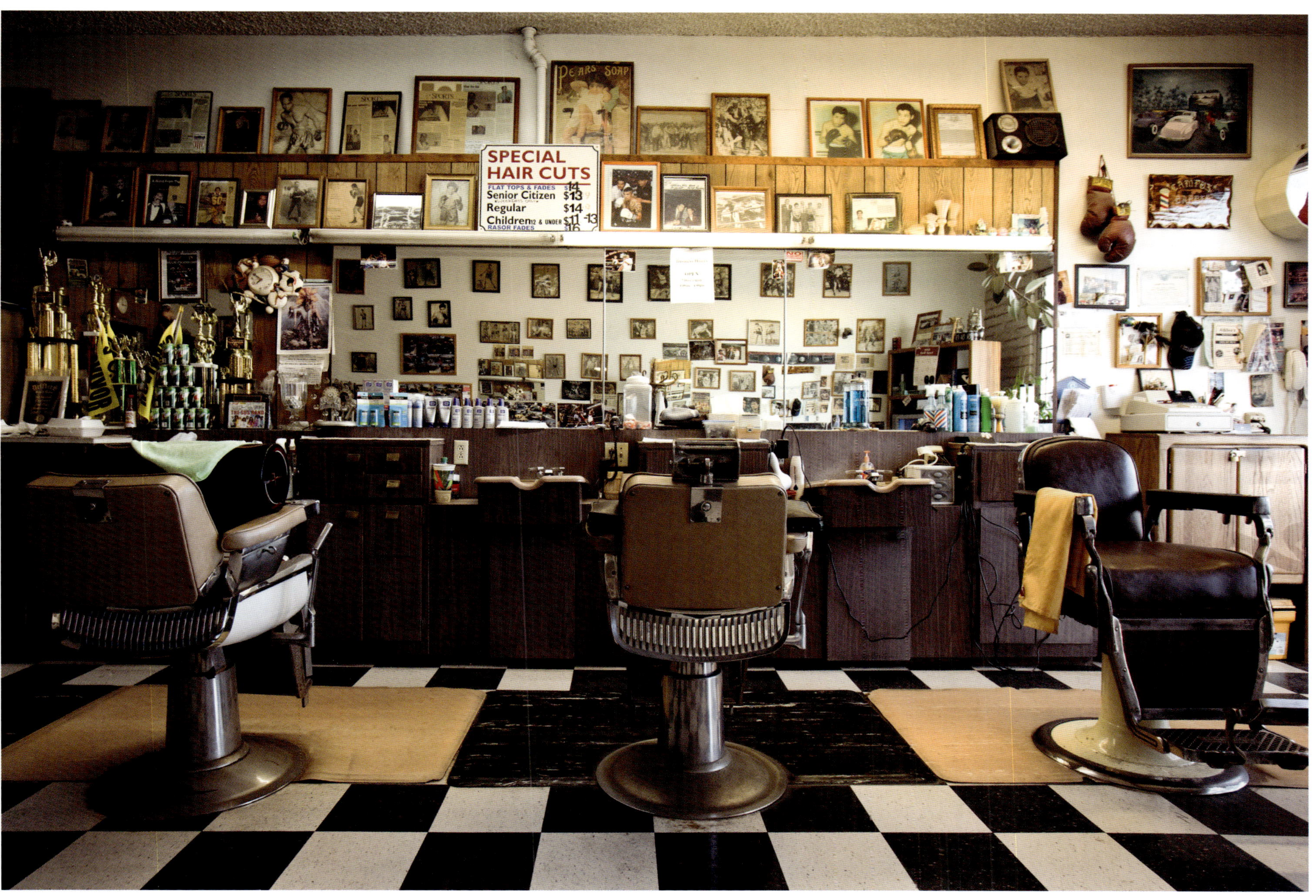

Unknown, Santa Maria, California

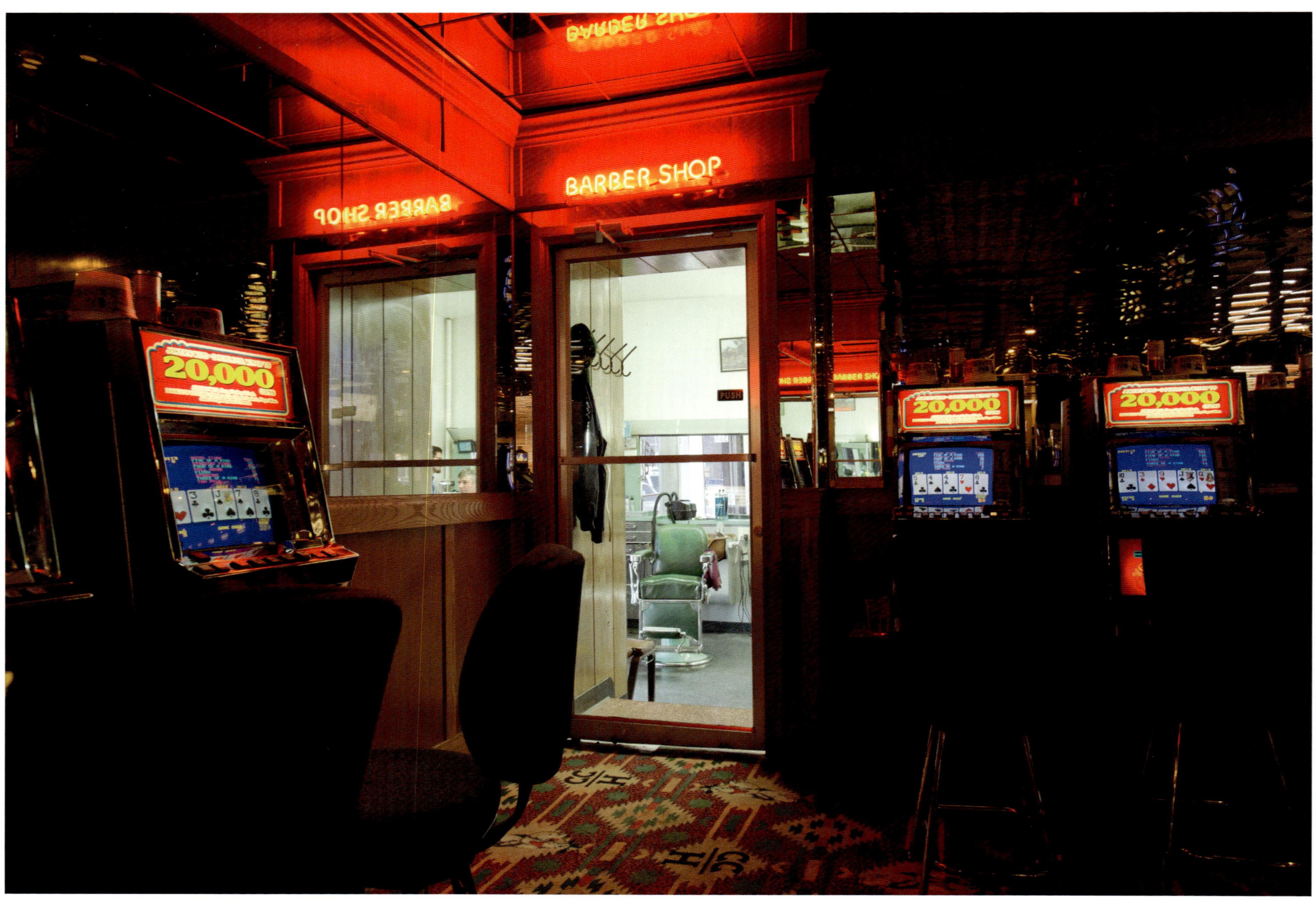

Commercial Barbershop, Elko, Nevada

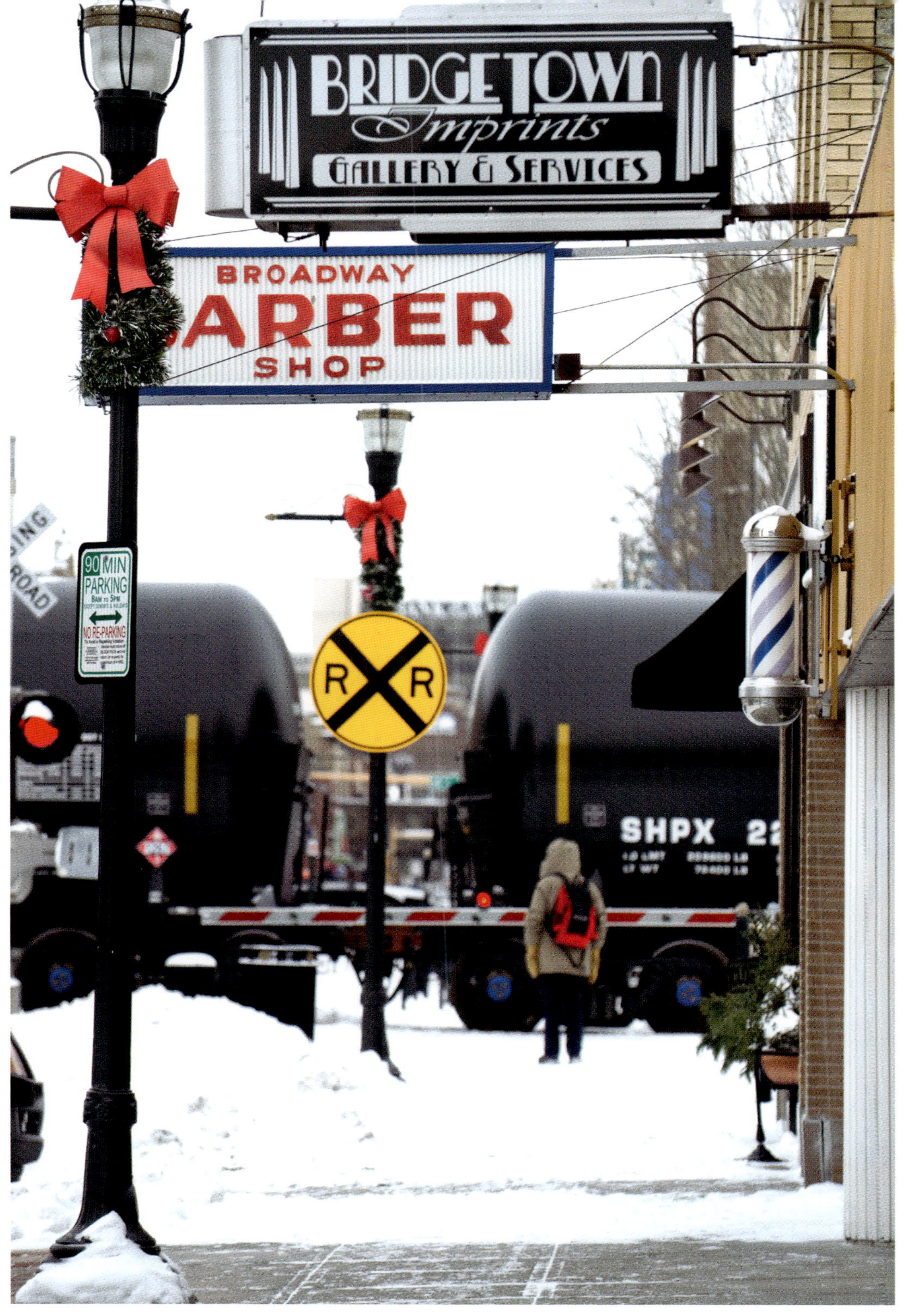

Broadway Barbershop, Anchorage, Alaska

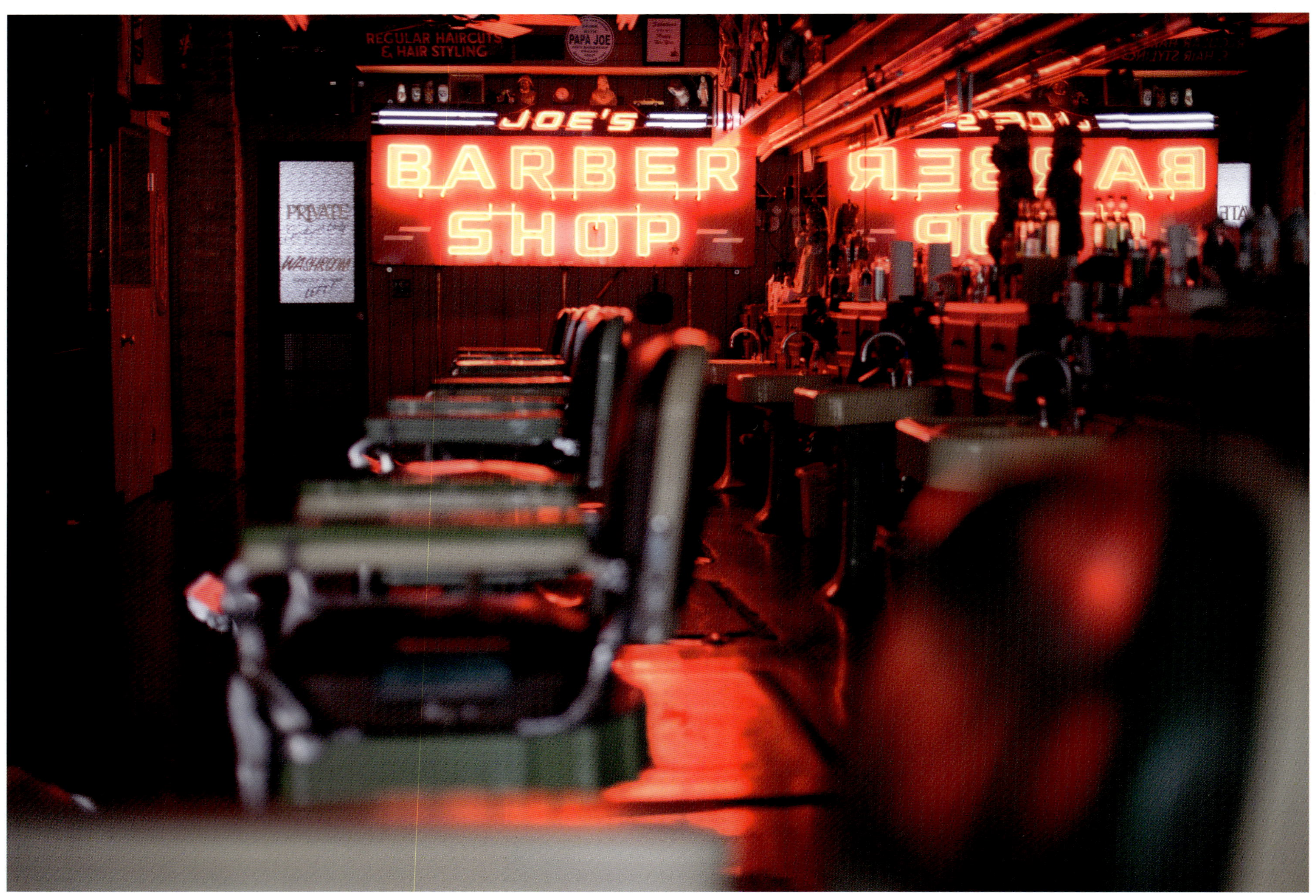

Joe's Barbershop, Chicago, Illinois

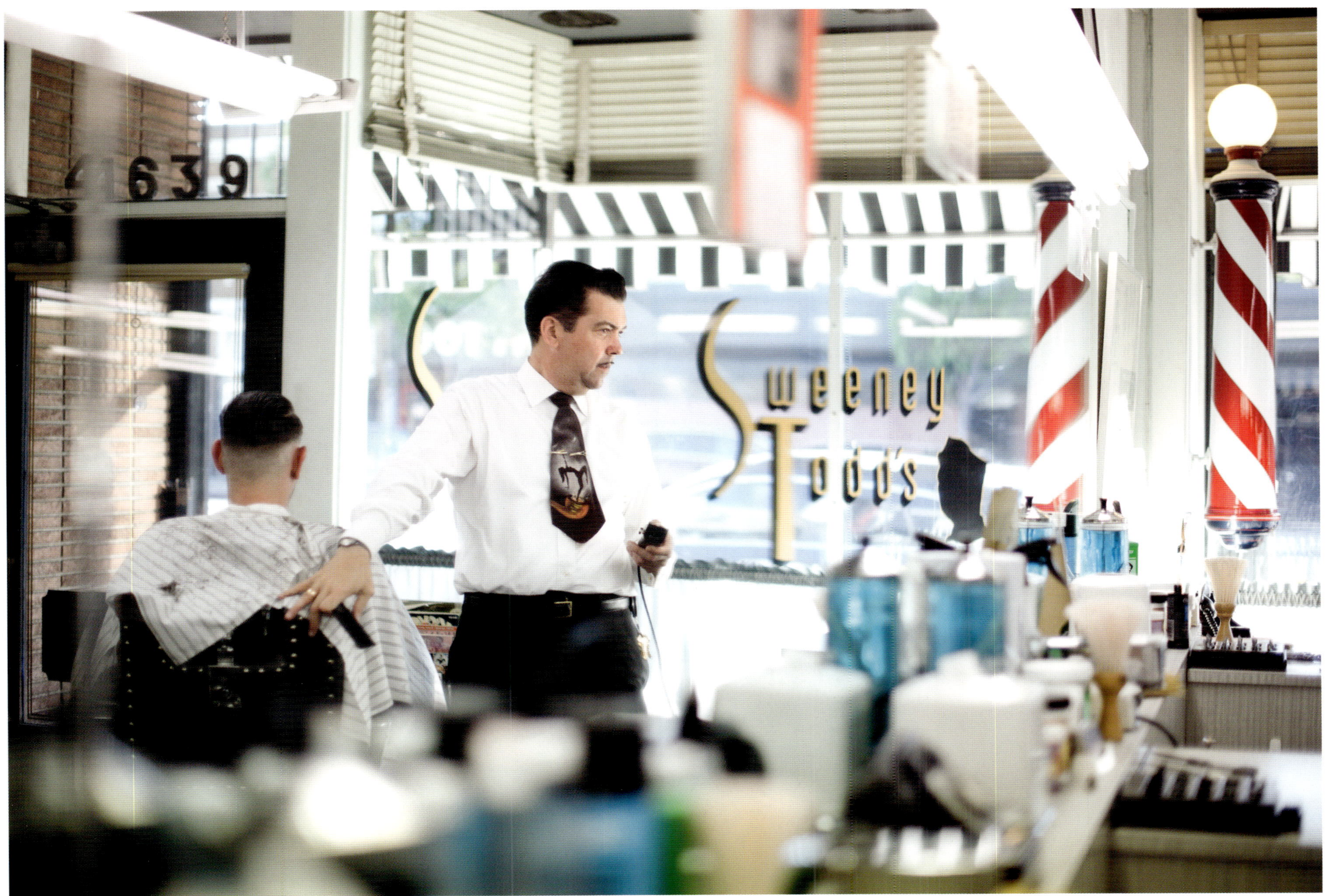

Sweeney Todd's Barbershop, Los Angeles, California

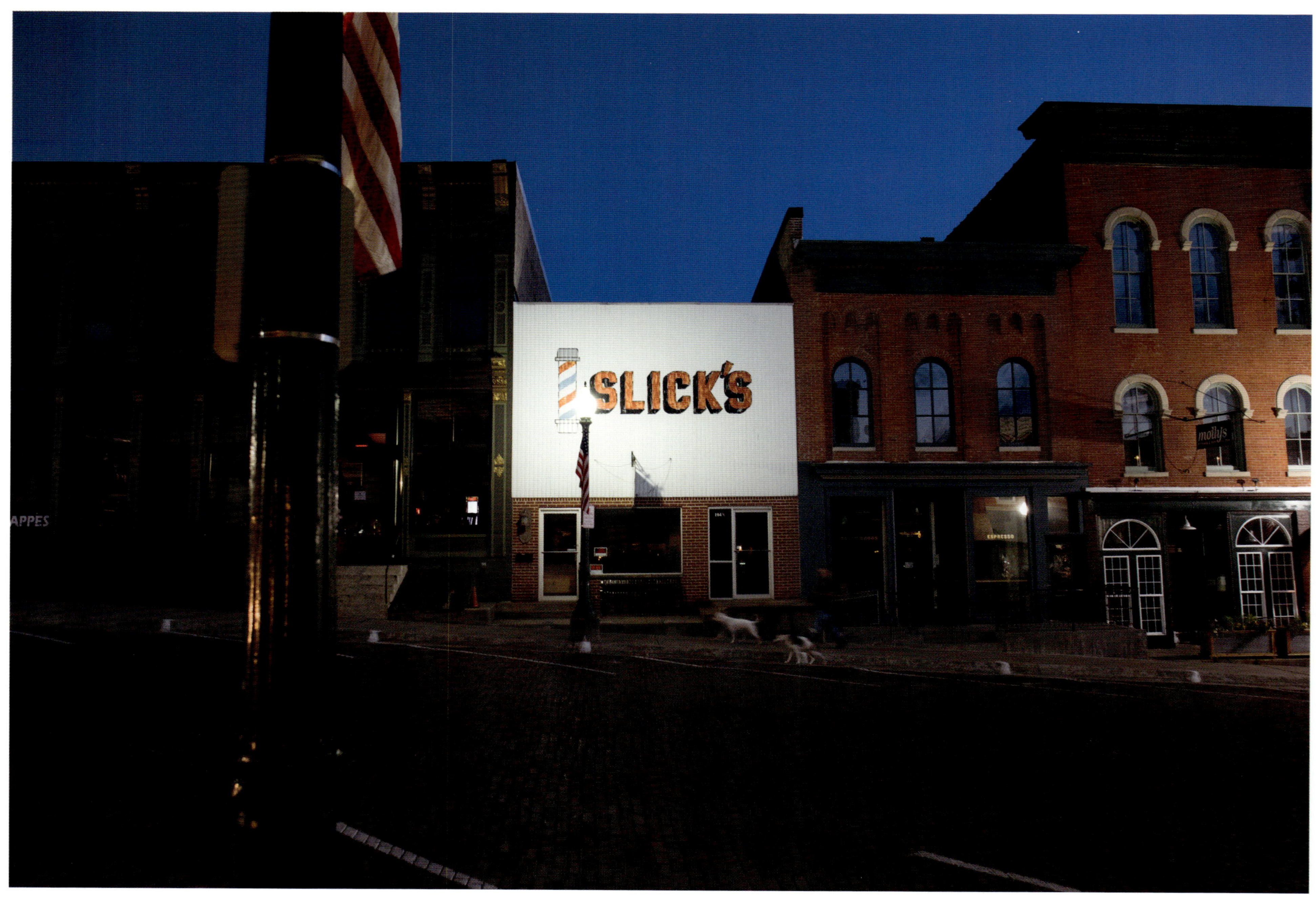

Slick's Barbershop, Mt. Carroll, Illinois

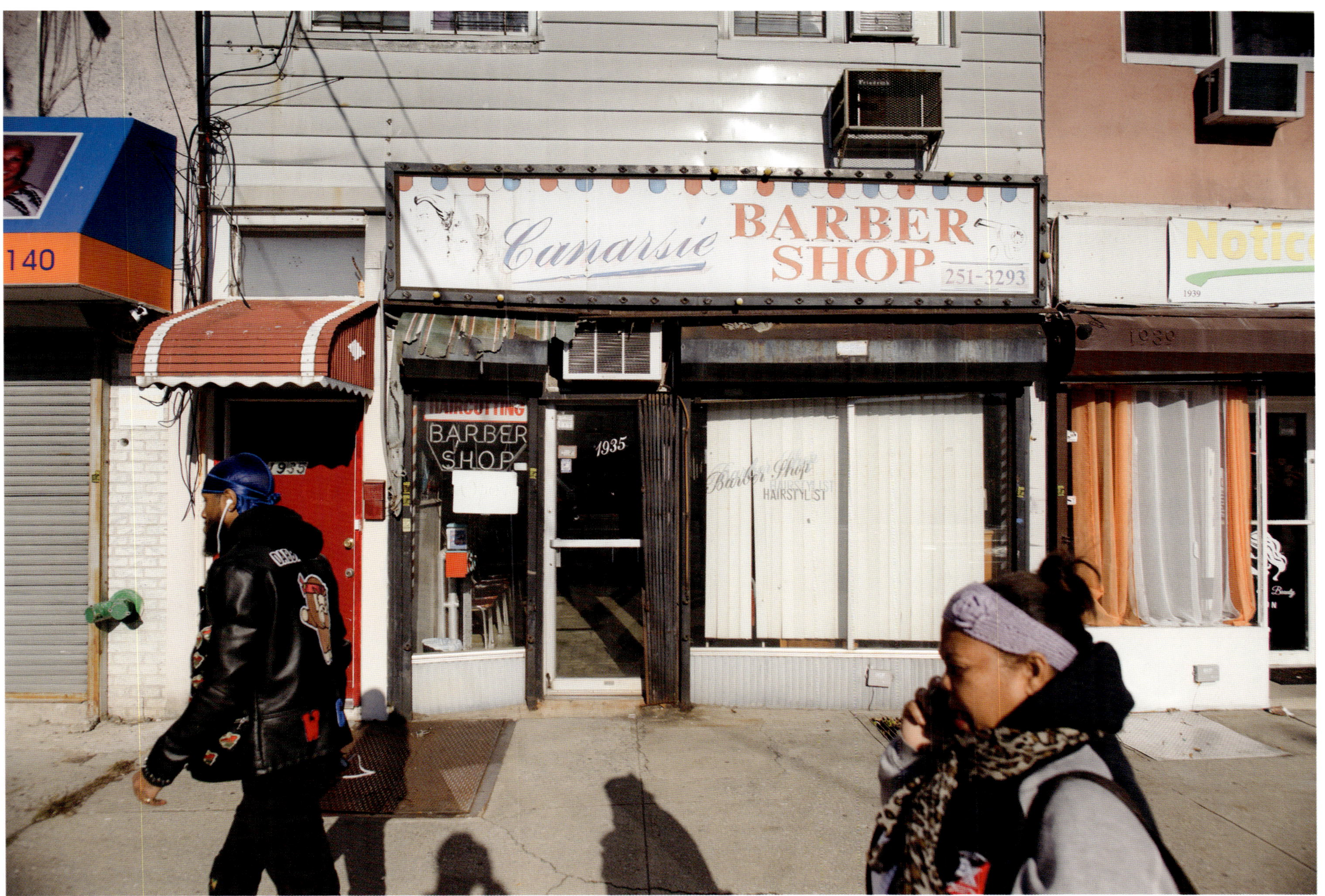

Canarsie Barbershop, Brooklyn, New York

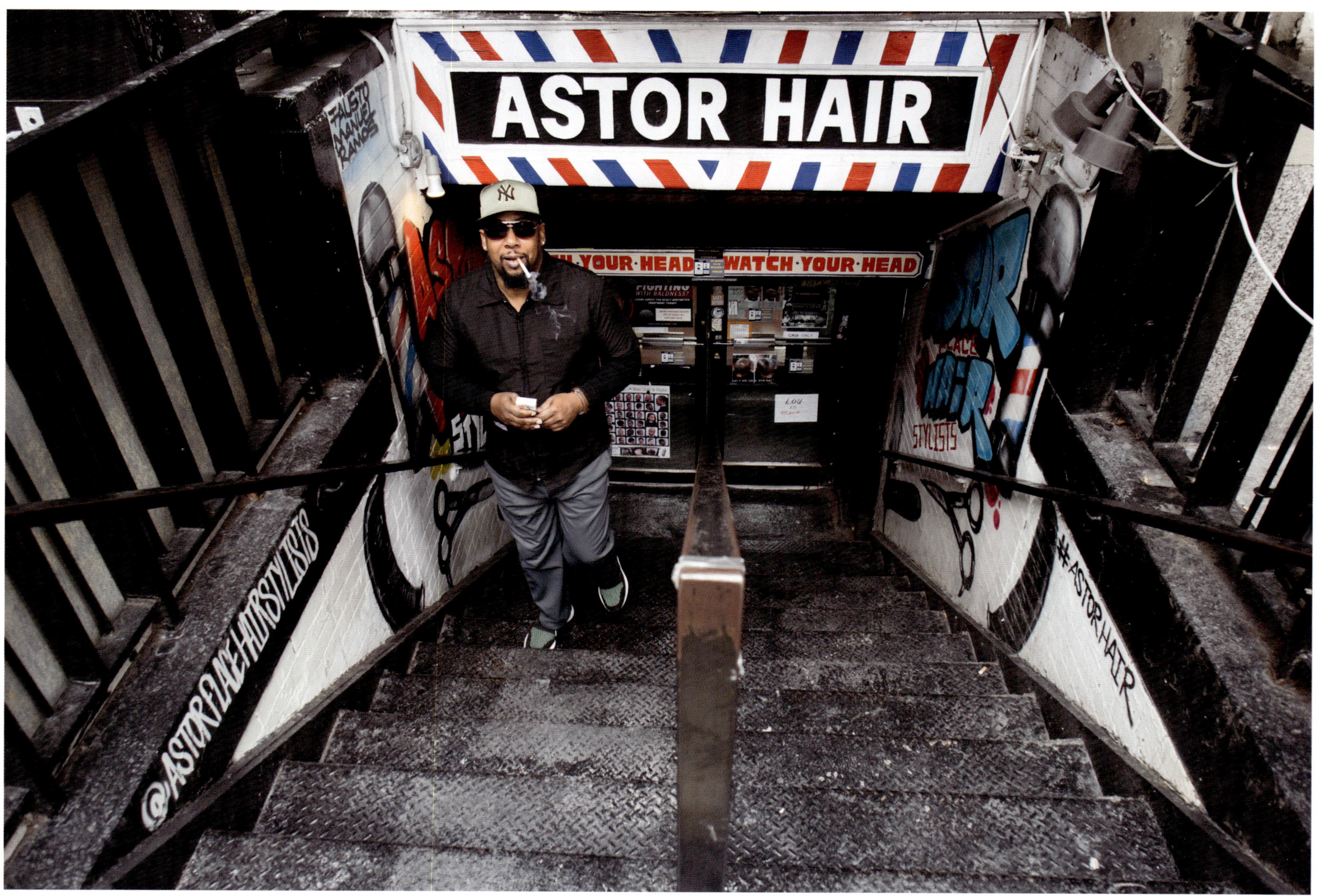

Astor Hair, New York City

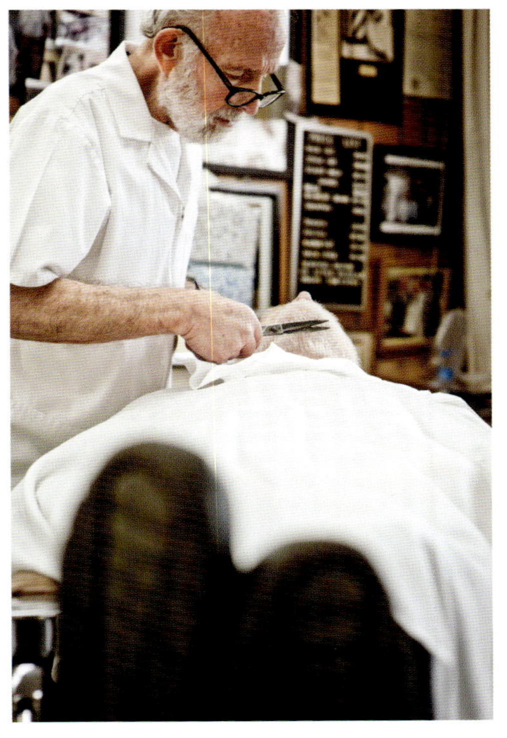

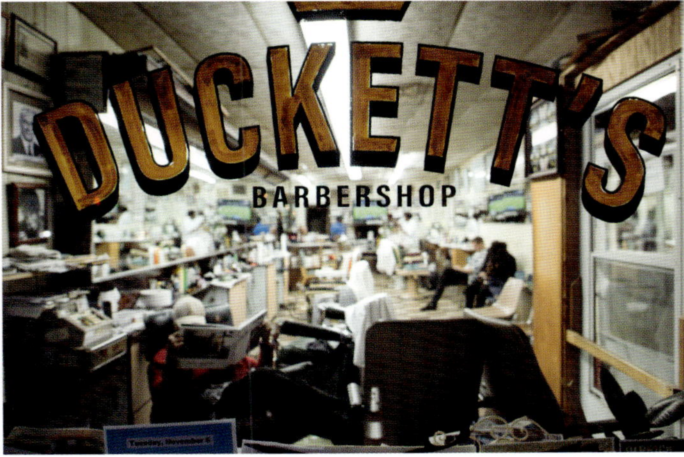

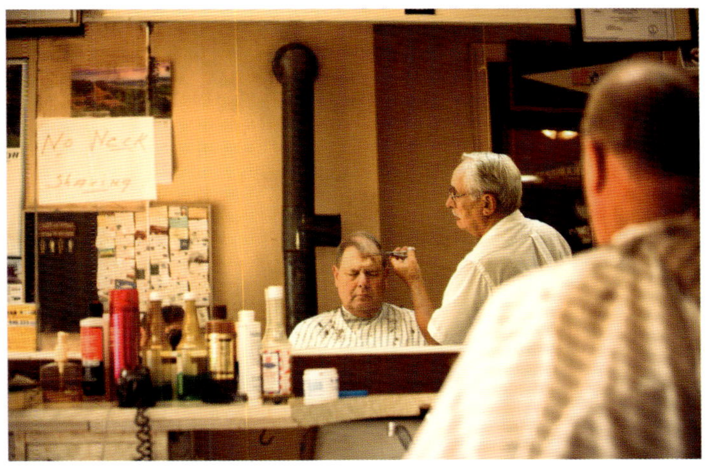

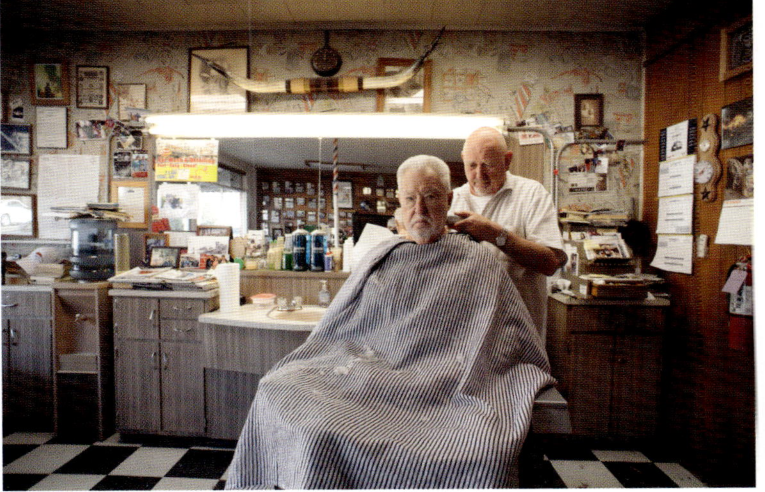

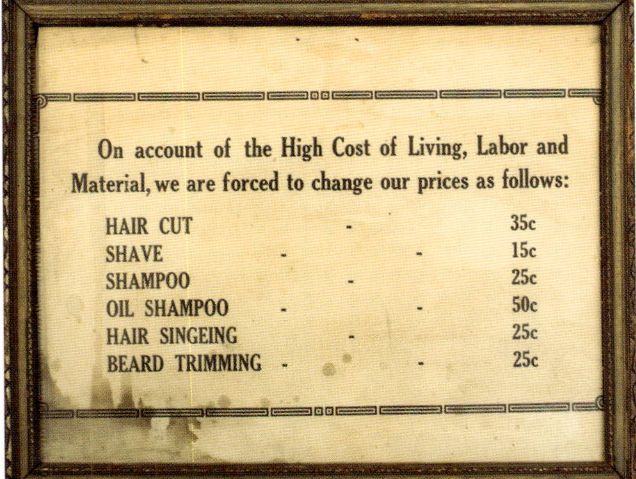
On account of the High Cost of Living, Labor and Material, we are forced to change our prices as follows:

HAIR CUT	35c
SHAVE	15c
SHAMPOO	25c
OIL SHAMPOO	50c
HAIR SINGEING	25c
BEARD TRIMMING	25c

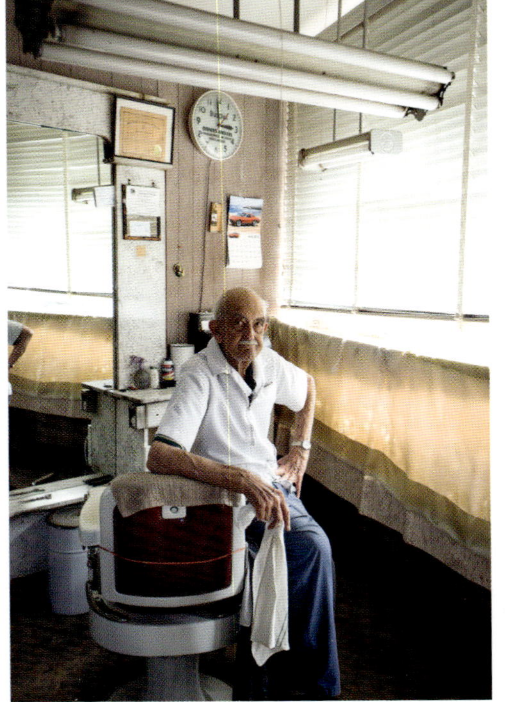

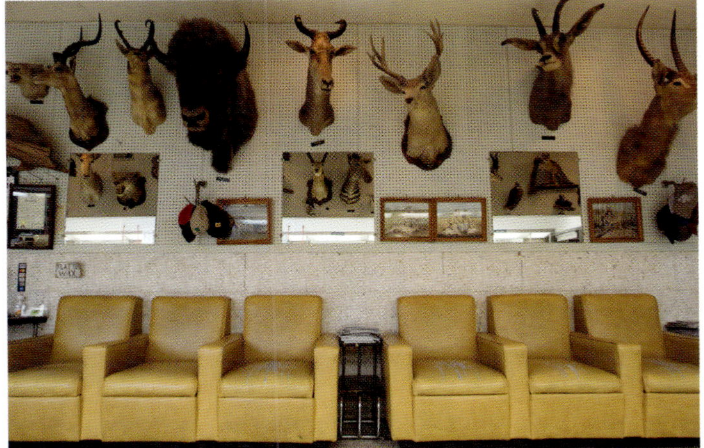

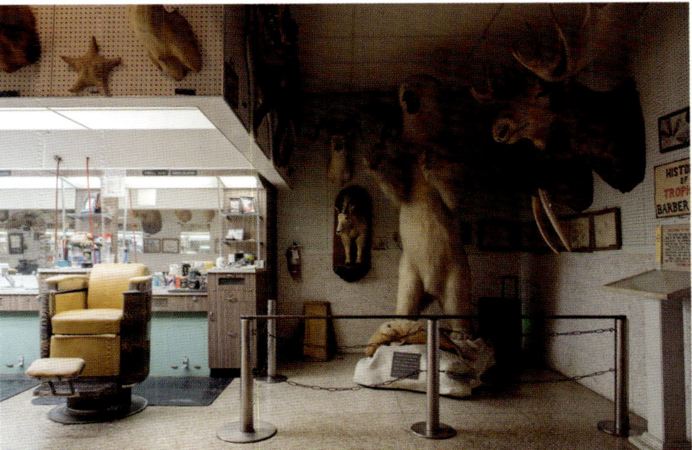

“I keep a file on my computer of all the stories he’s told me.”

– Customer, Fausto Ferrari Barbershop, Cincinnati, Ohio

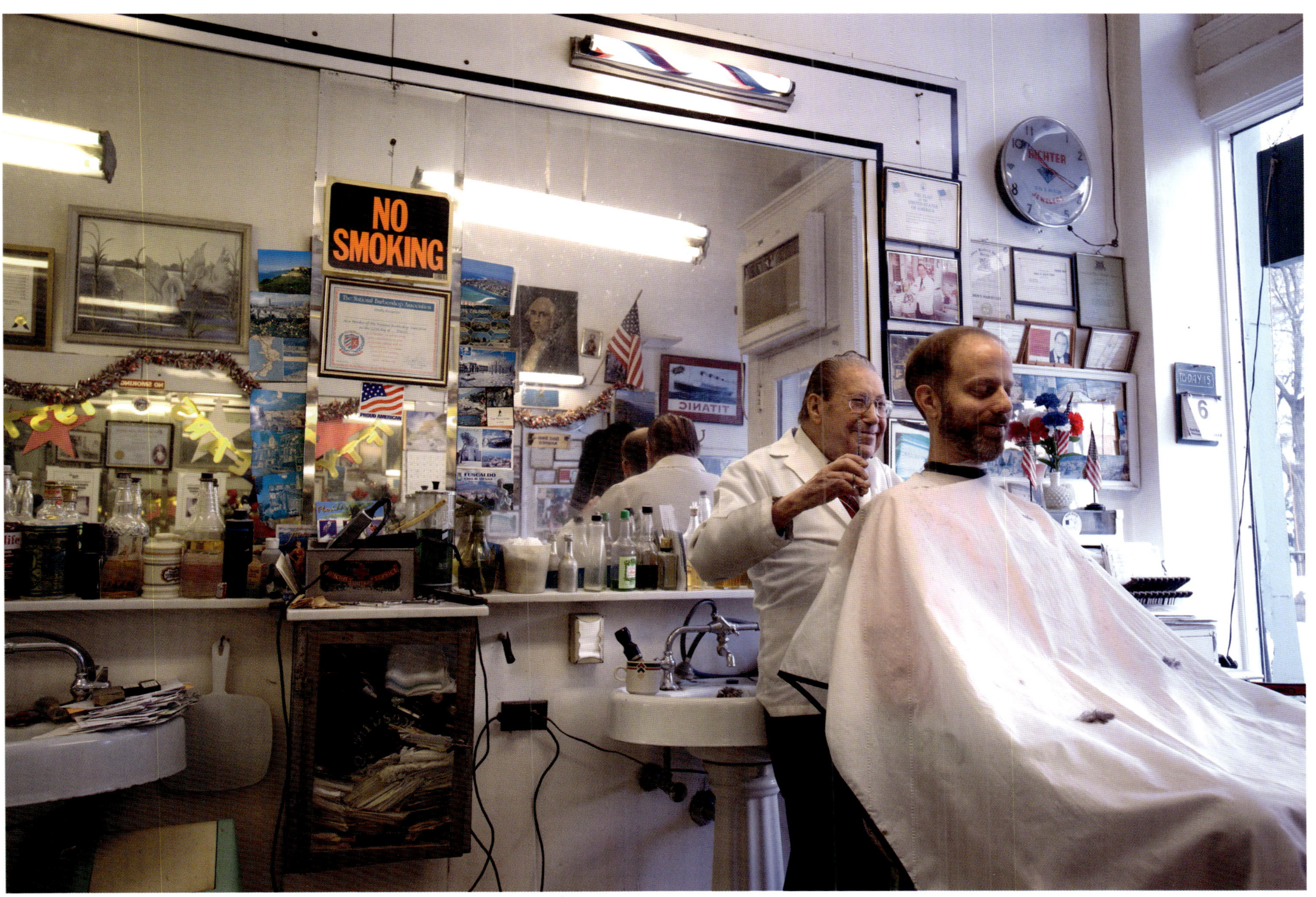

Fausto Ferrari Barbershop, Cincinnati, Ohio

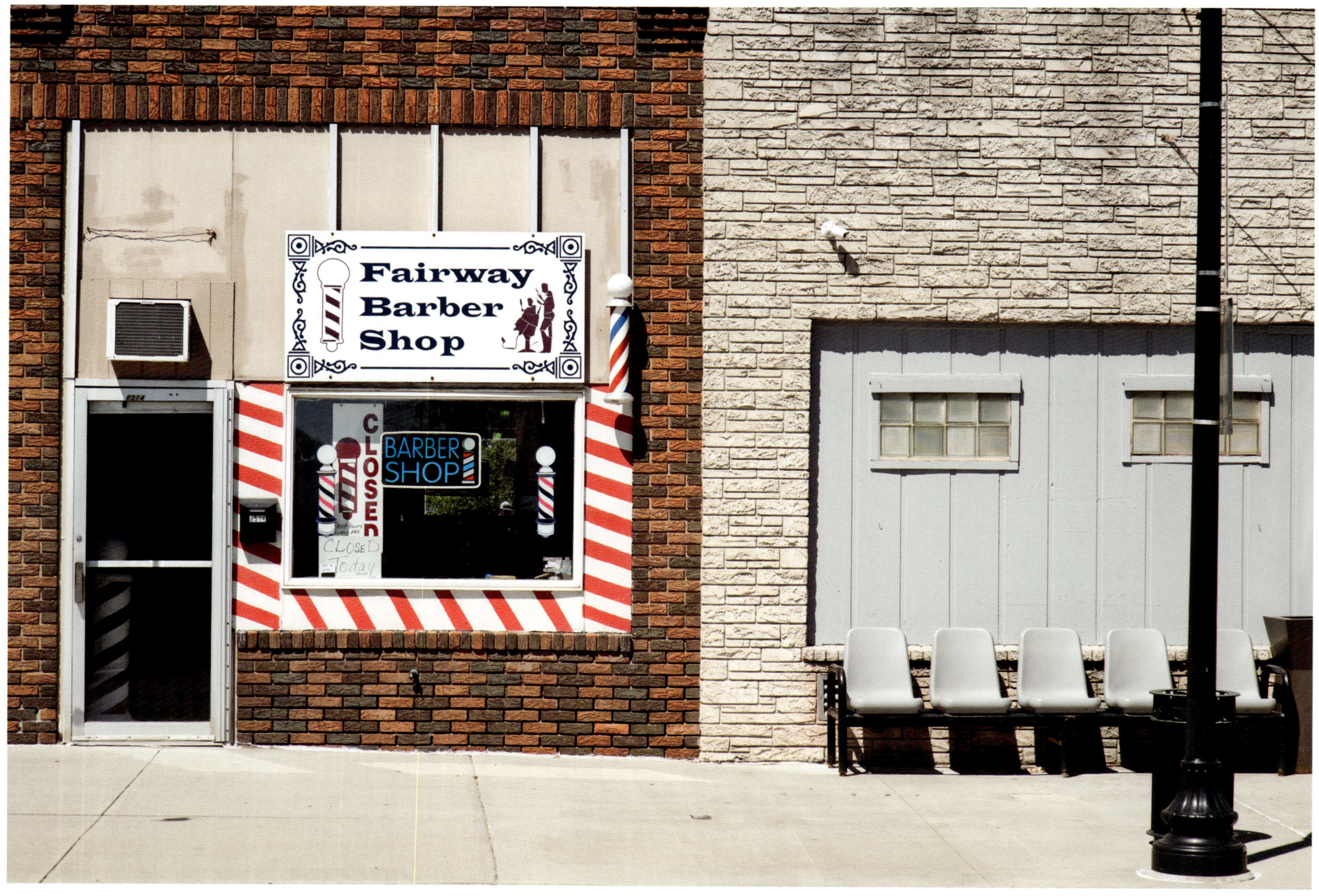

Fairway Barbershop, Omaha, New England

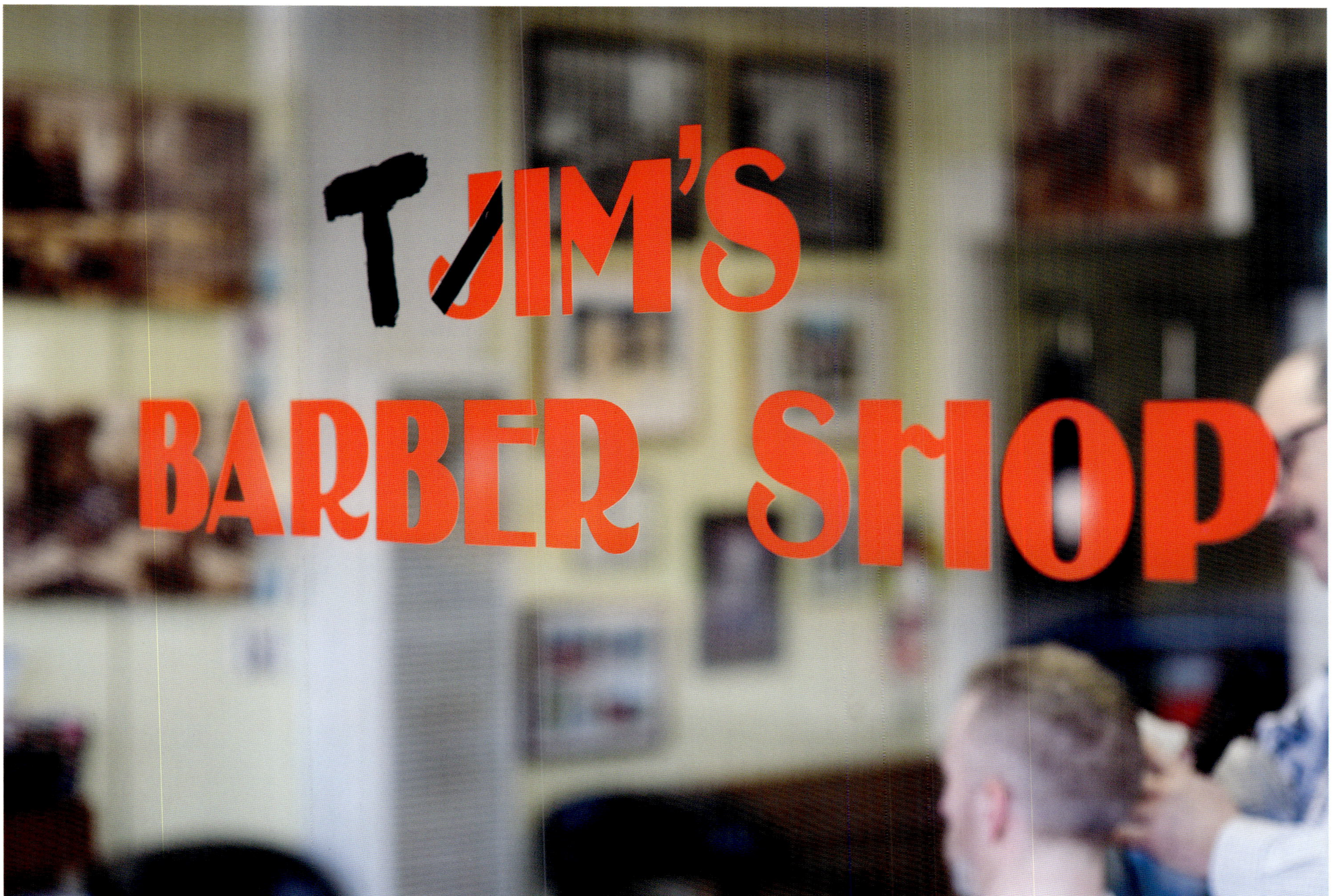

Tim's Barbershop, Portland, Oregon

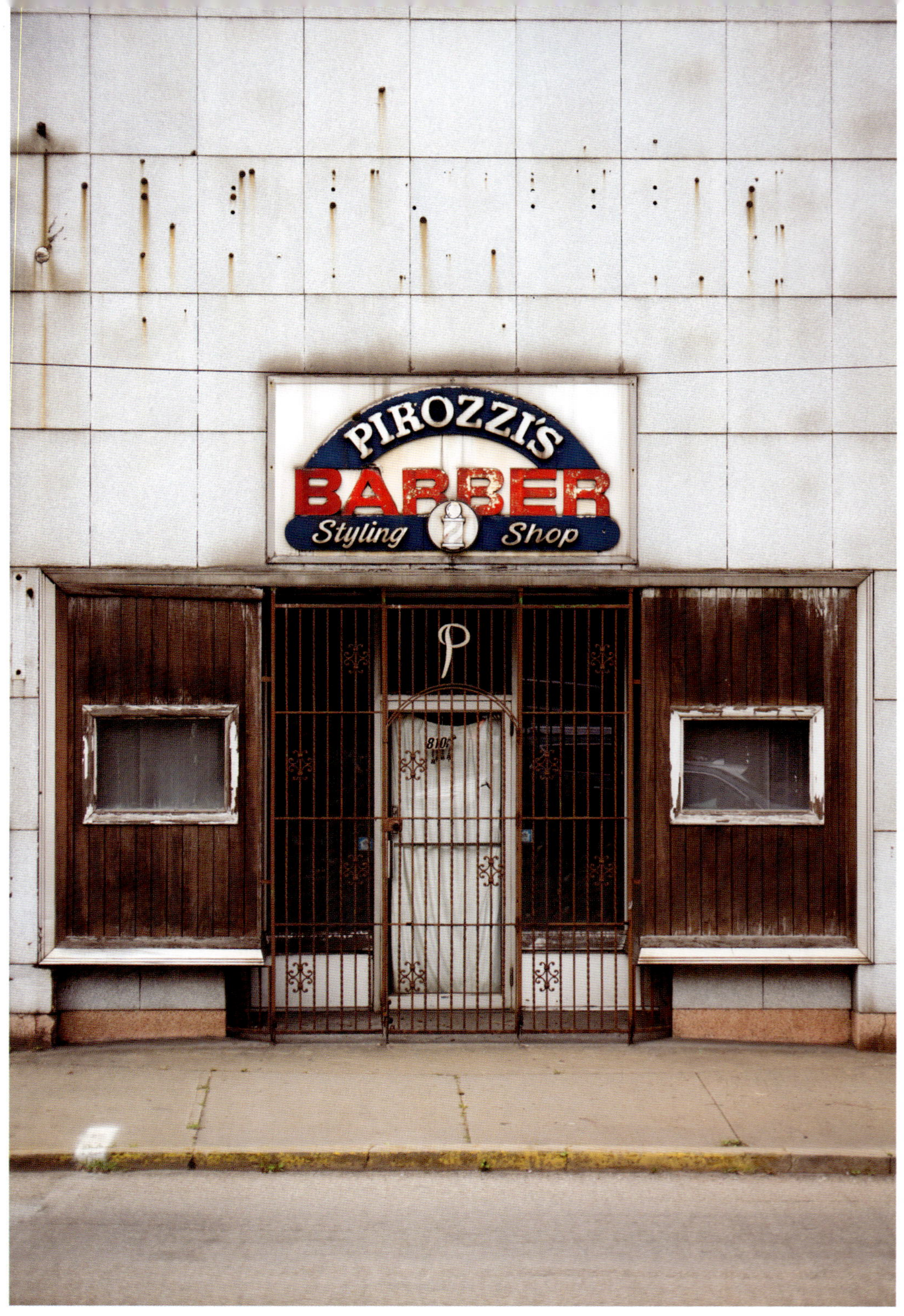

Pirozzi's Barbershop, Braddock, Pennsylvania

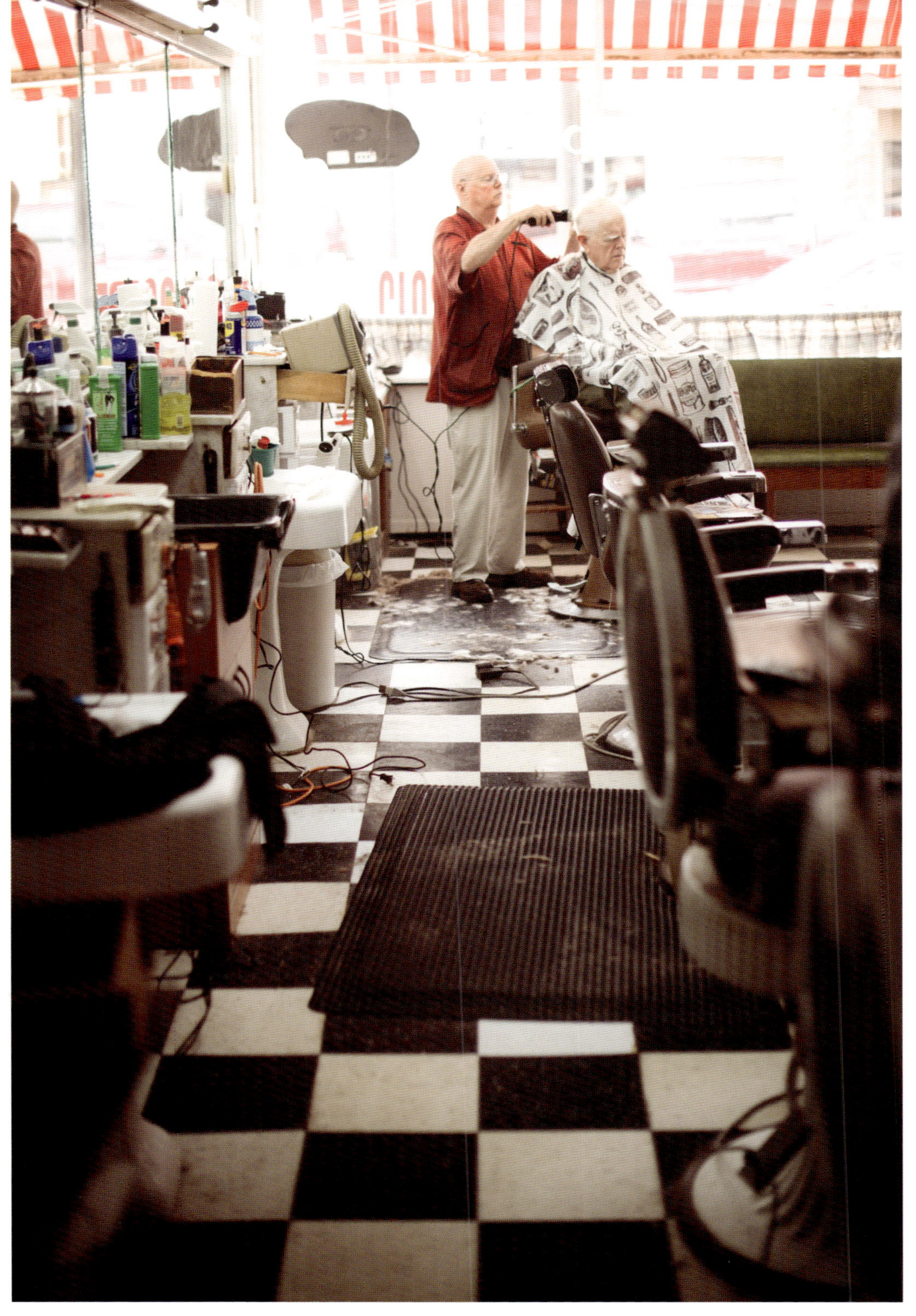

Ron's Barbershop, Mexico, Missouri

Bird
LARRY
Indiana
Pacers
RAY'S
BARBER & STYLE
SHOP
OPEN
TUE WED&FRI 9-5
SAT 9-1
CLOSED SUN MON&THUR
APPOINTMENTS ONLY
REG. HAIRCUTS 14.00
REG. BURR 11.00
STYLECUTS 18.00
BEARD TRIM 7.00
ROCK N BOWL
TUESDAY NIGHT MEN'S LEAGUE
CHAMPIONS
JEFF LYONS, DICK SHIPMAN SR.
ANDY SHIPMAN, CURT STEPHENSON,
RICK LOTT & RAY MEEHAN
SPONSOR:
RAY'S BARBER & STYLE SHOP
WHEATIES
WARNING
— NO —
TRESPASSING
VIOLATORS
WILL BE SHOT
SURVIVORS
WILL BE SHOT
AGAIN!

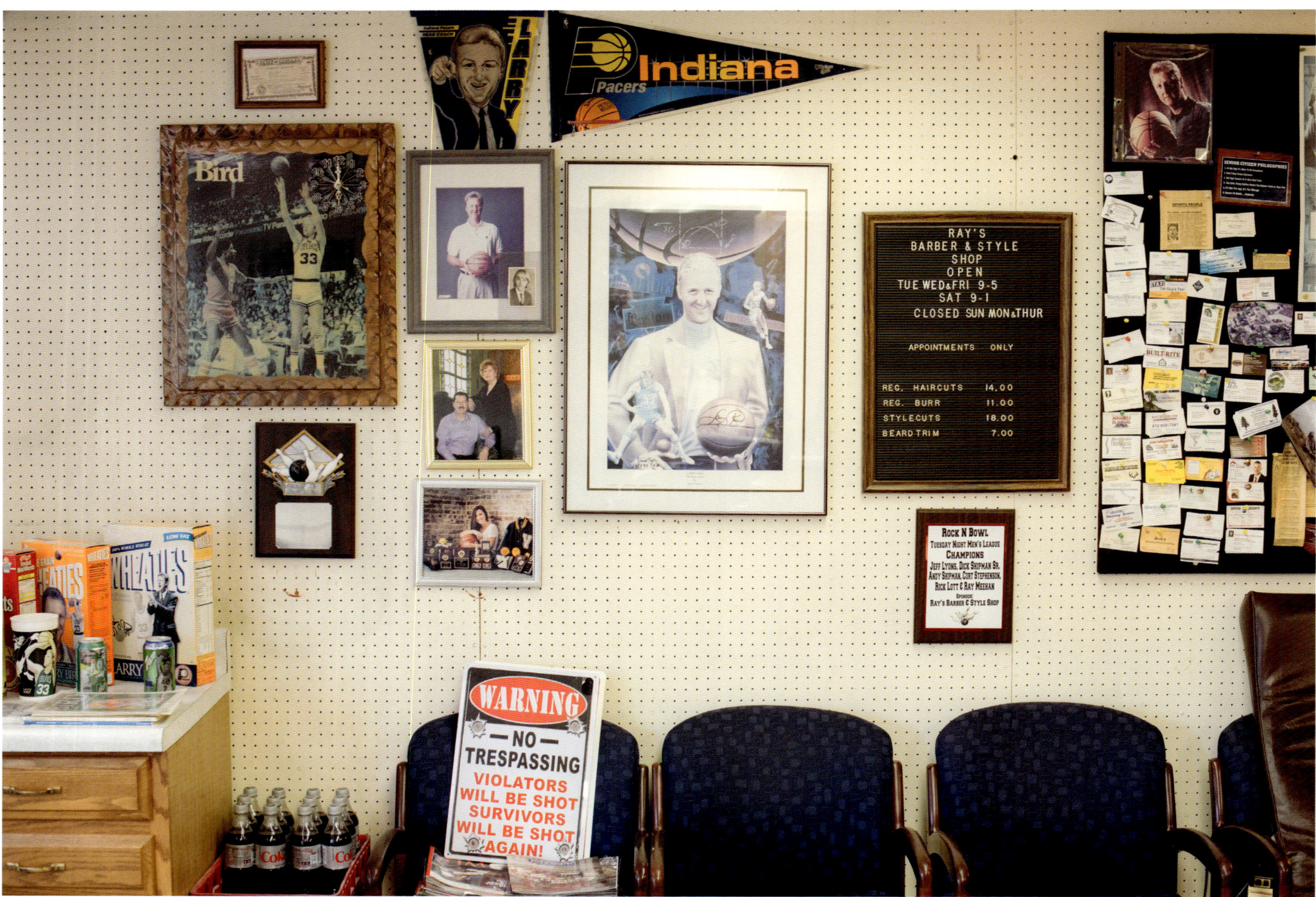

Ray's Barbershop, French Lick, Indiana

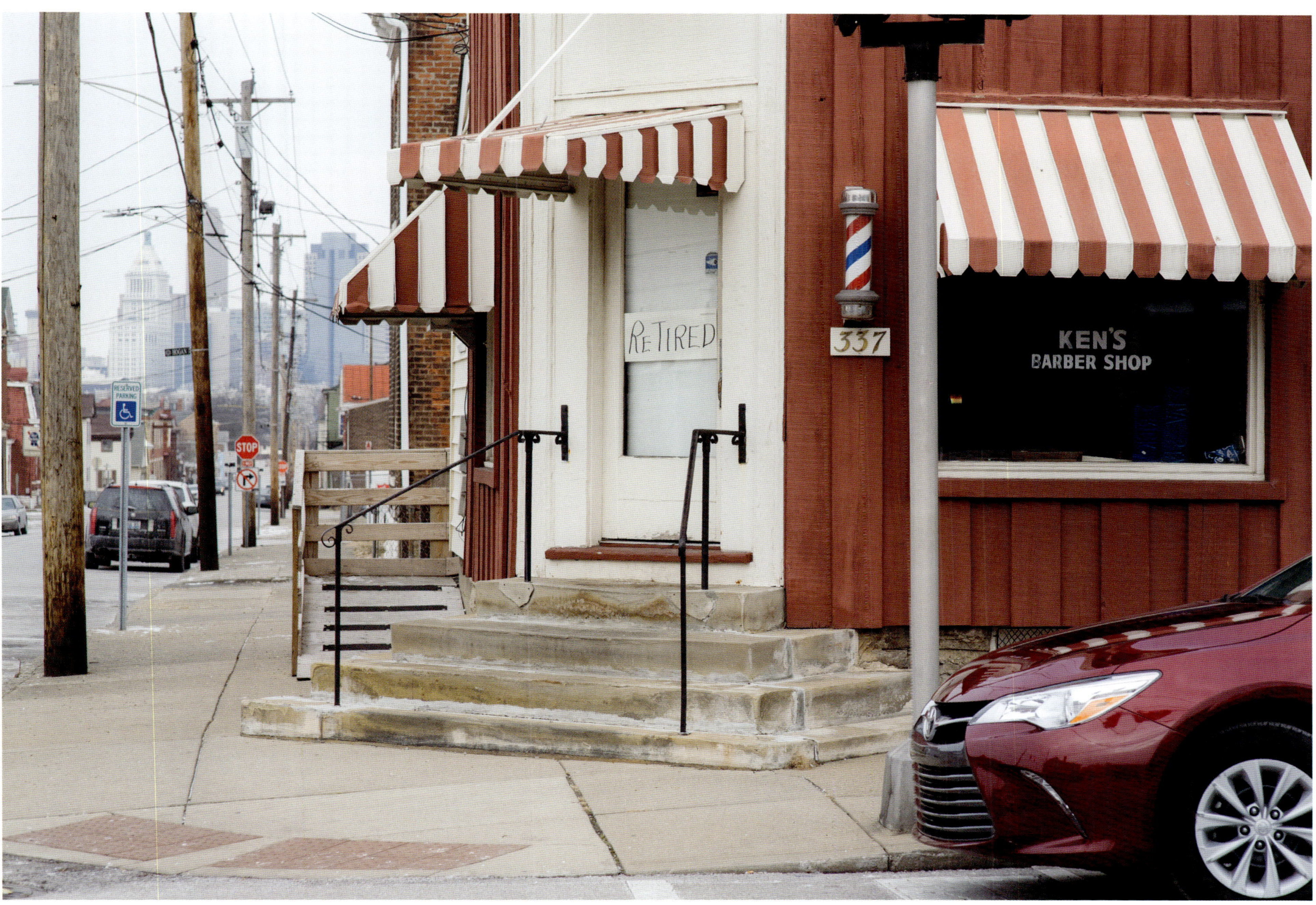

Ken's Barbershop, Newport, Kentucky

NEXT GENERATION

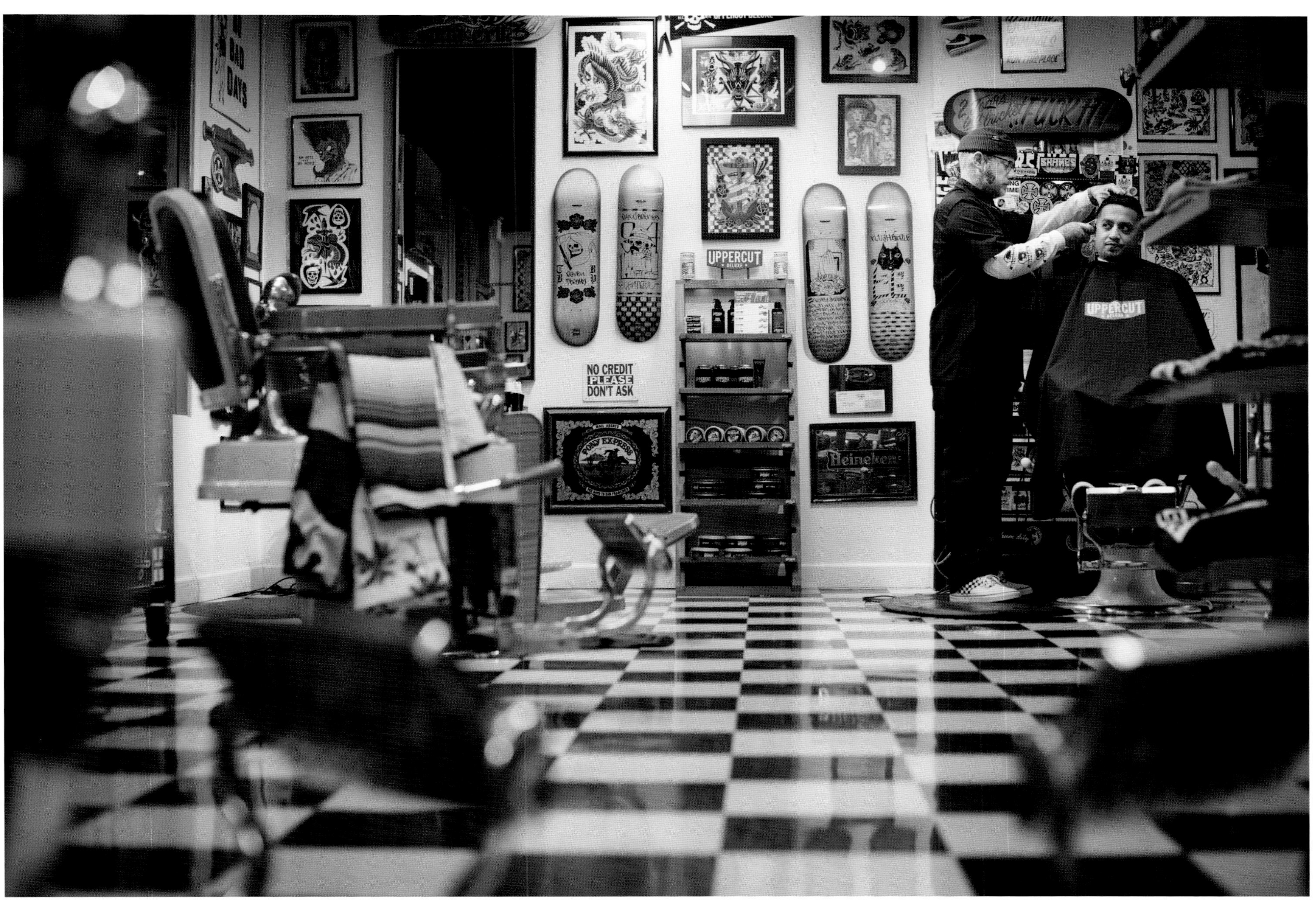

Shane's Barbershop, San Mateo, California

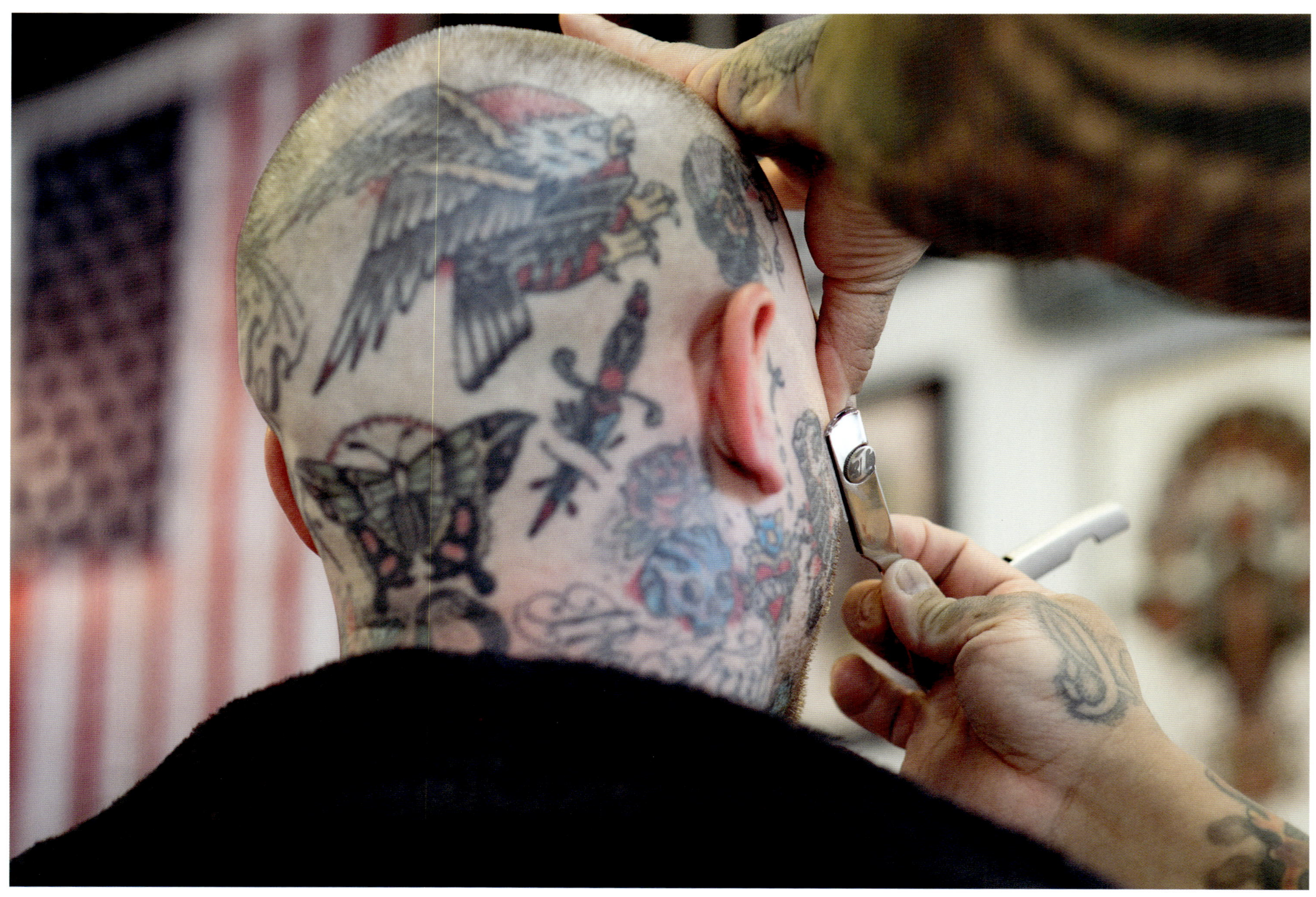

Shane's Barbershop, San Mateo, California

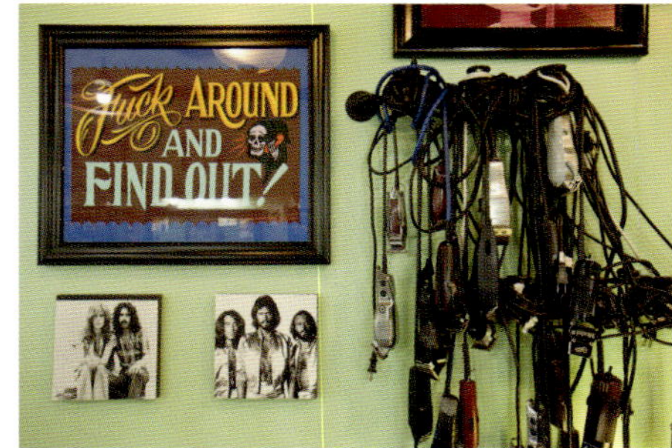
Fuck Around
AND
FIND OUT!

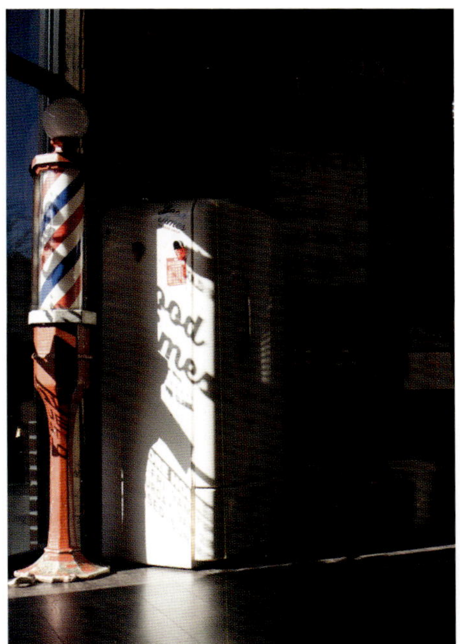

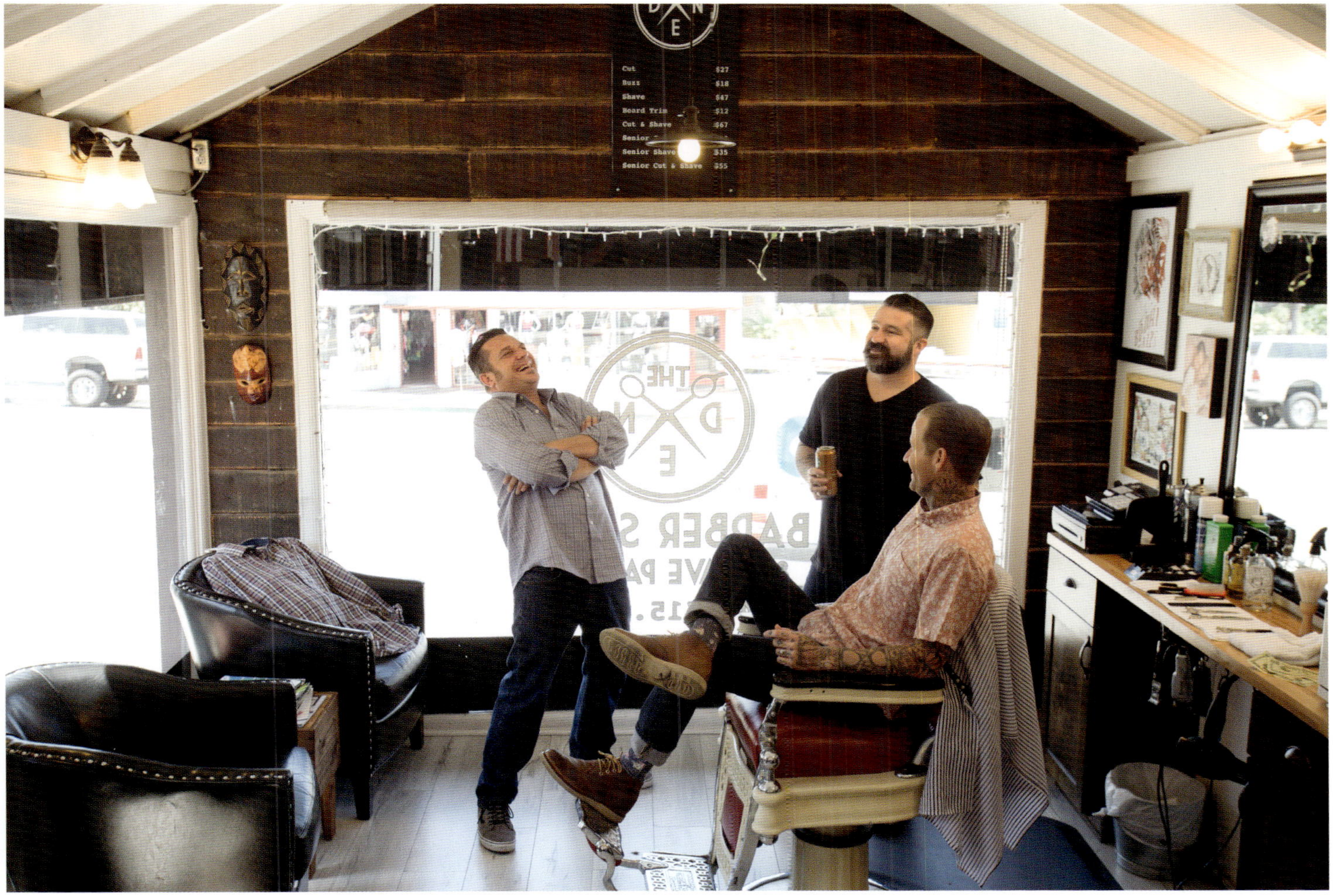

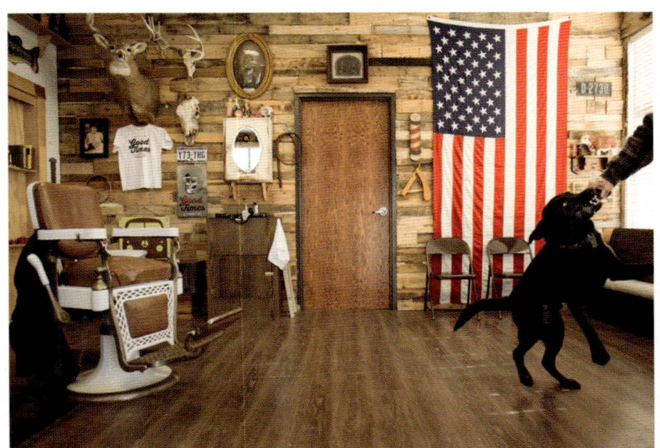

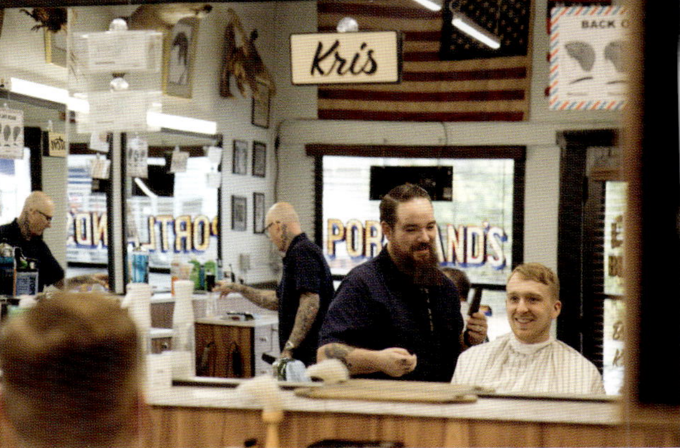
Kris

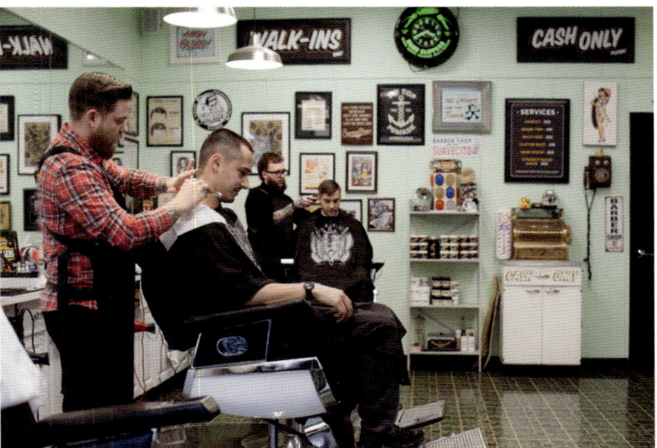
WALK-INS
CASH ONLY
SERVICES

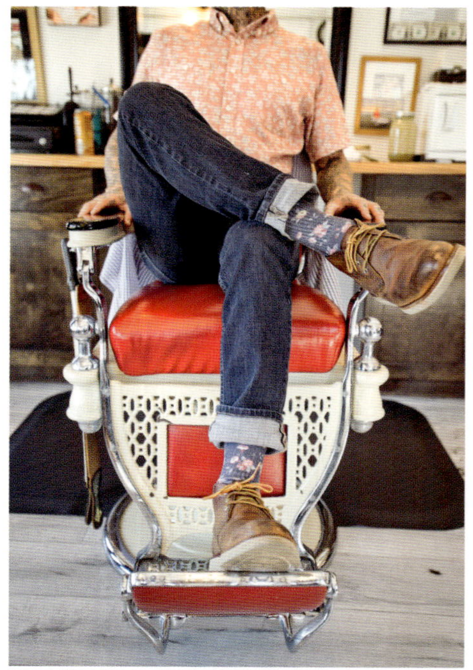

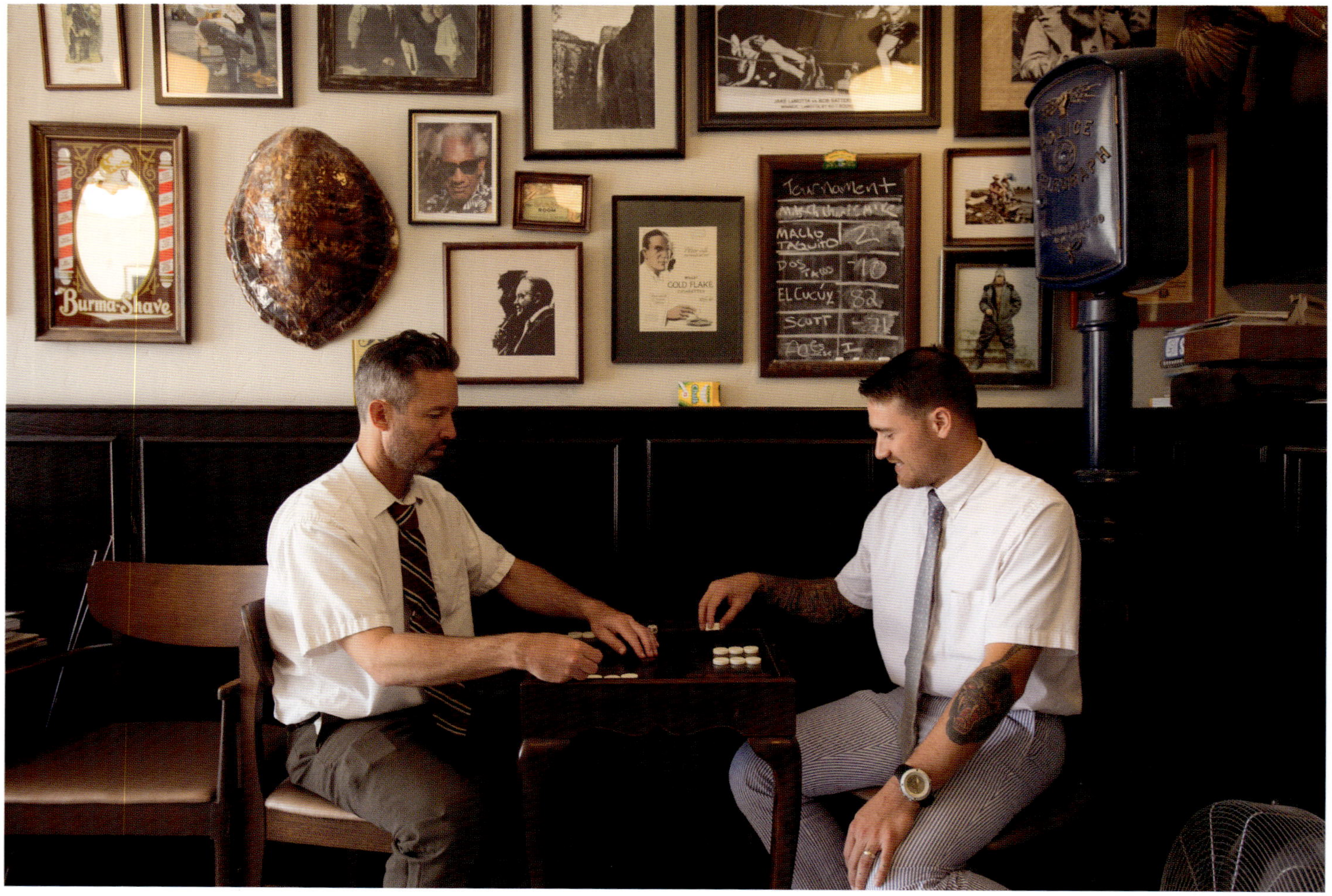

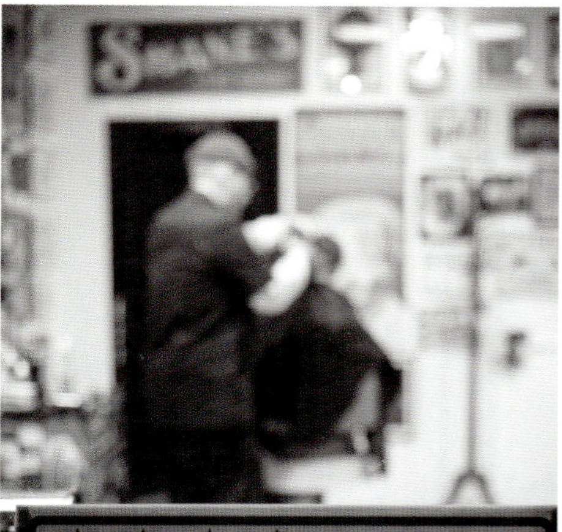

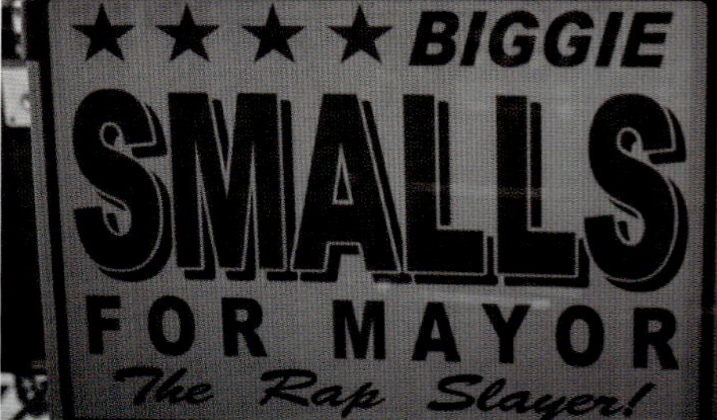
★★★★ BIGGIE
SMALLS
FOR MAYOR
The Rap Slayer!

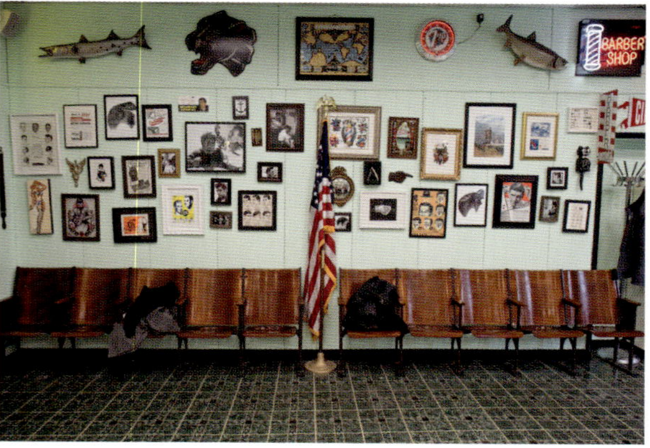
BARBER SHOP

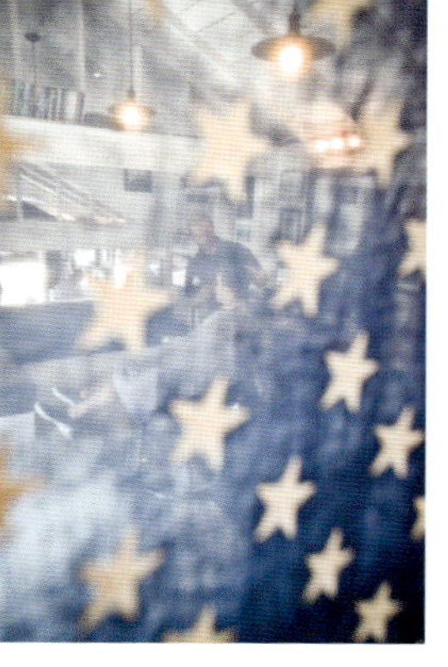

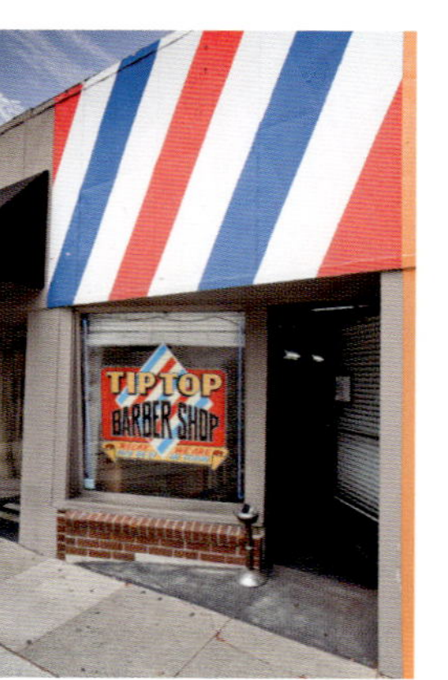
TIPTOP
BARBER SHOP

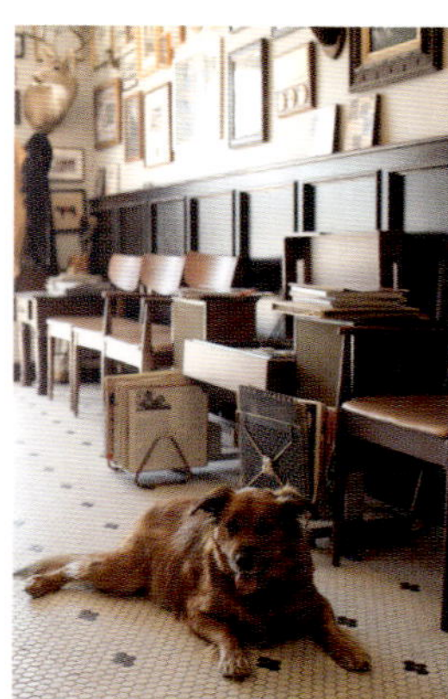

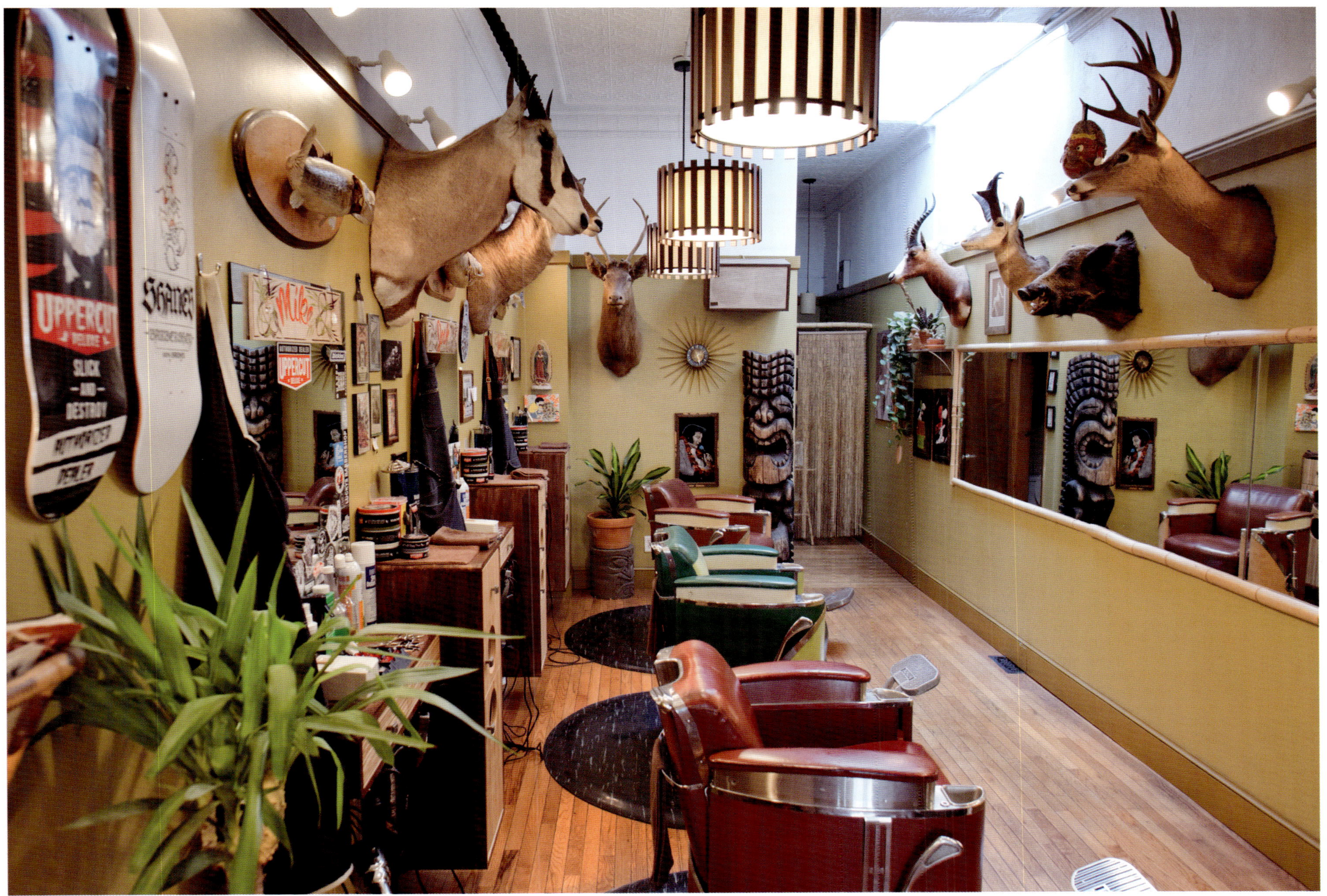

Pugsly's SideShow Barbershop, Kingston, New York

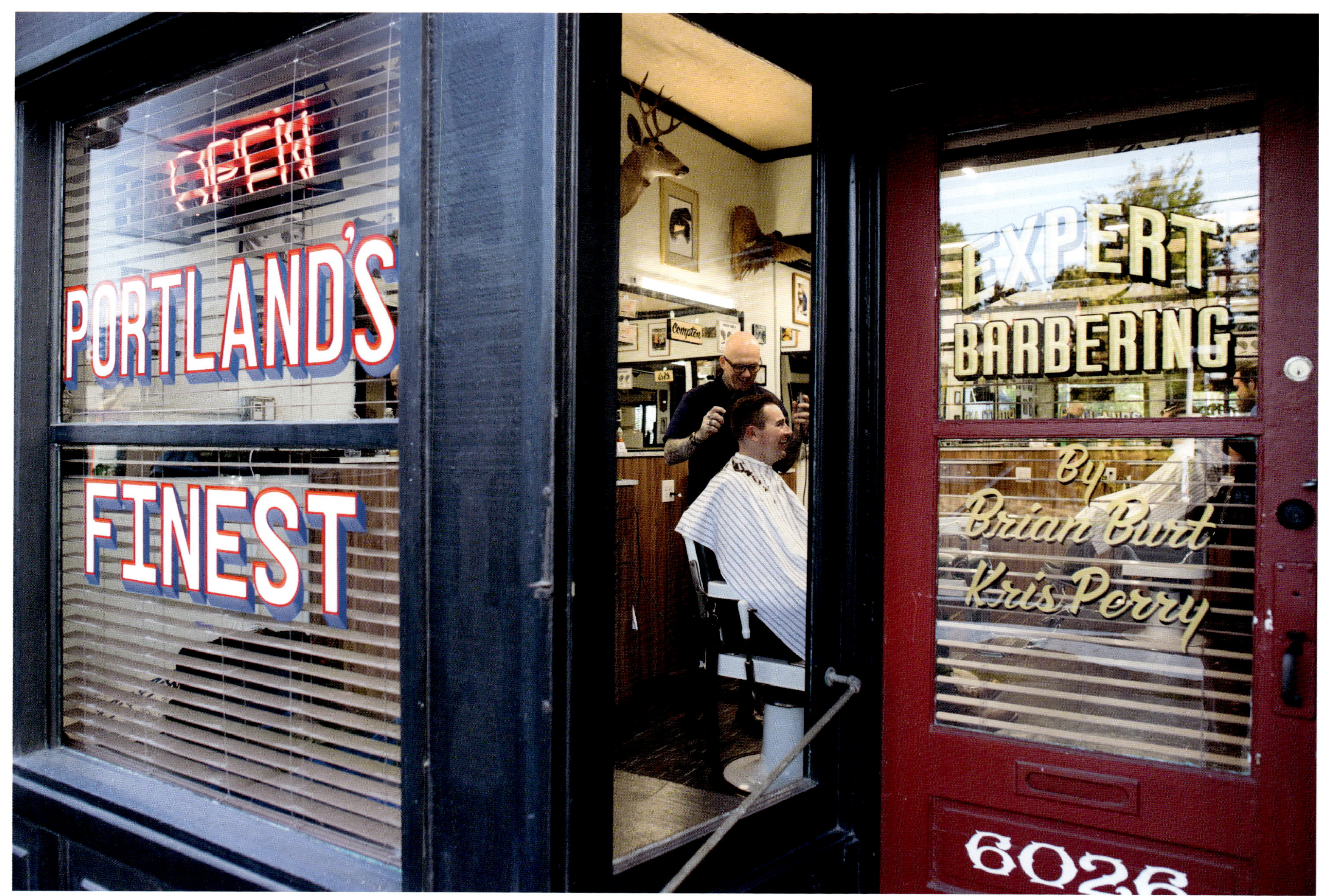

Lyle's Barbershop, Portland, Oregon

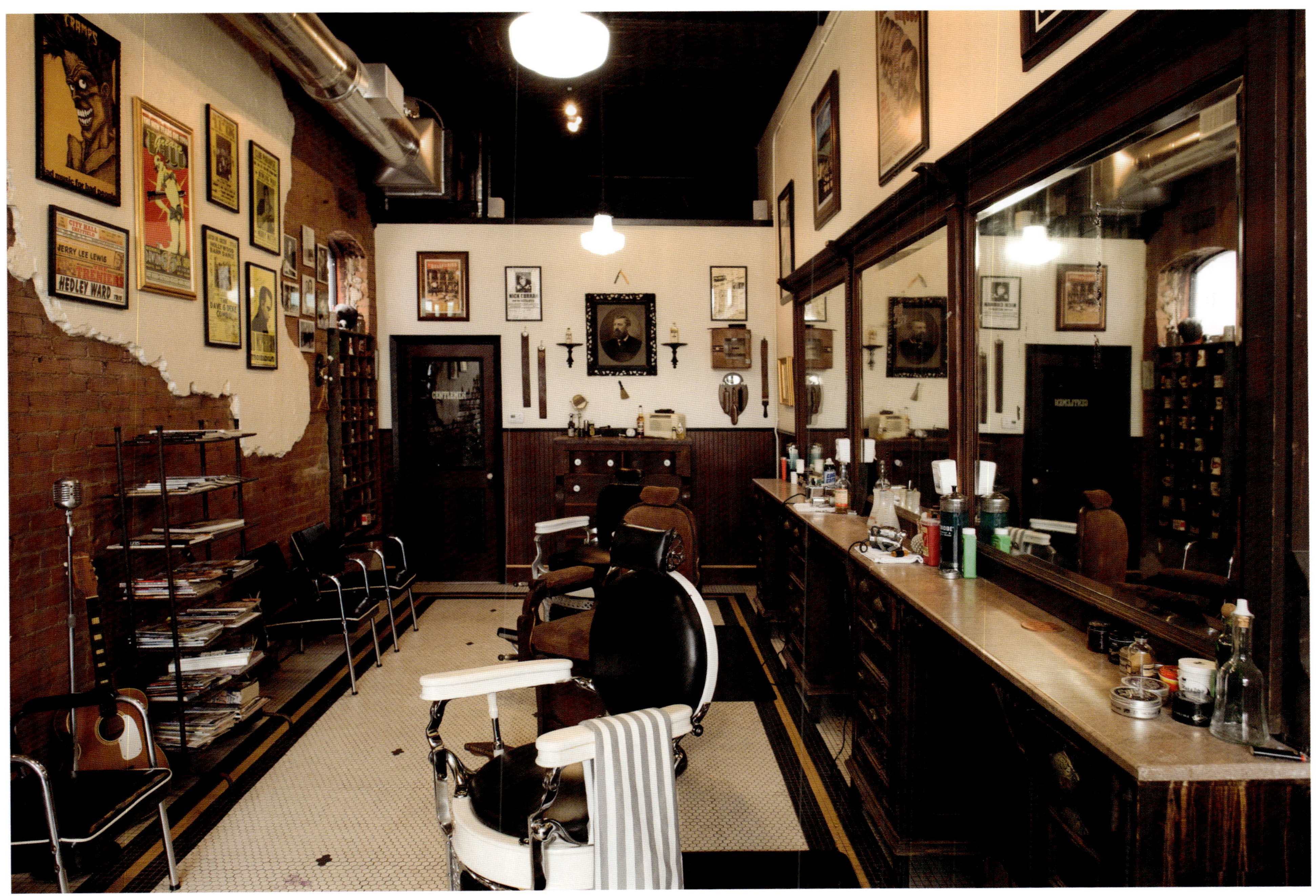

Rob's Chop Shop, Dallas, Texas

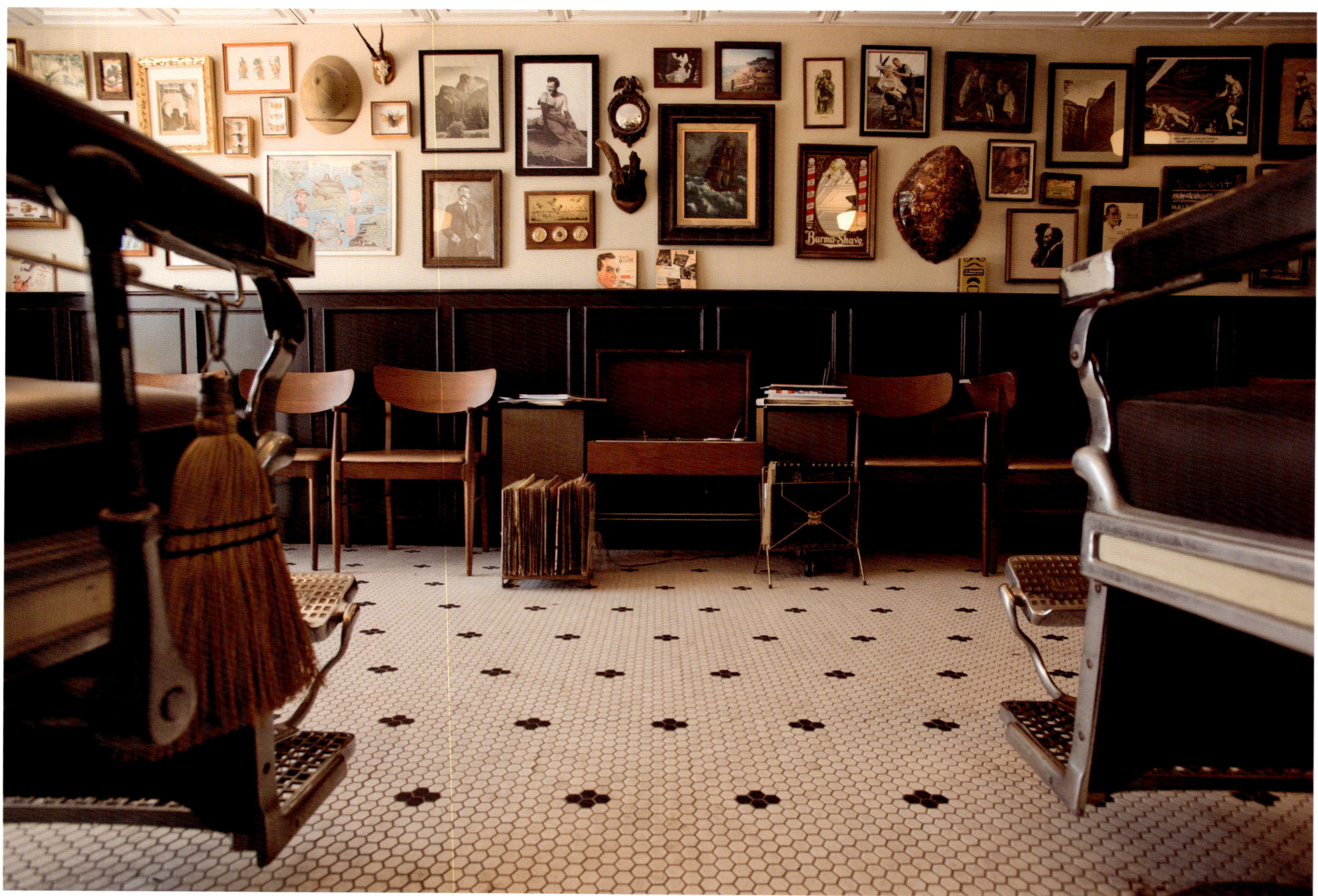

The King's Club Barbershop, Dana Point, California

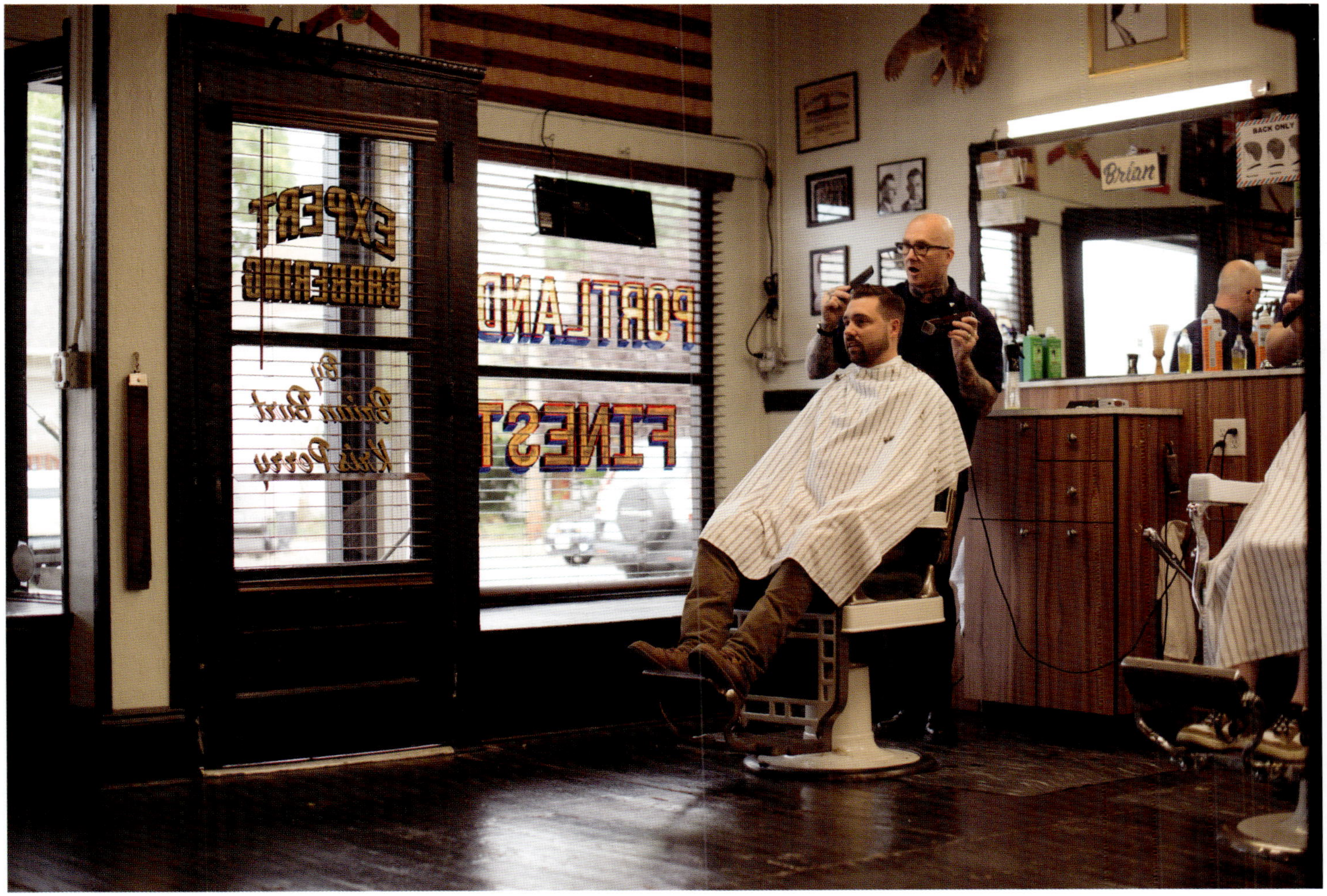

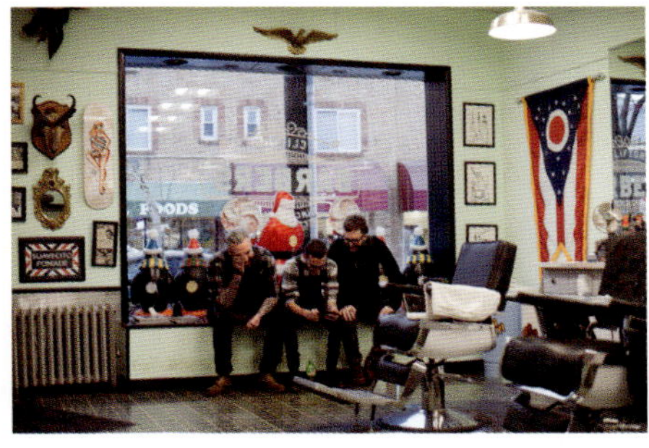

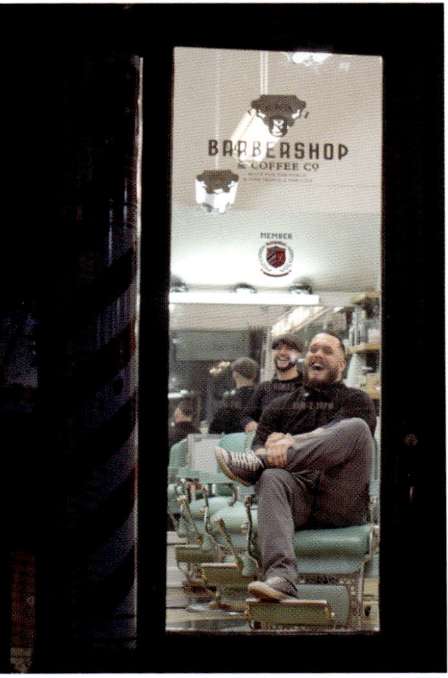
BARBERSHOP
& COFFEE CO
MEMBER

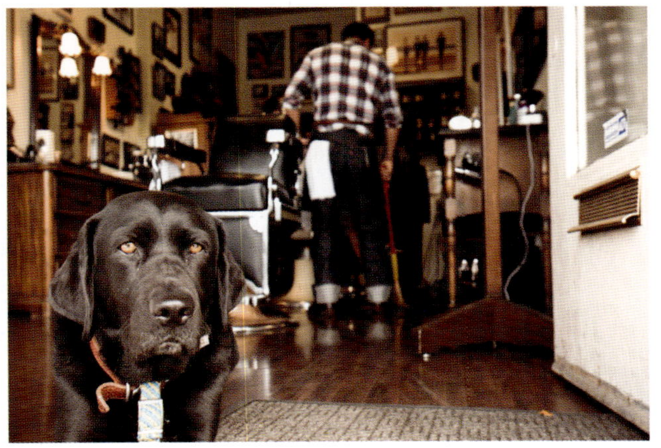

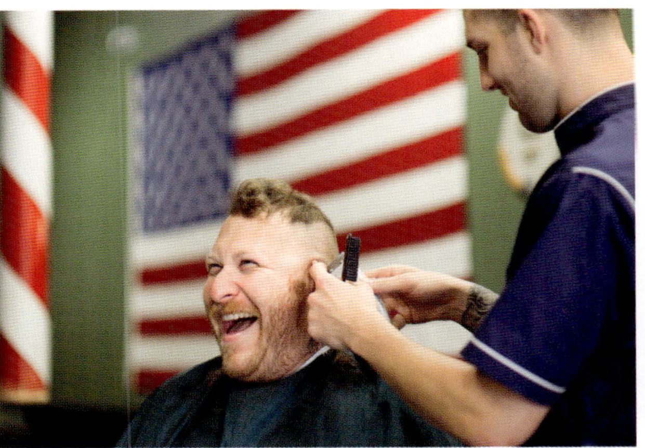

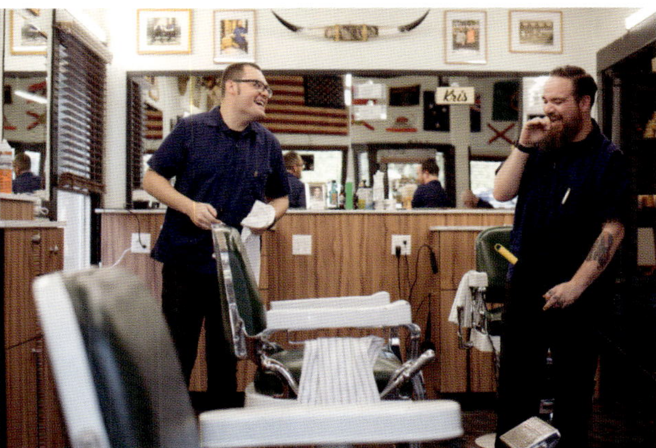

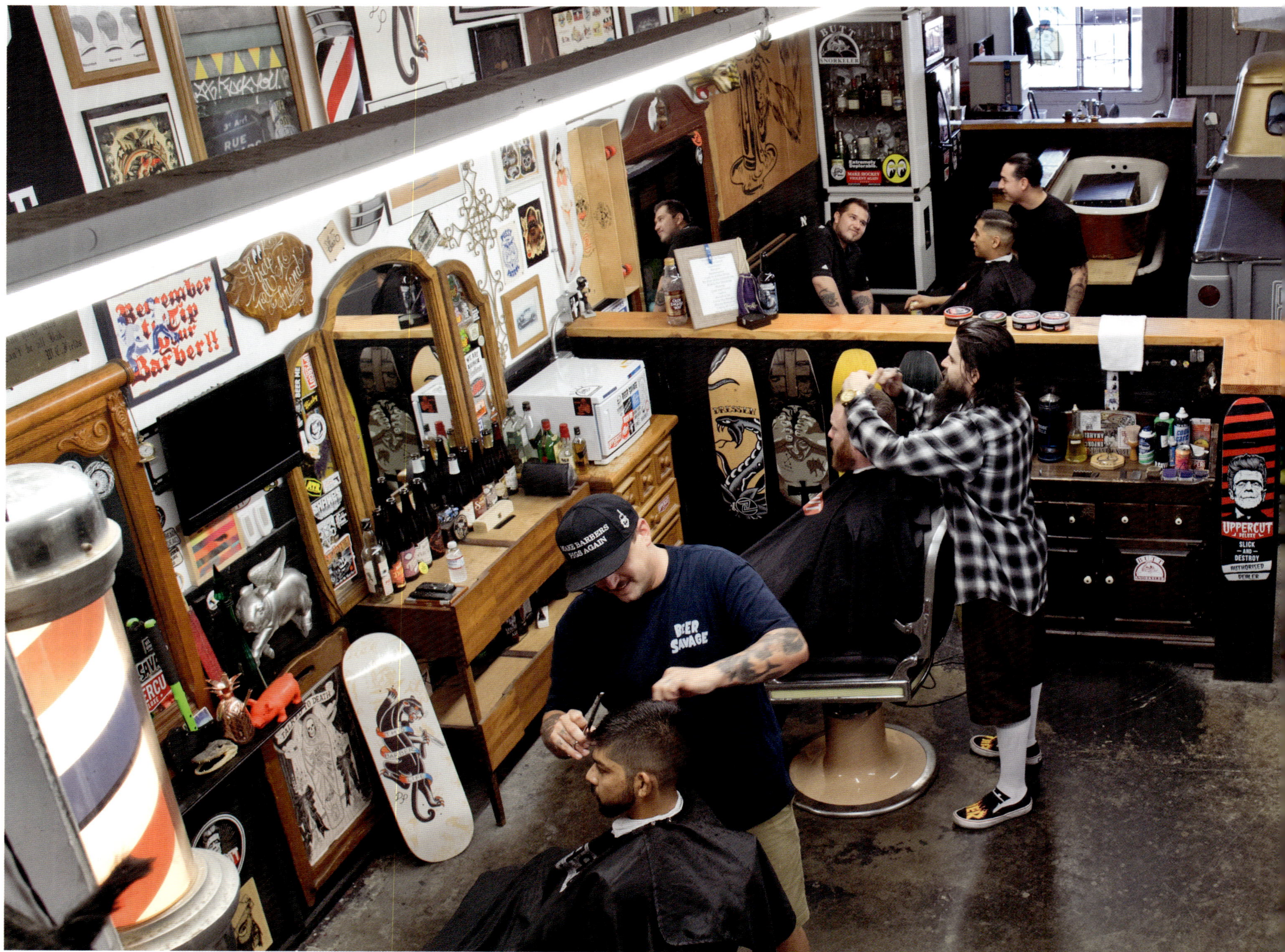
MAKE BARBERS PIGS AGAIN
BEER SAVAGE
UPPERCUT DELUXE
SLICK AND DESTROY
AUTHORISED DEALER
BUTT SNORKELER

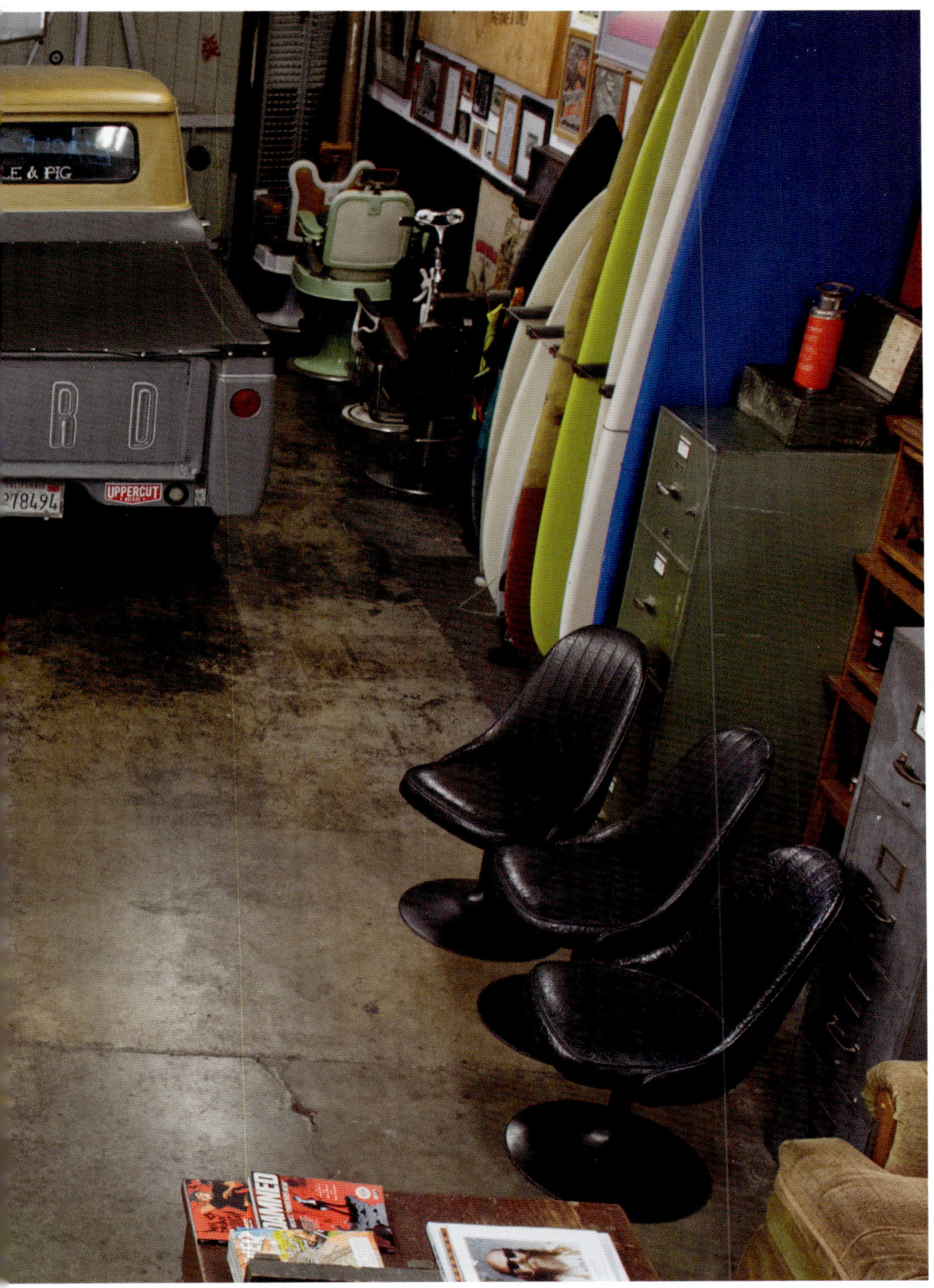

Eagle & Pig Barbershop, Costa Mesa, California

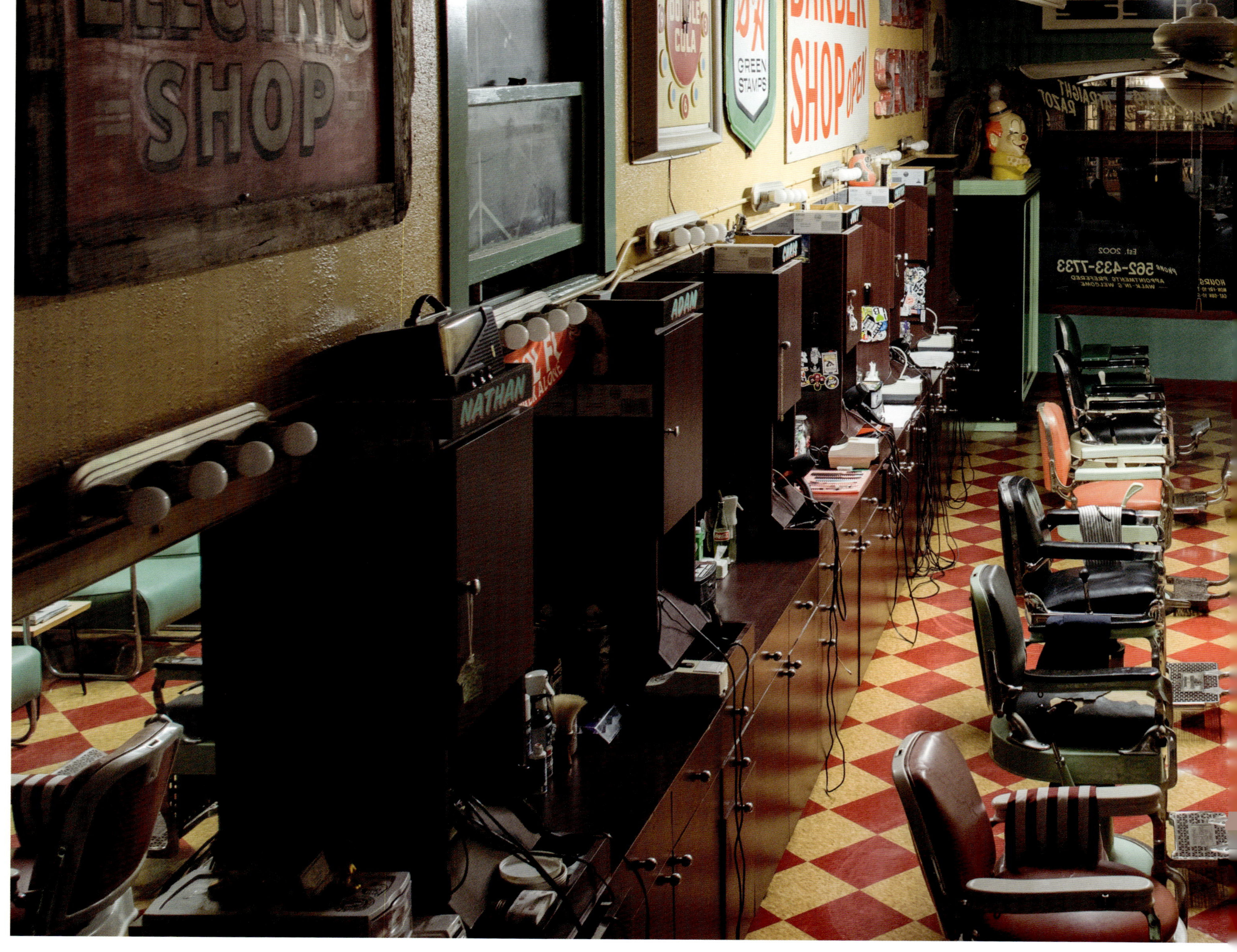

SHOP
DOUBLE COLA
GREEN STAMPS
SHOP OPEN
NATHAN
ADAM

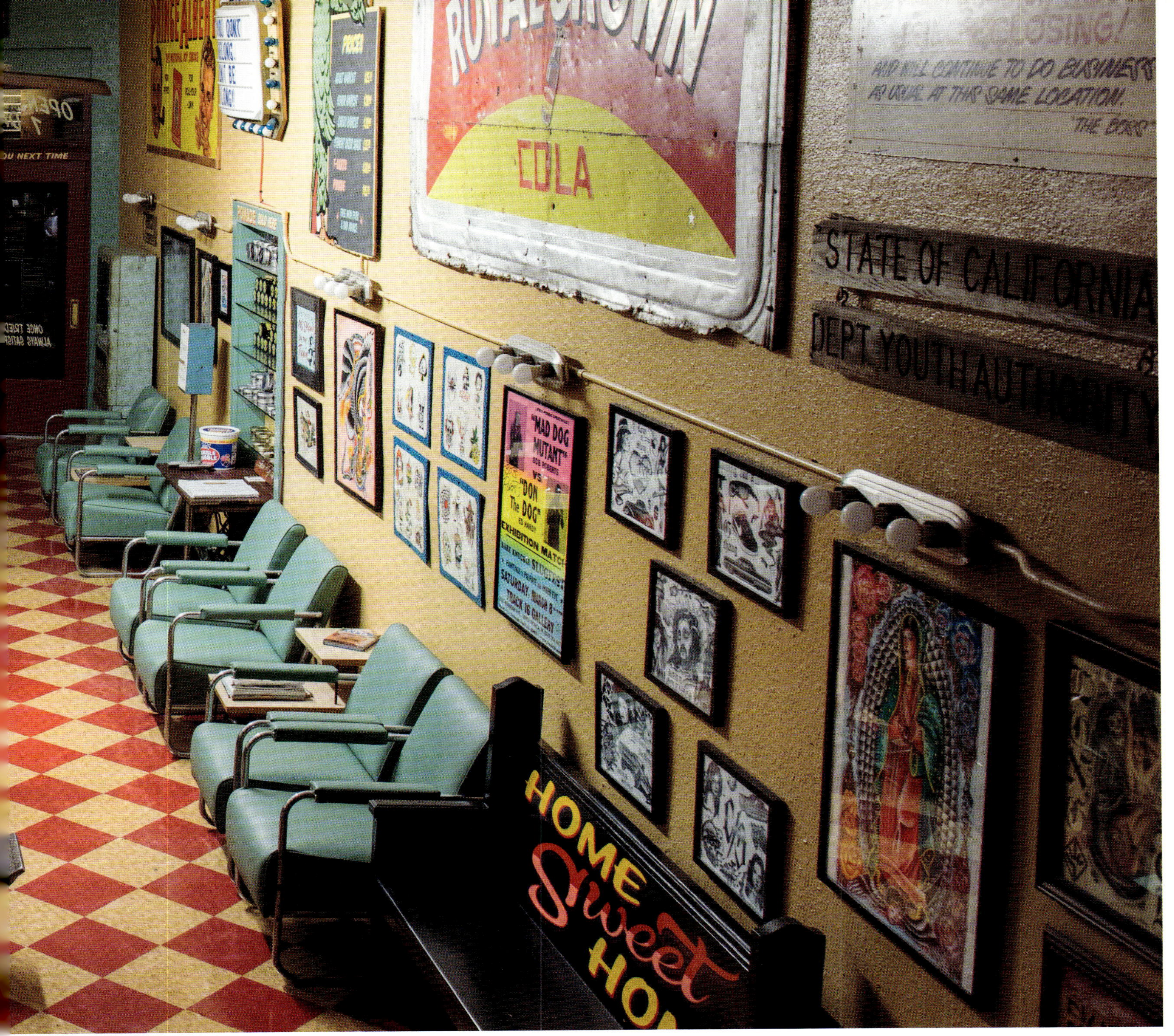

Syndicate Barbershop, Long Beach, California

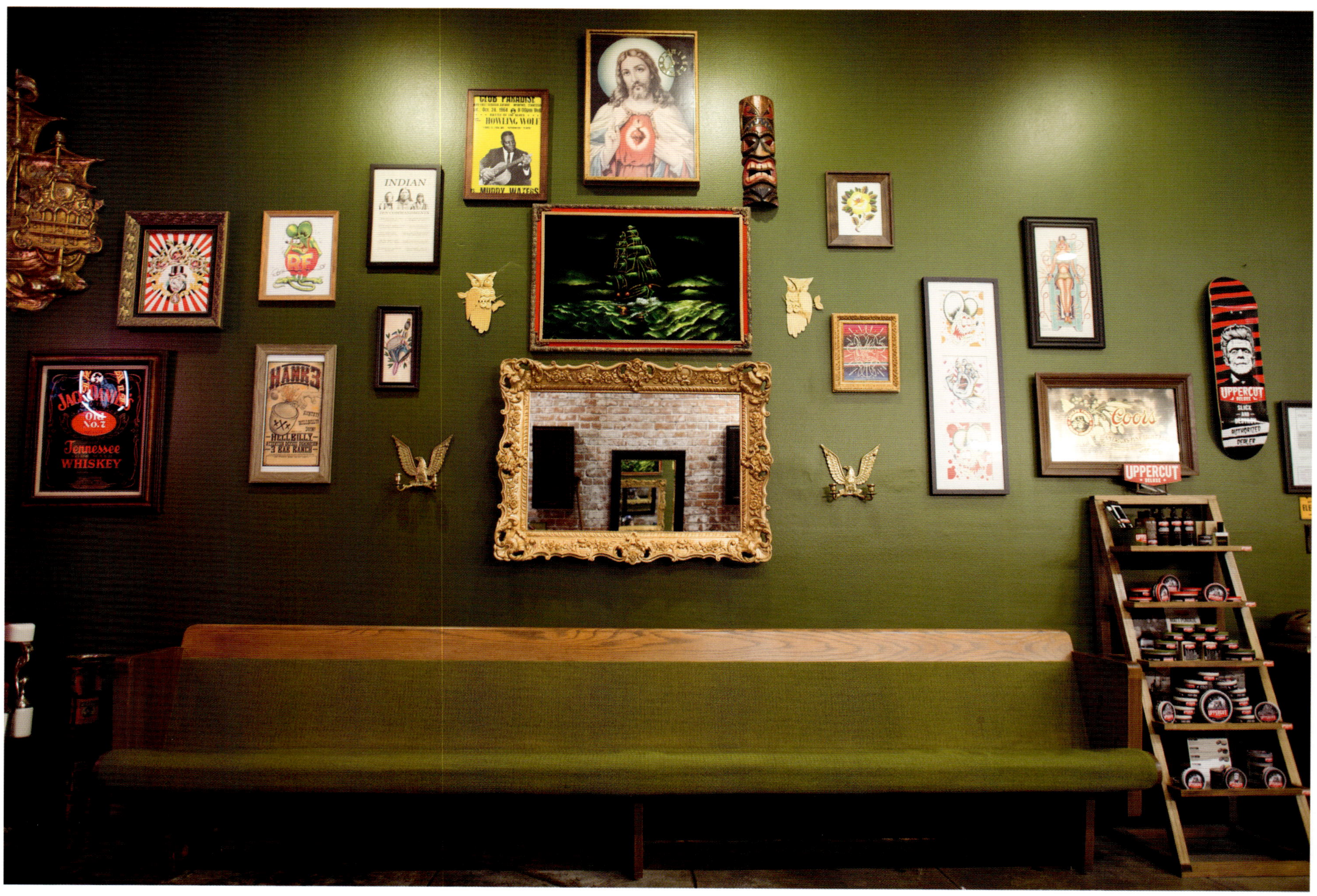

Electric Barbershop, Riverside, California

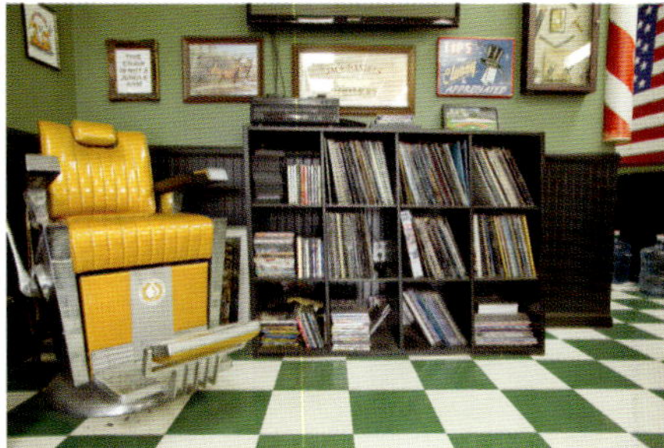

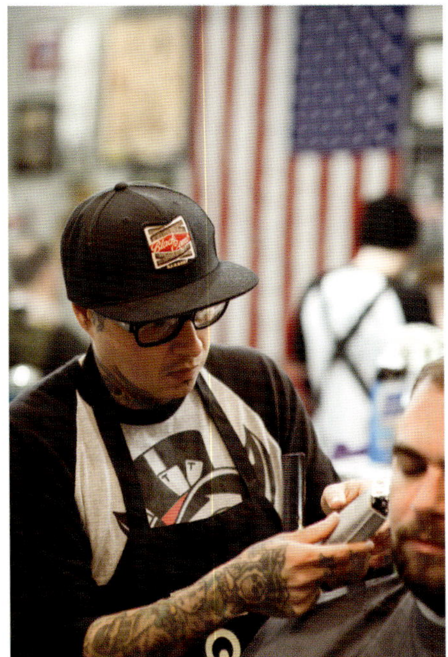

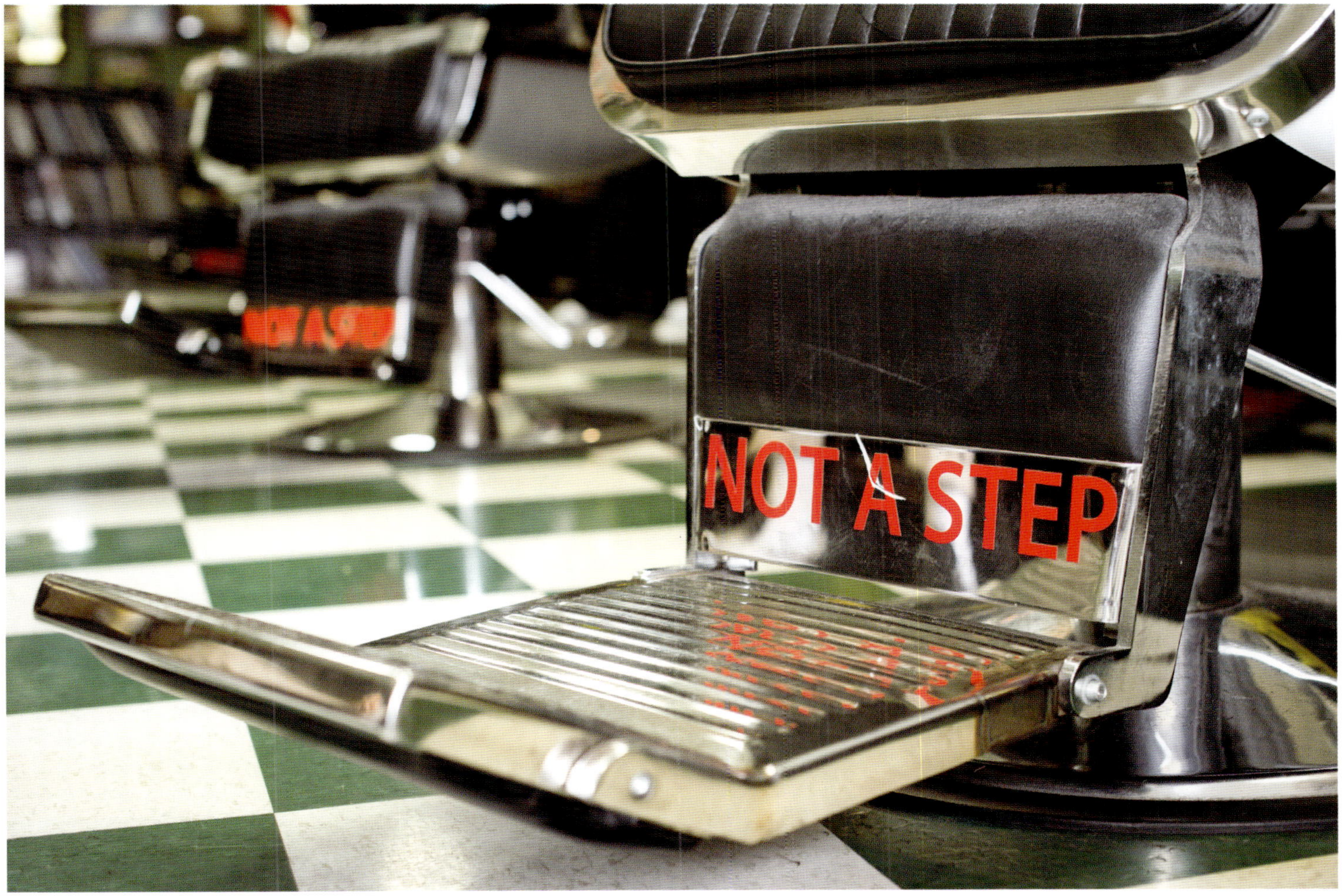

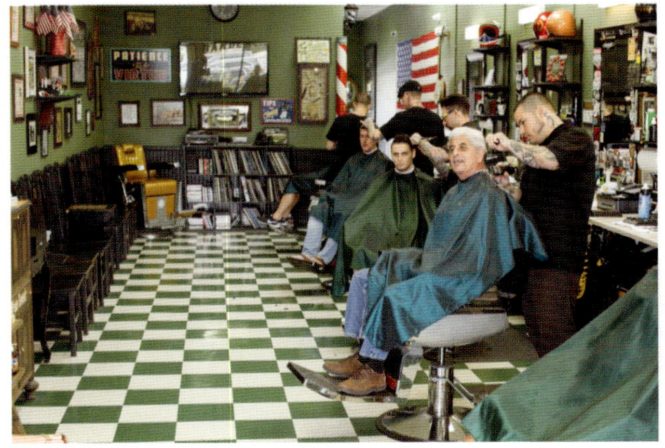
PATIENCE

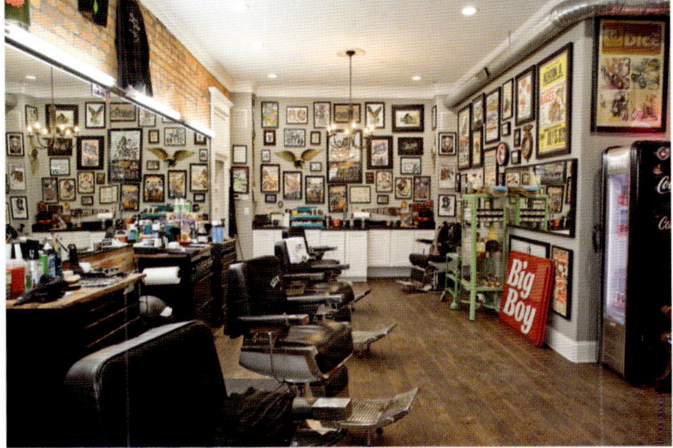
Big Boy

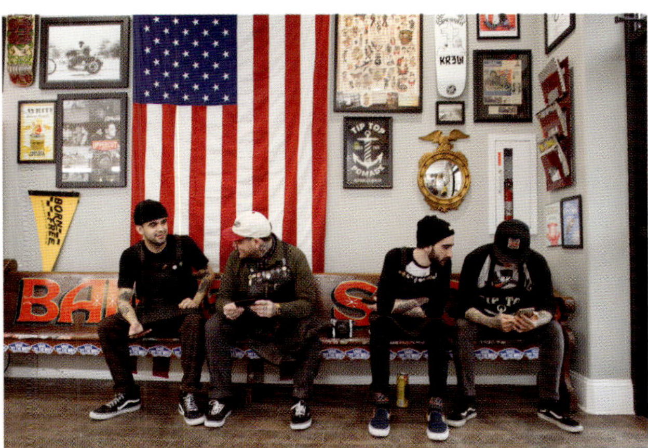

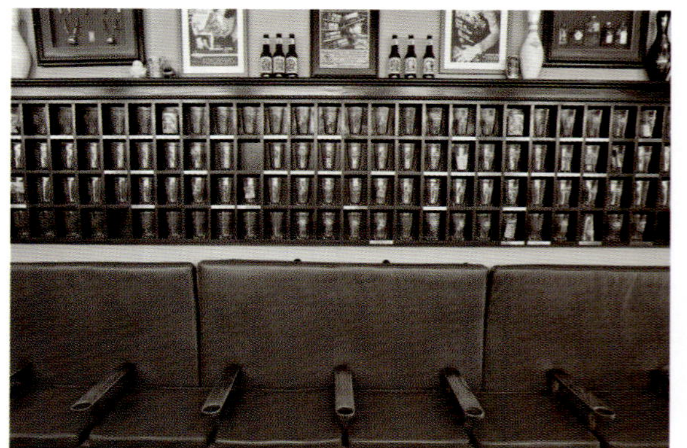

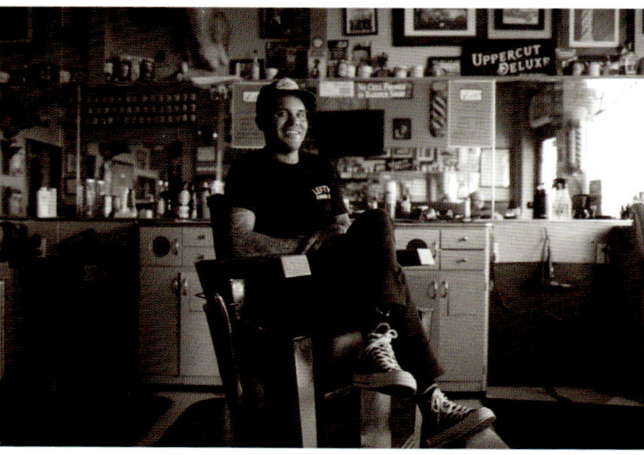
UPPERCUT DELUXE

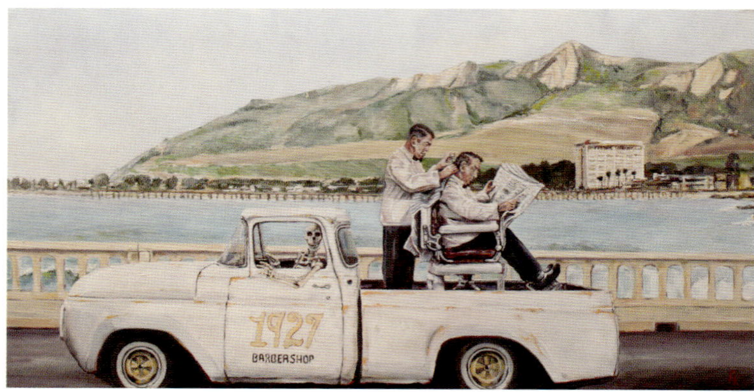
1927
BARBERSHOP

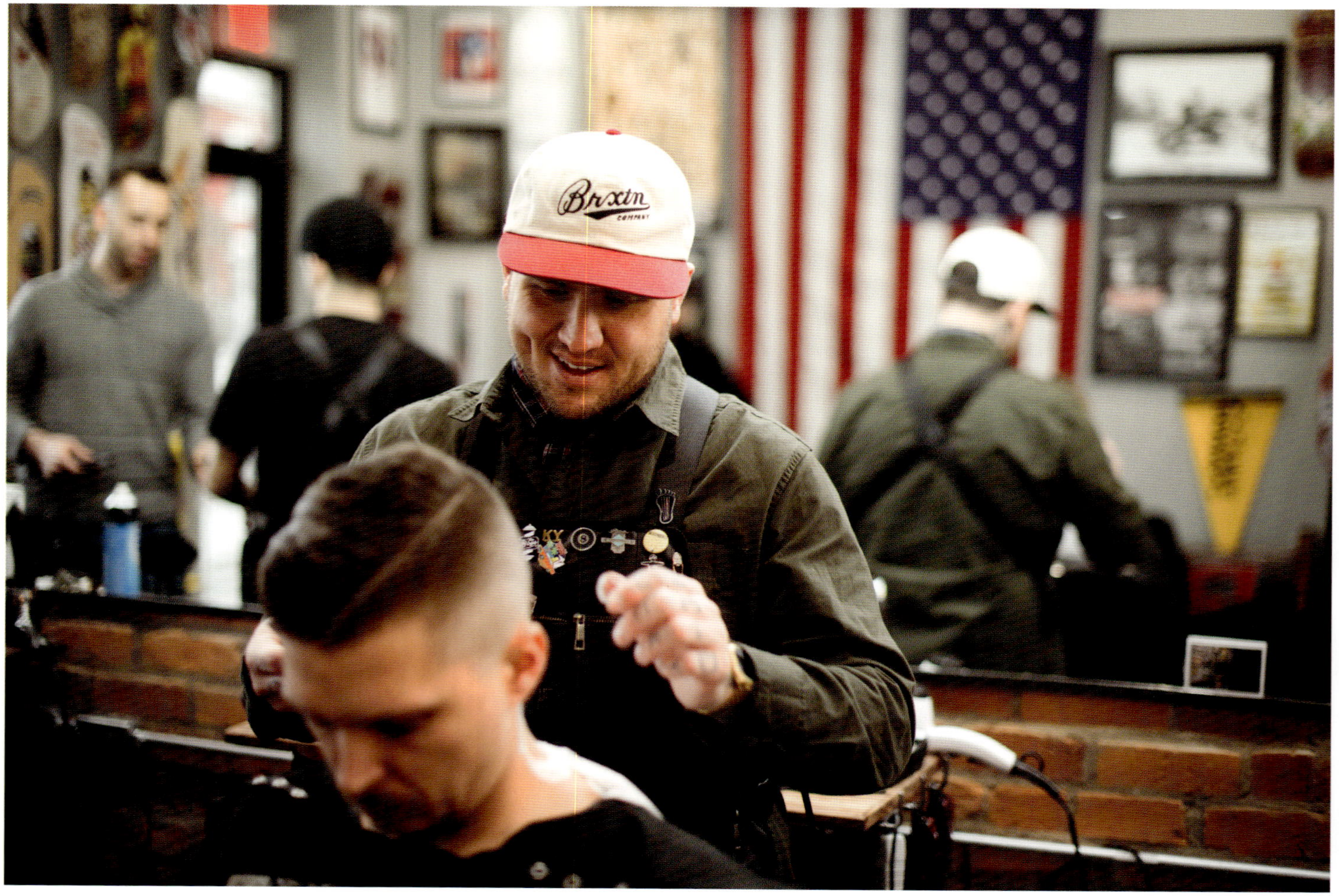

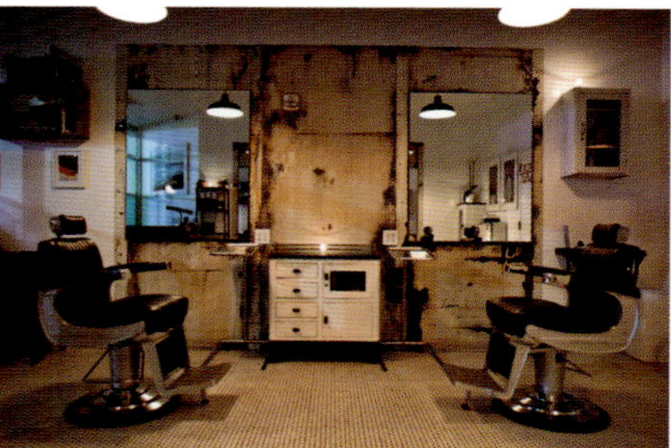

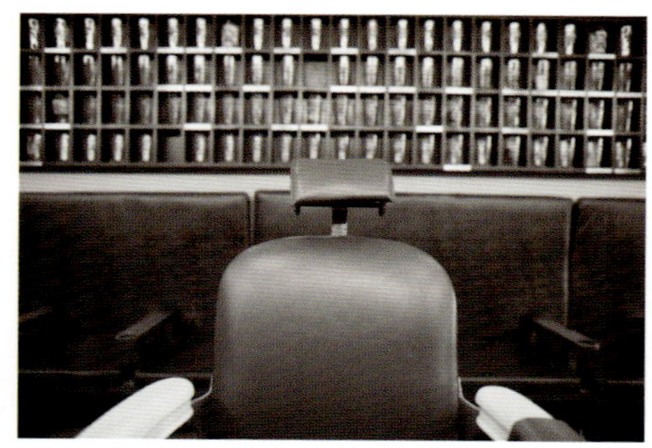

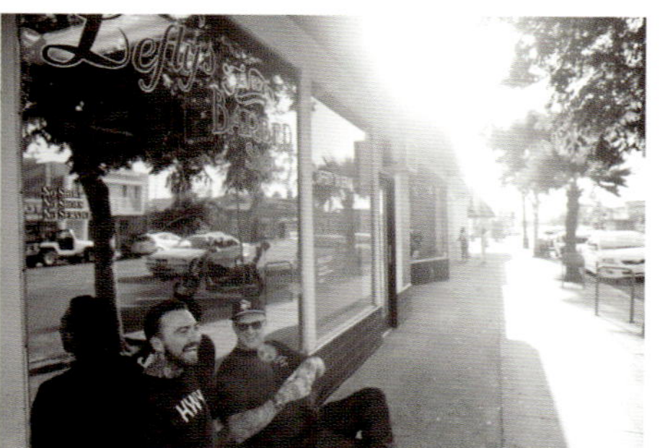

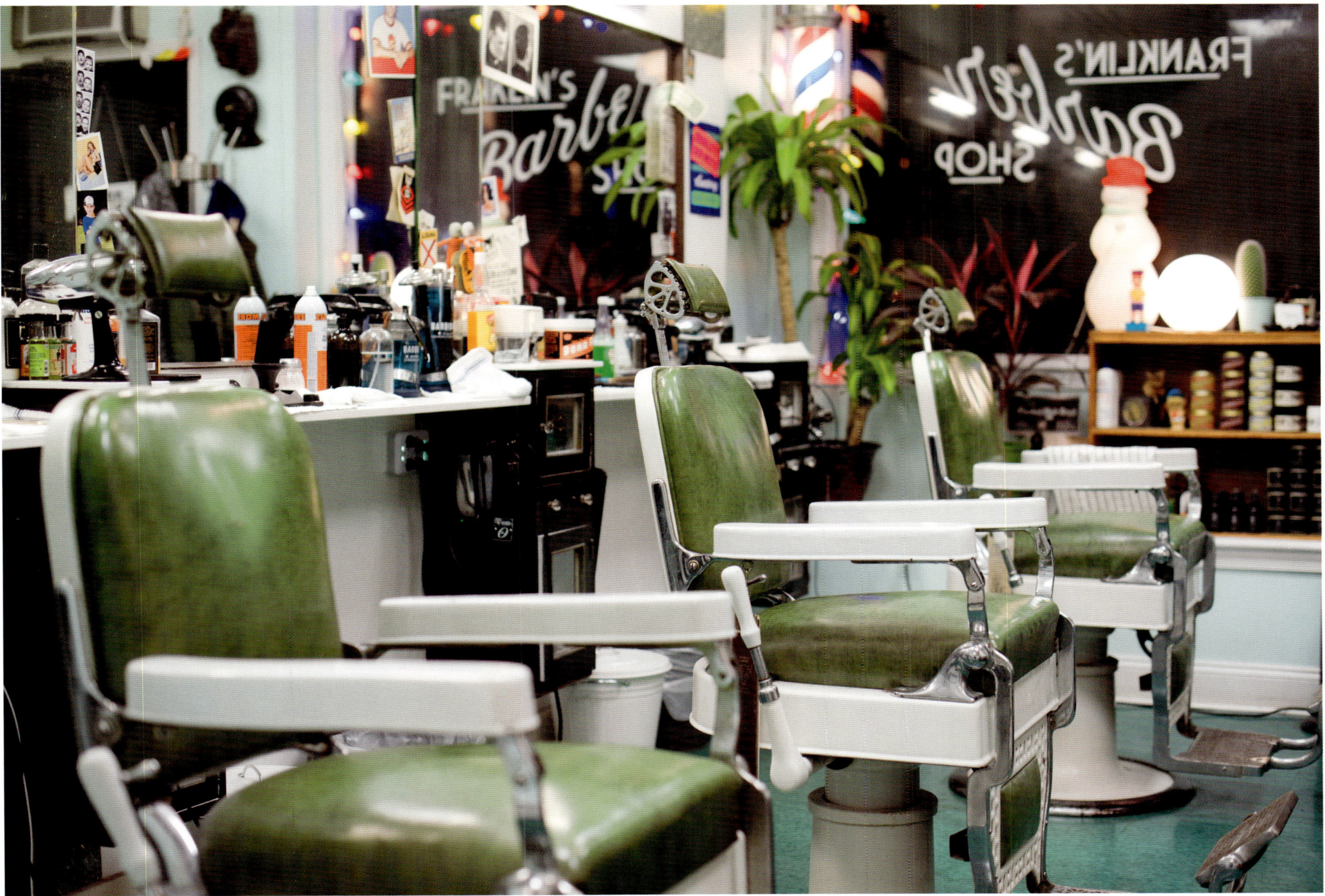

Franklin's Barbershop, Philadelphia, Pennsylvania

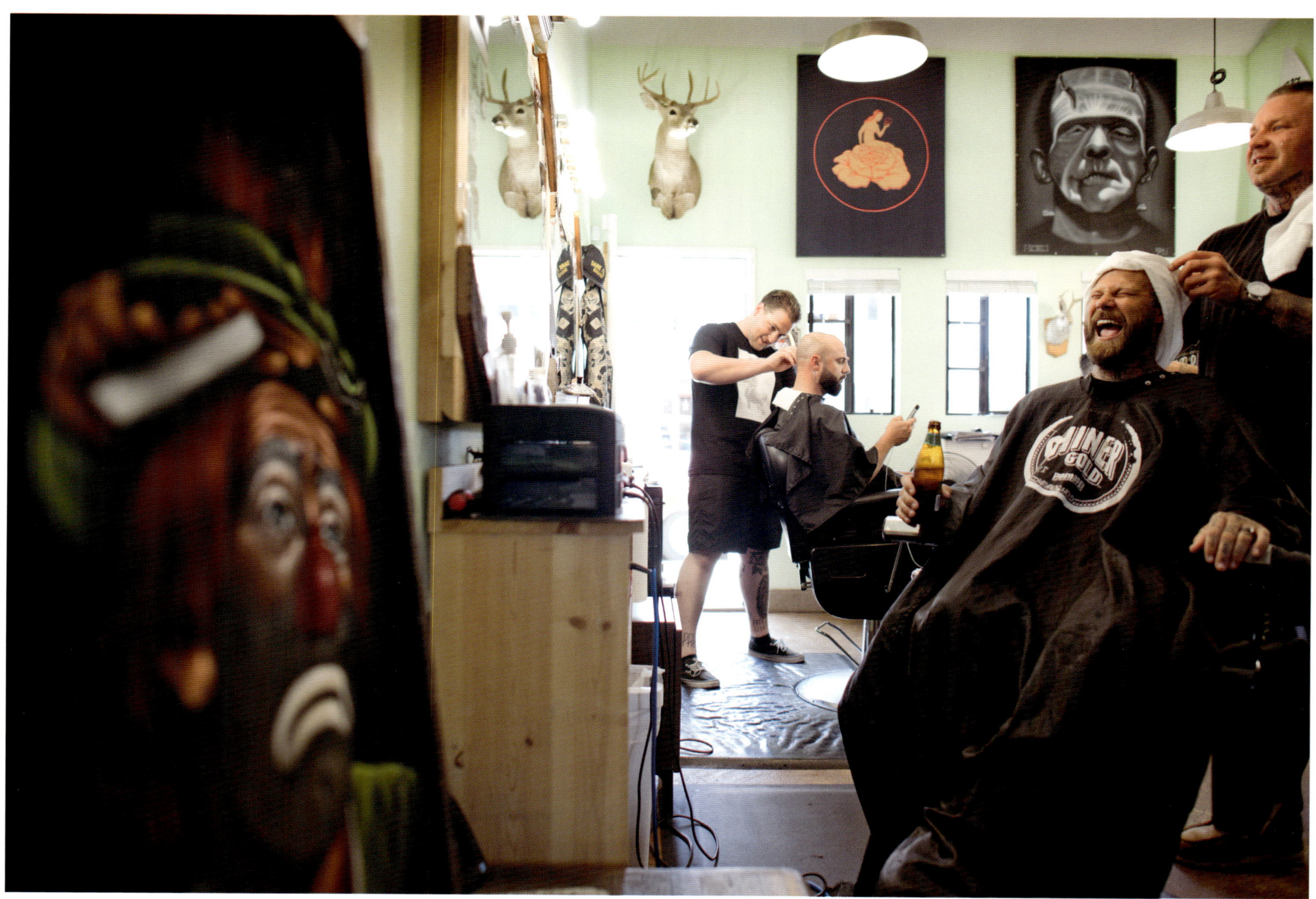

1927 Barbershop, Ventura, California

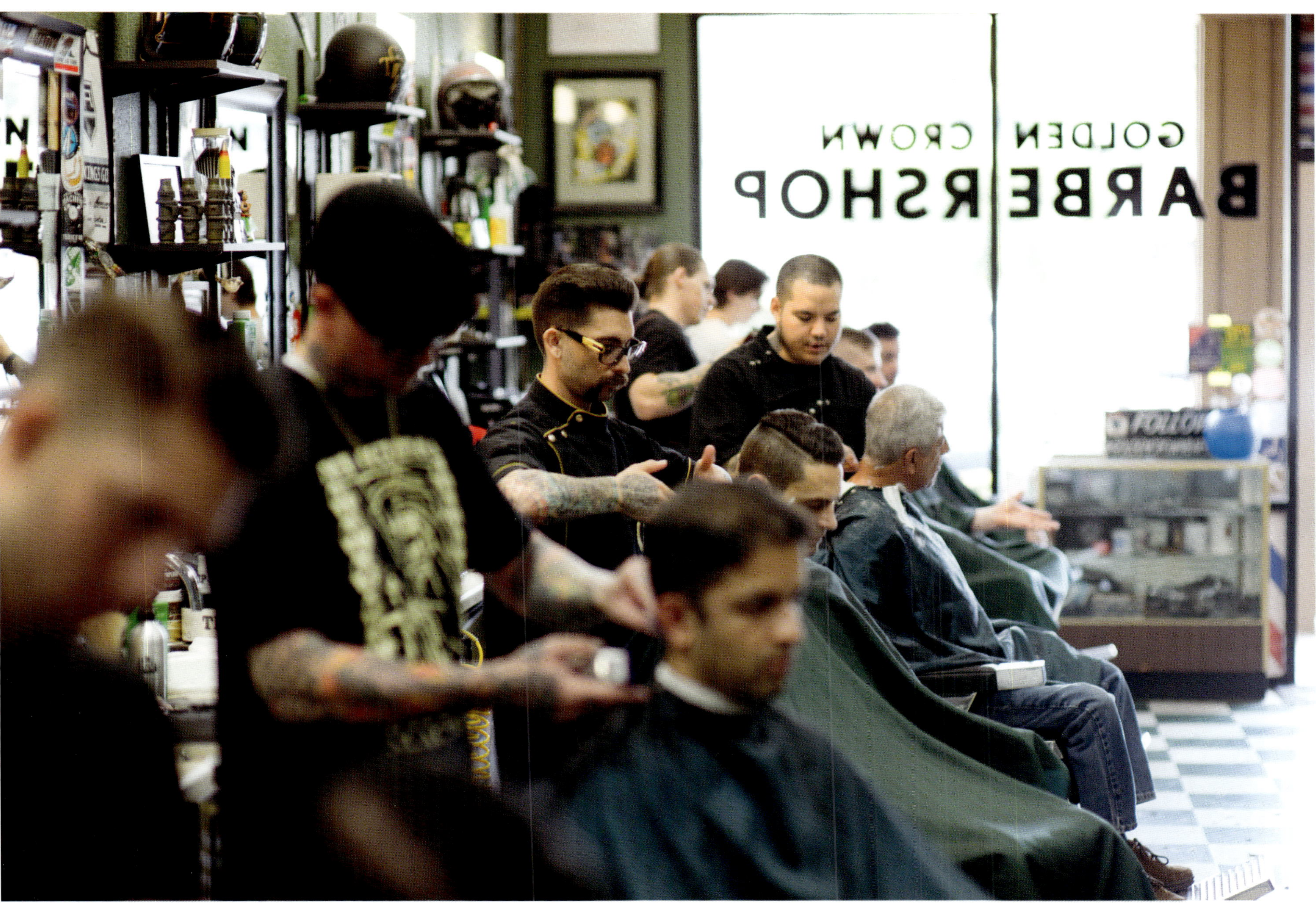

Golden Crown Barbershop, Laguna Niguel, California

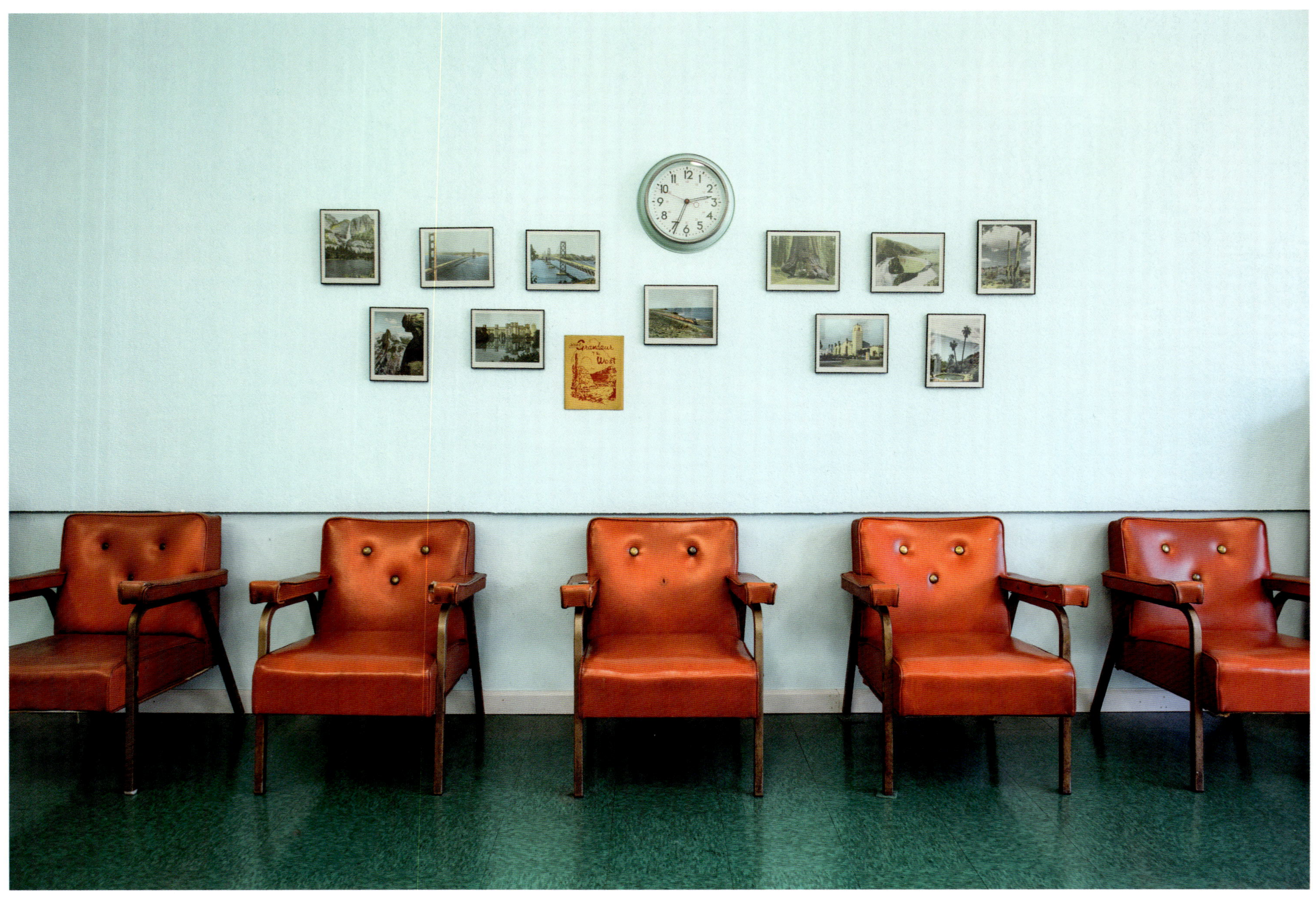

Nate's Barbershop, Atascadero, California

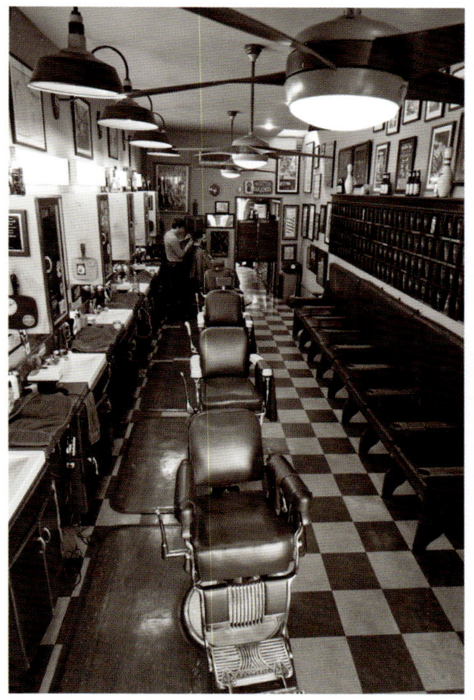

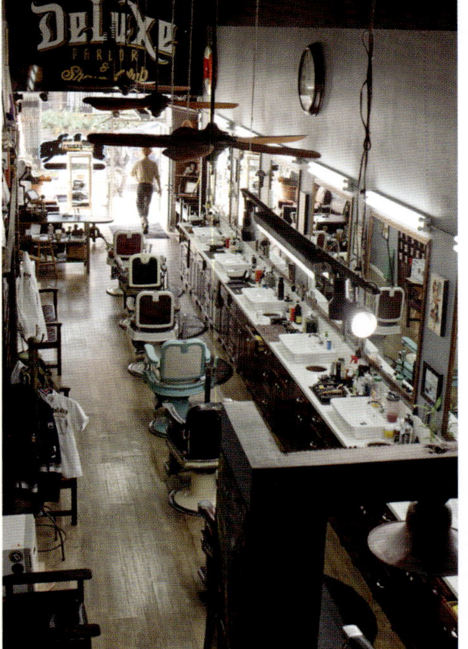
DeLuxe

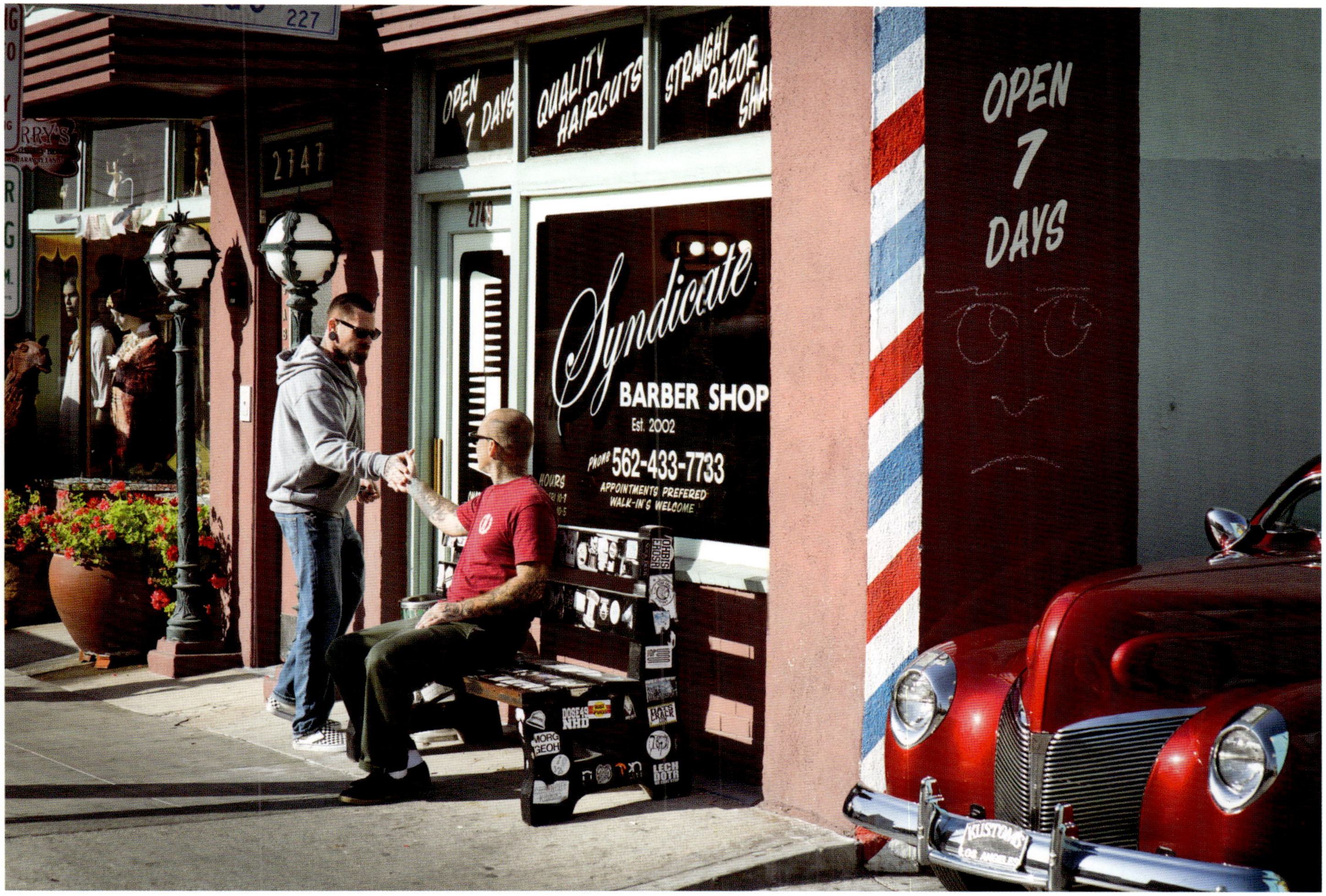

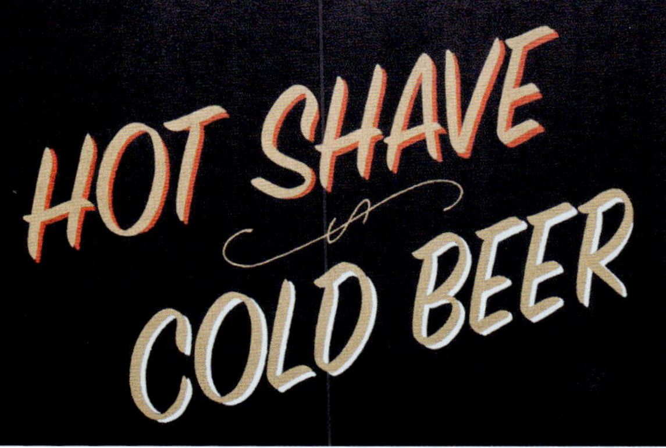
HOT SHAVE
COLD BEER

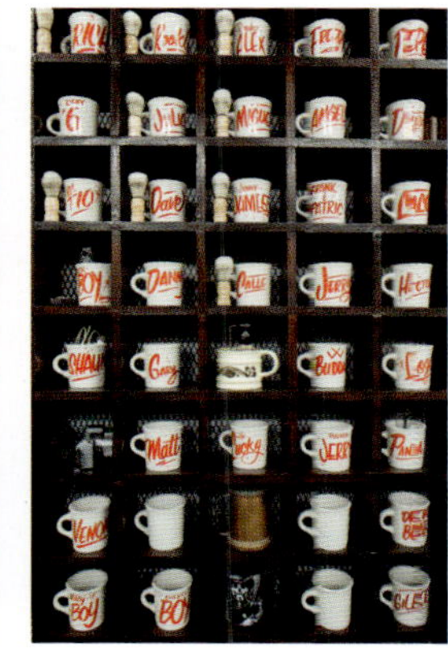

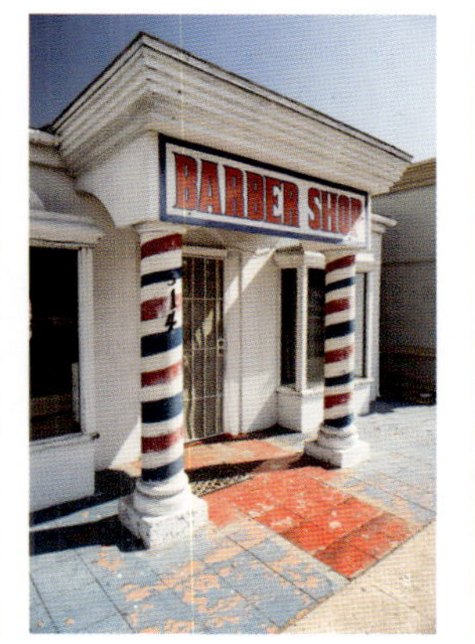
BARBER SHOP

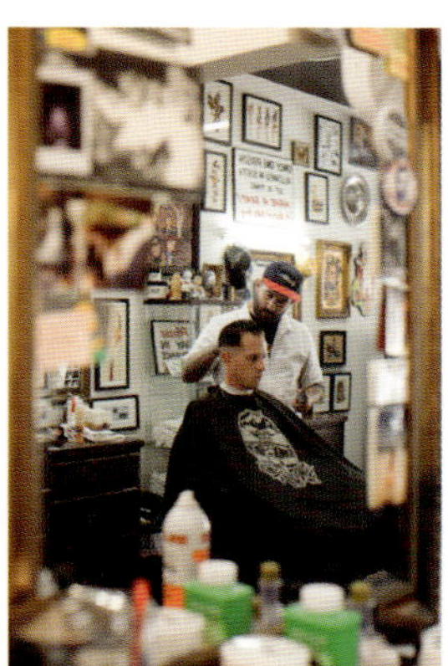

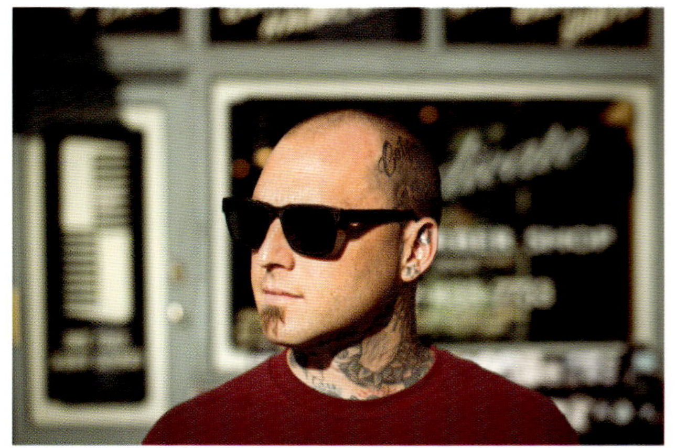

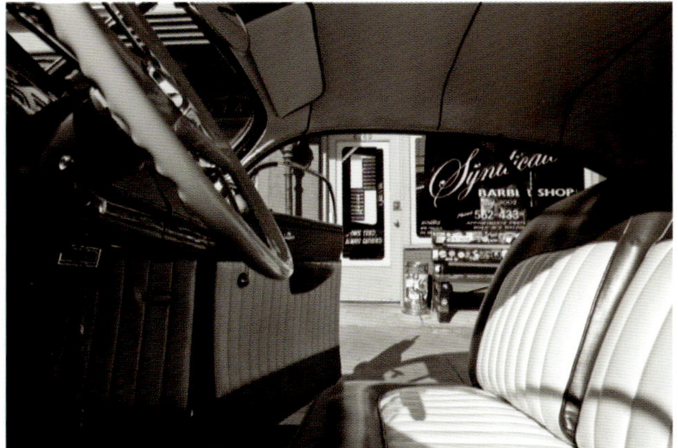
SHOP

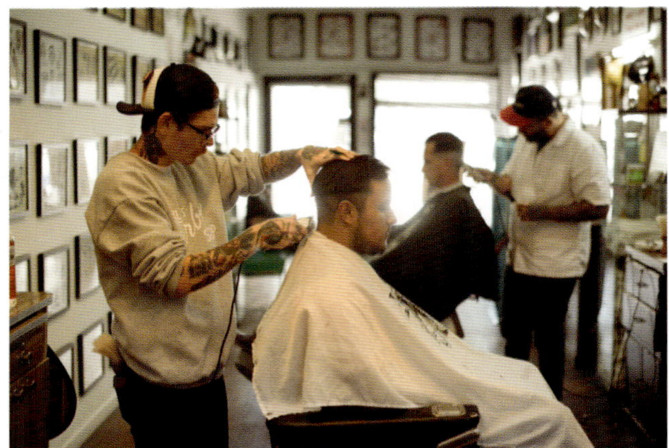

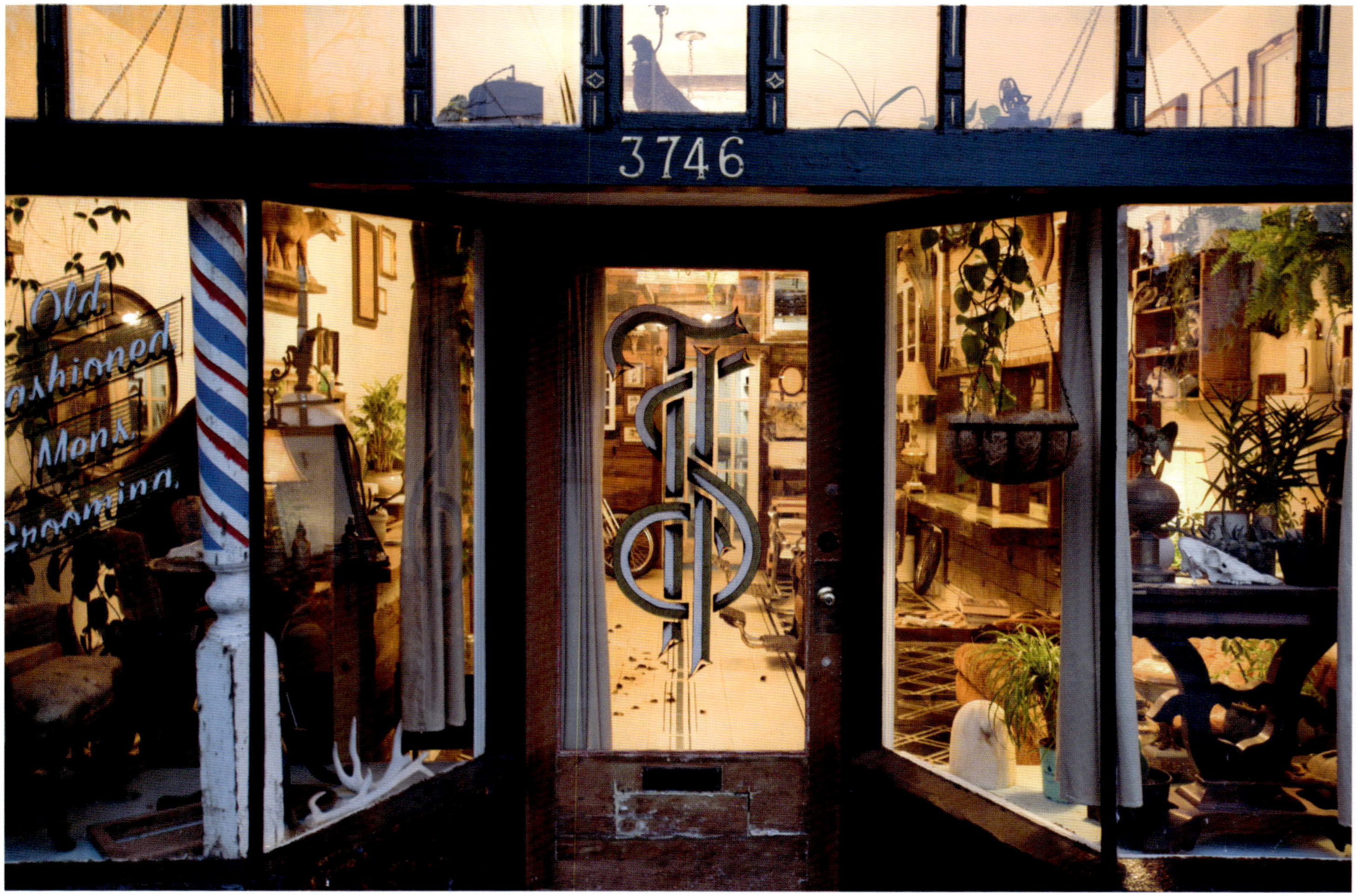

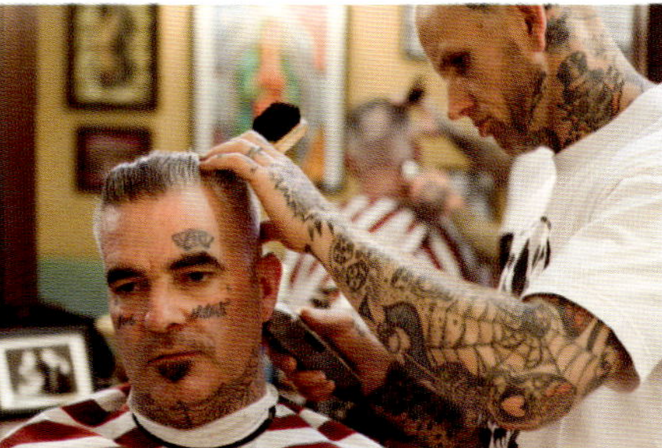

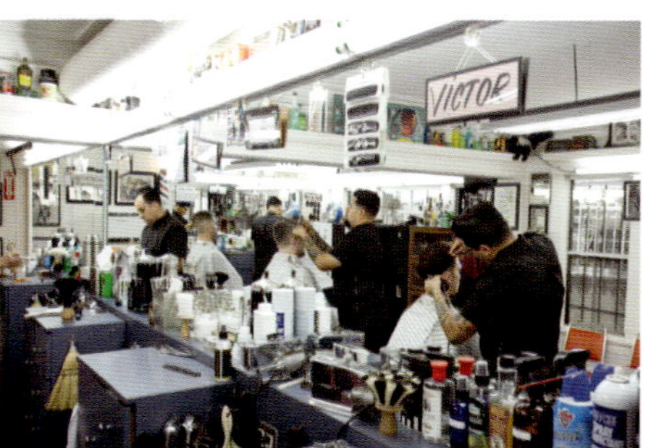
VICTOR

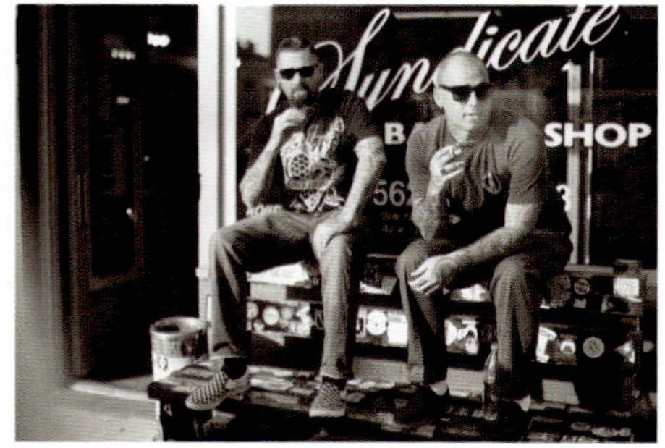
SHOP

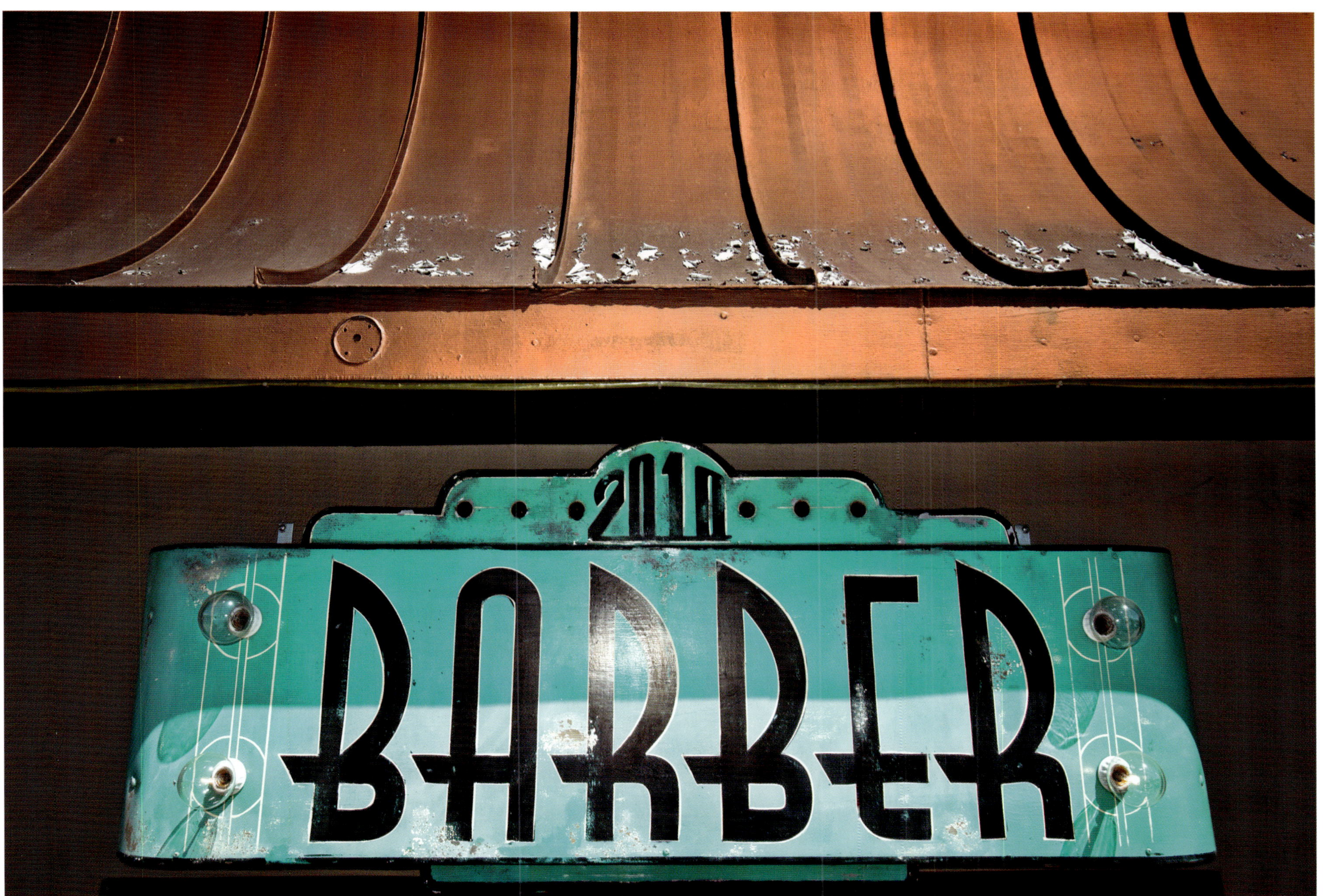

Pappy's Barbershop, San Diego, California

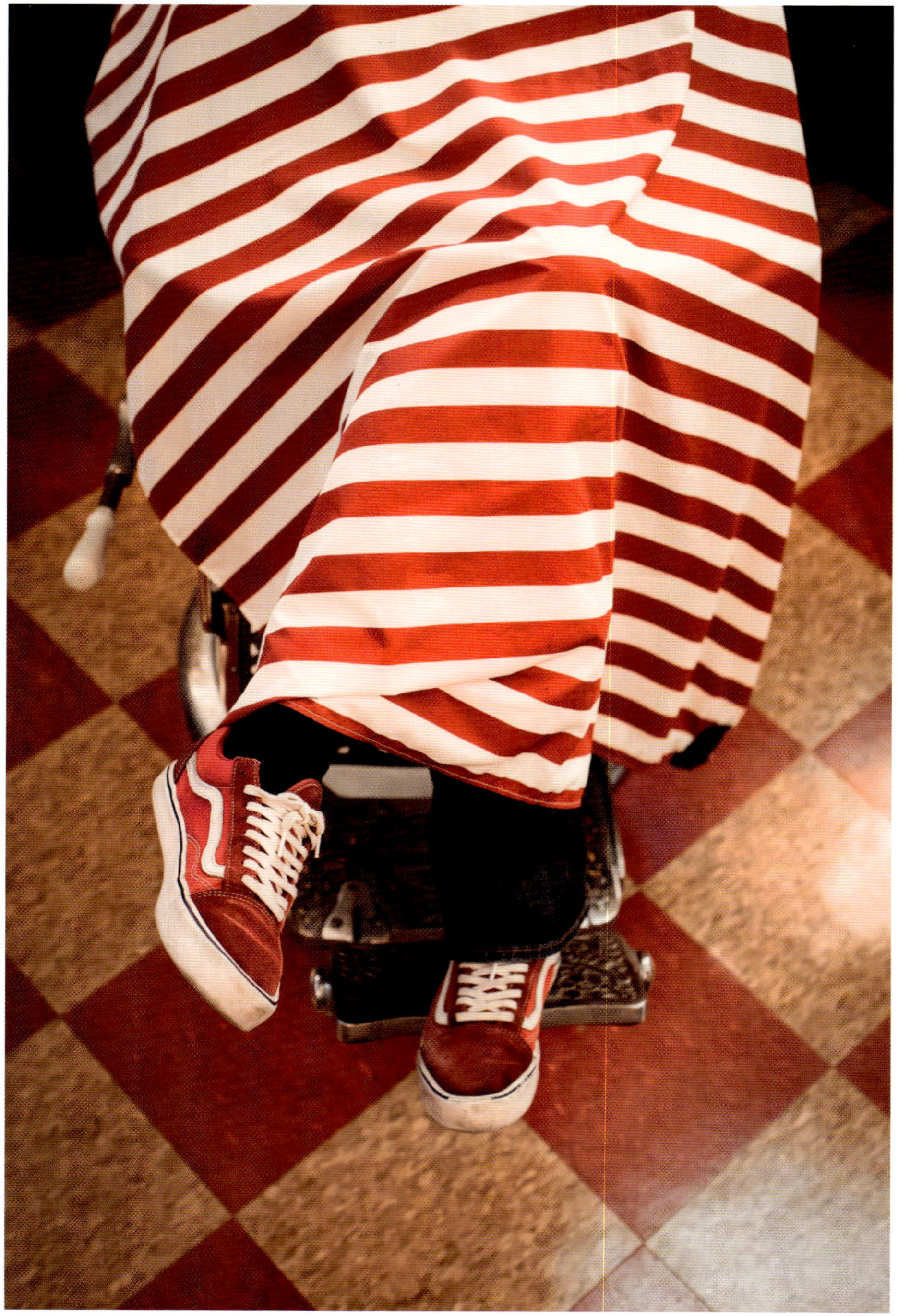

Syndicate Barbershop, Long Beach, California

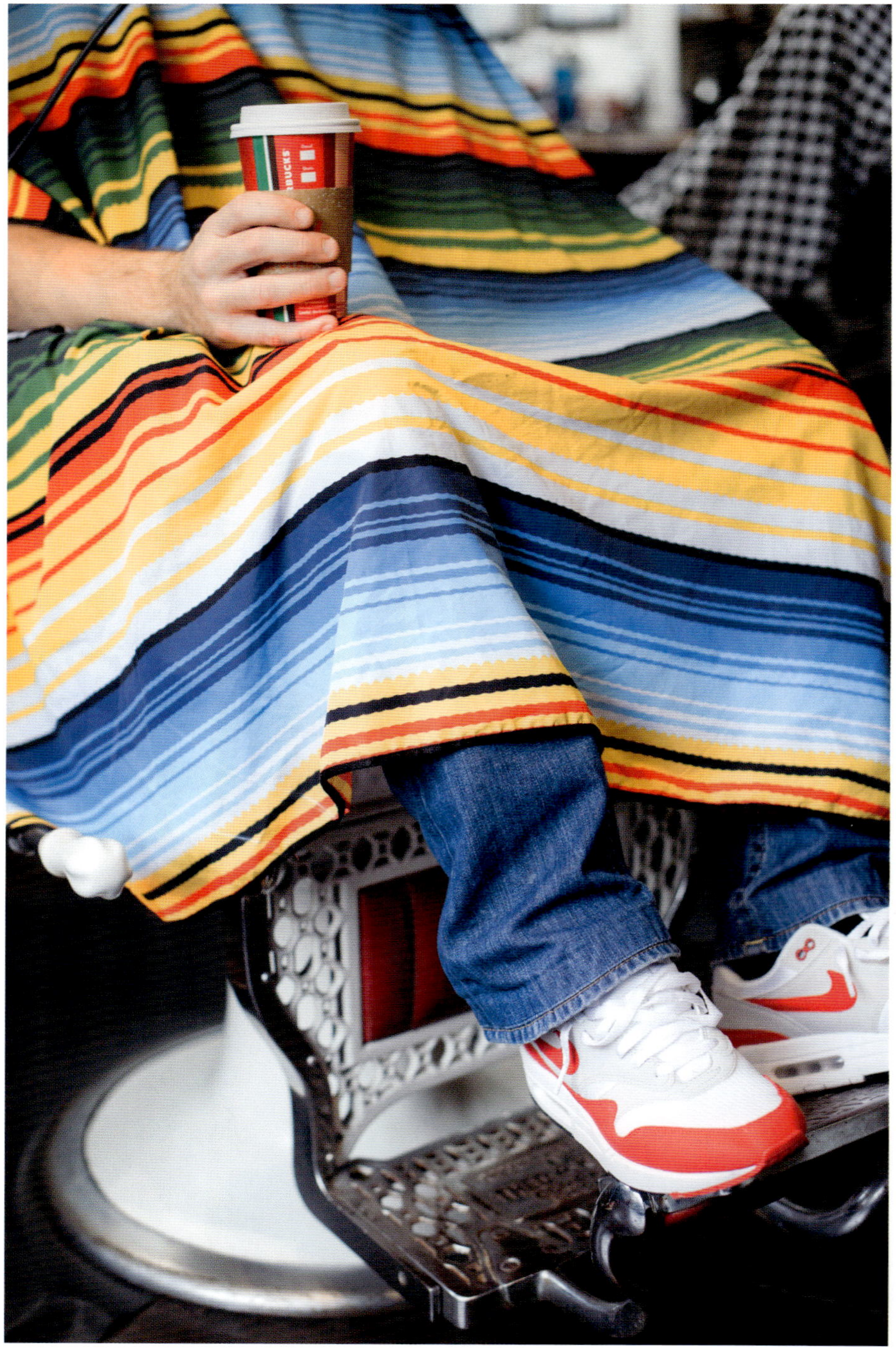

The Black Comb, Lancaster, Pennsylvania

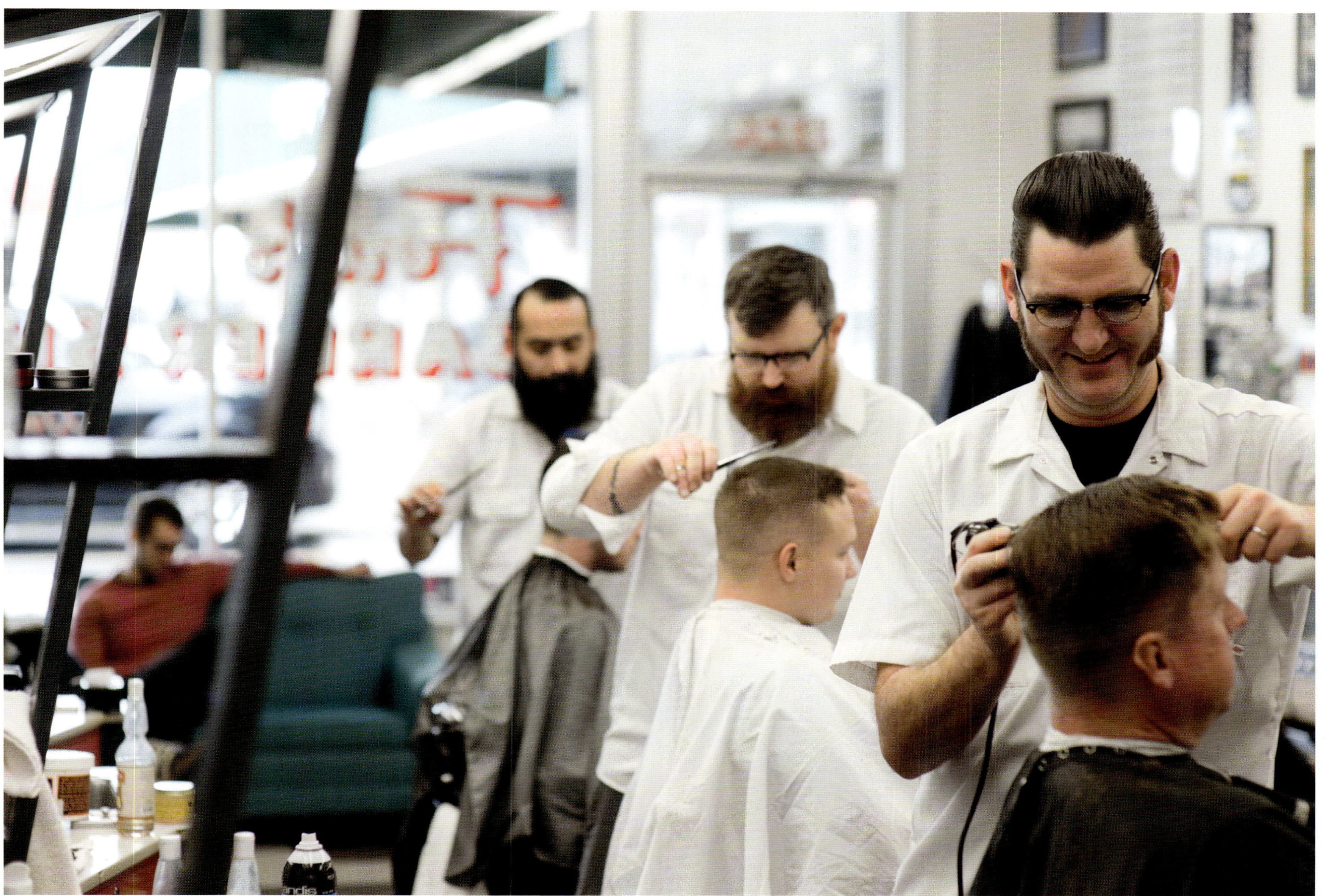

Ford's Barbershop, Tulsa, Oklahoma

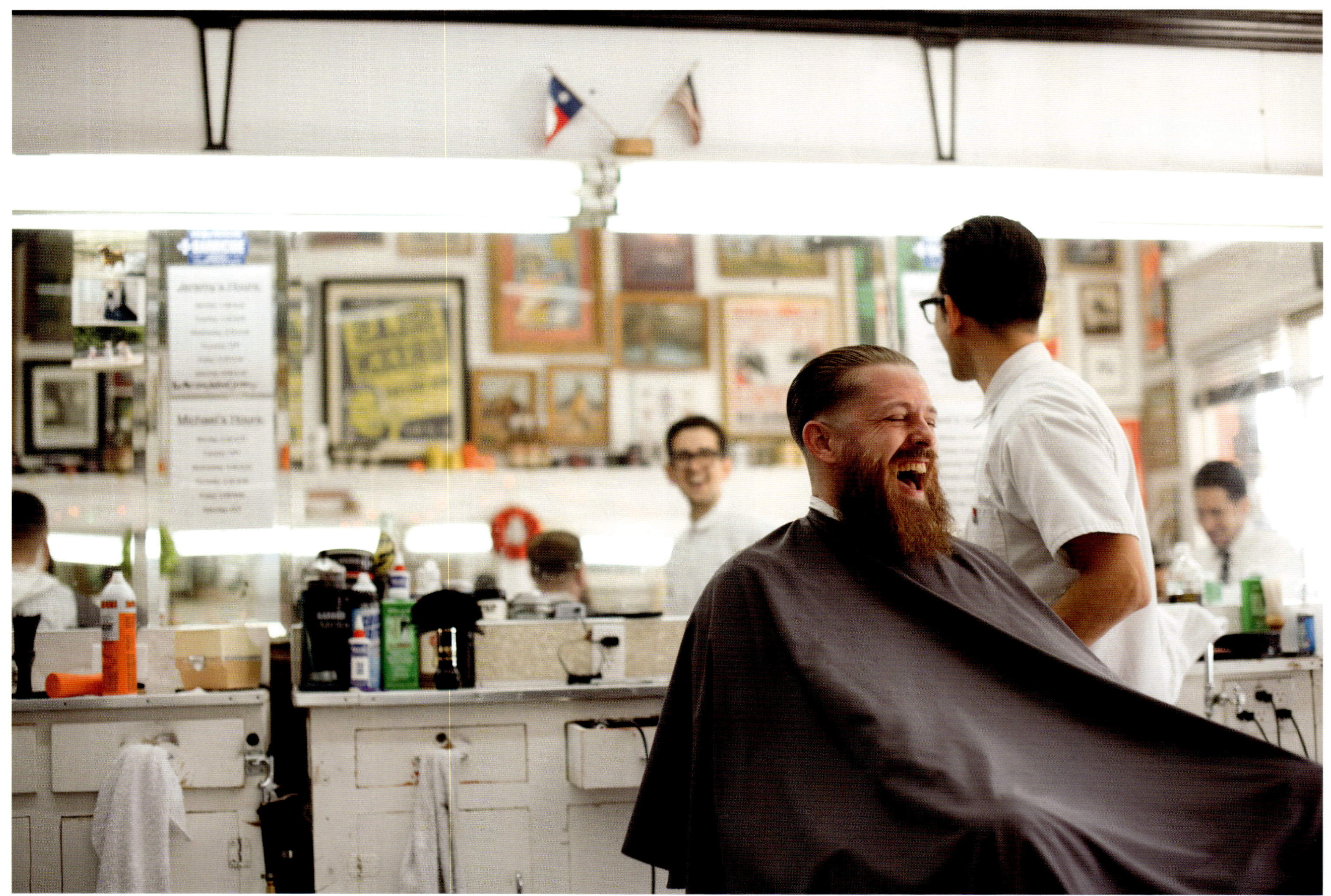

Avenue Barbershop, Austin, Texas

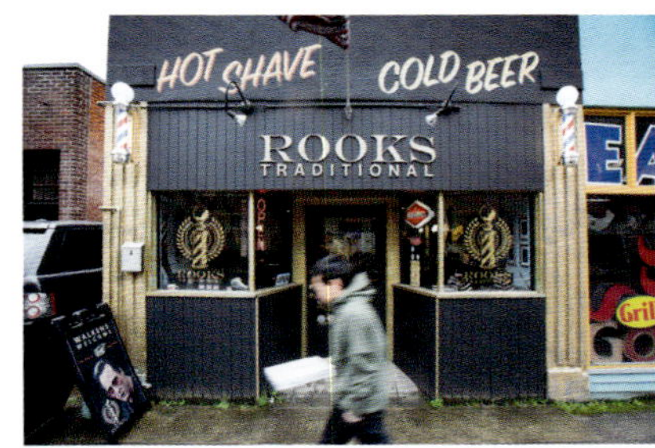
HOT SHAVE
COLD BEER
ROOKS
TRADITIONAL

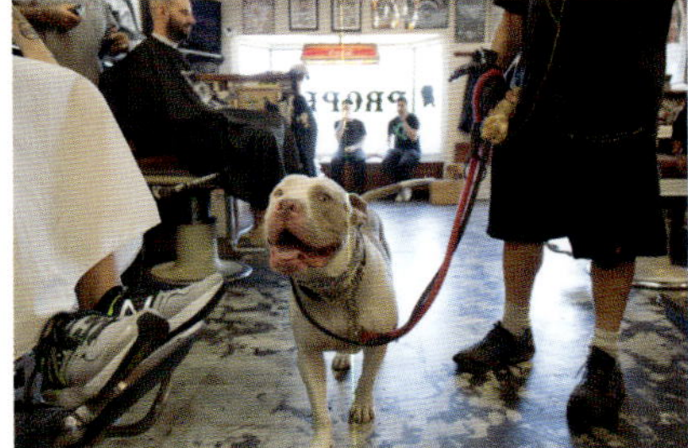

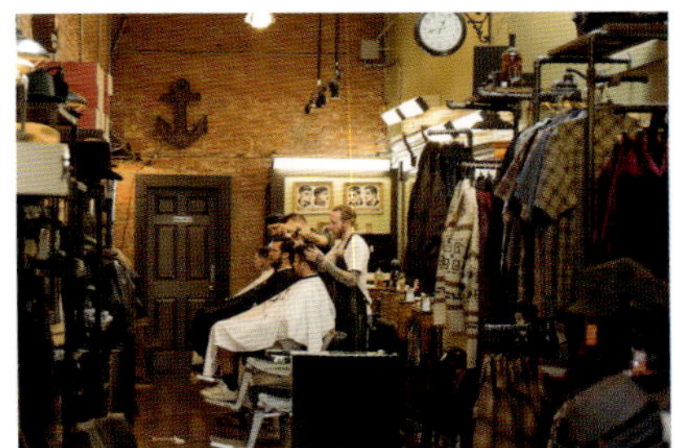

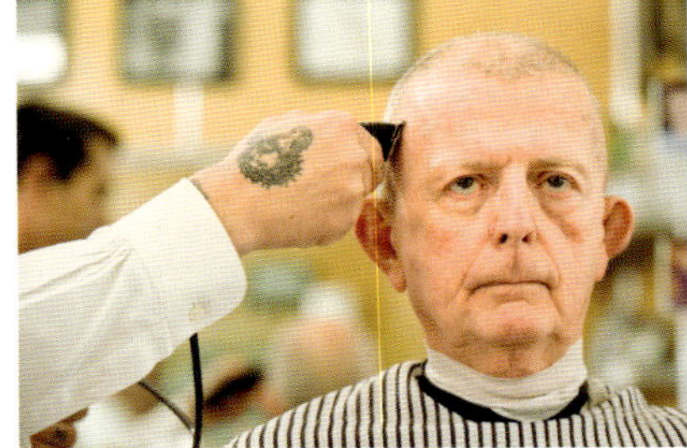

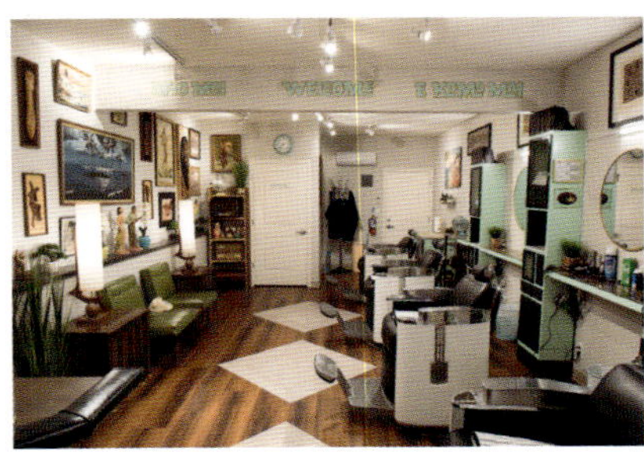

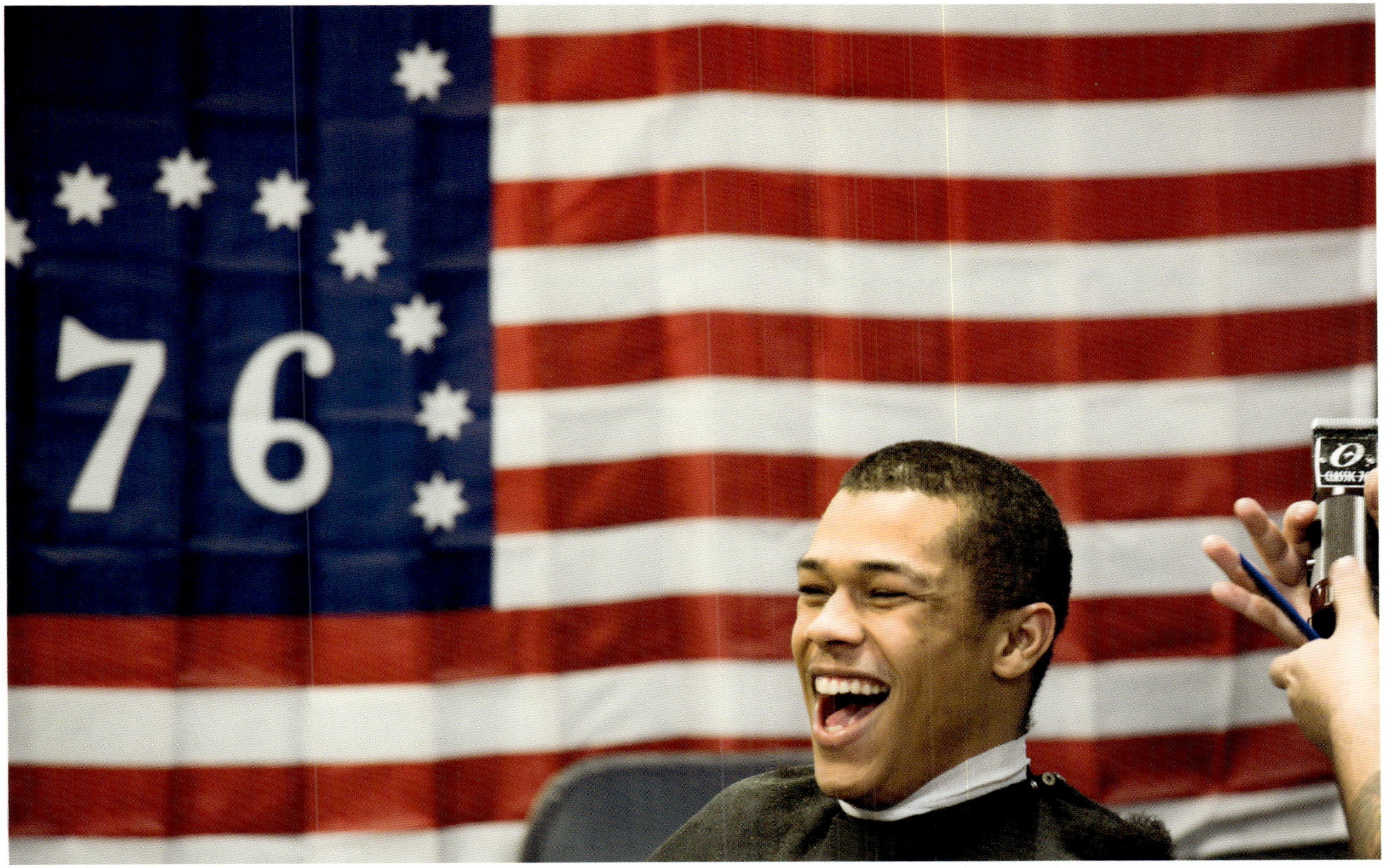

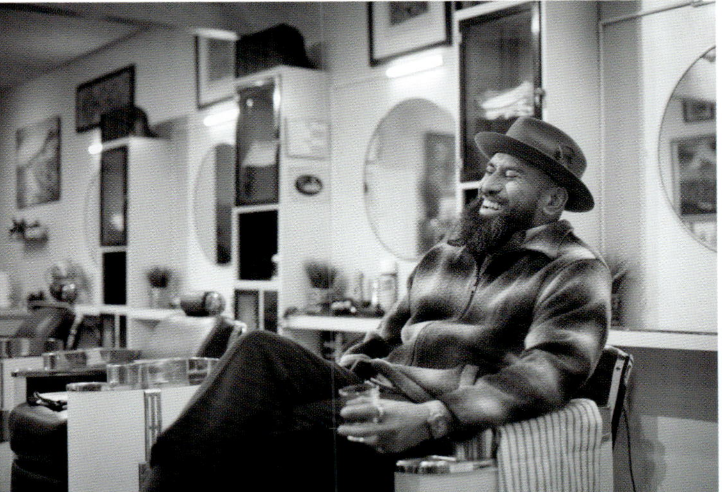

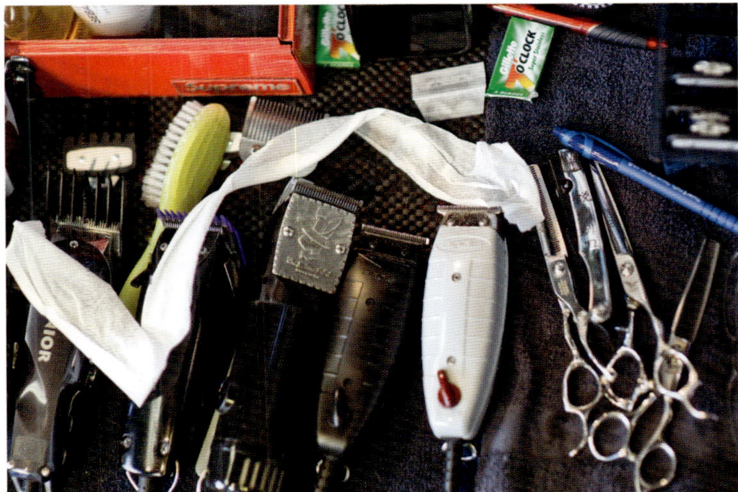

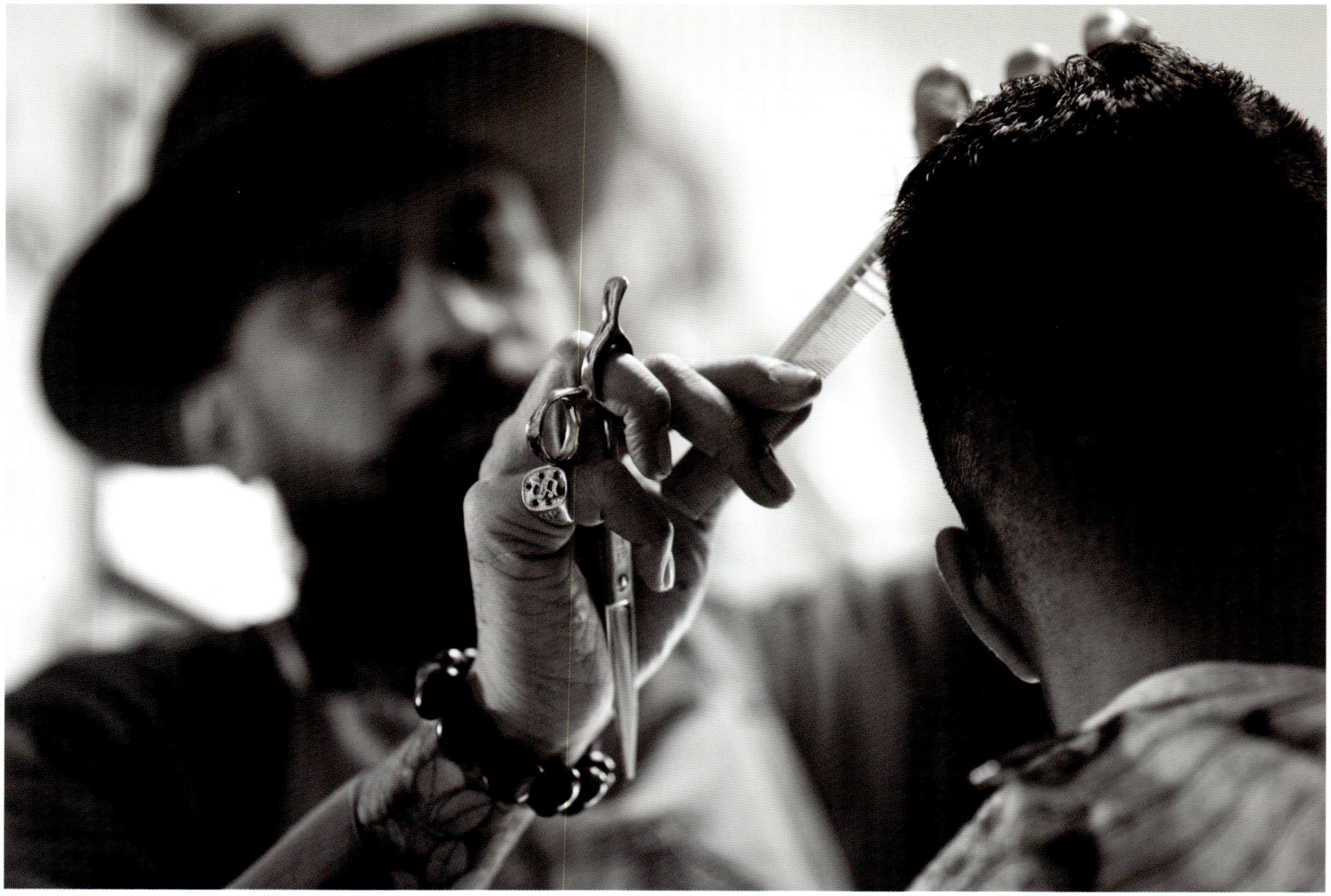

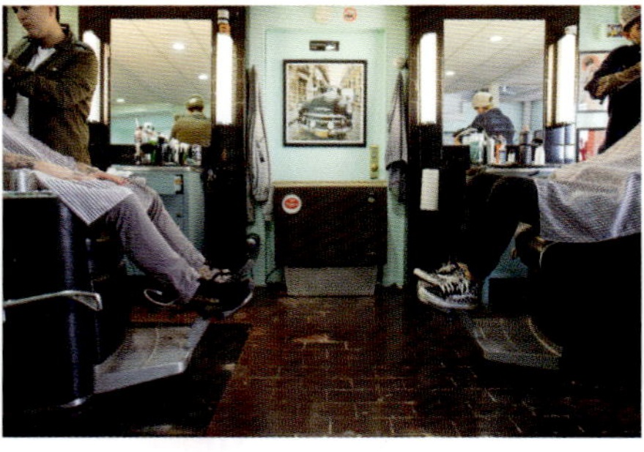

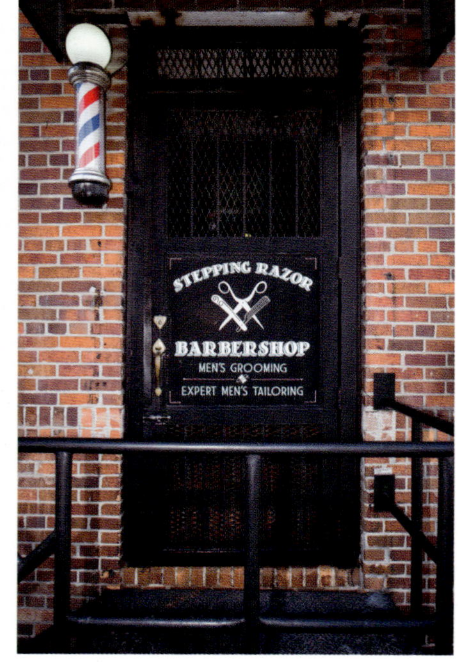
STEPPING RAZOR
BARBERSHOP
MEN'S GROOMING
EXPERT MEN'S TAILORING

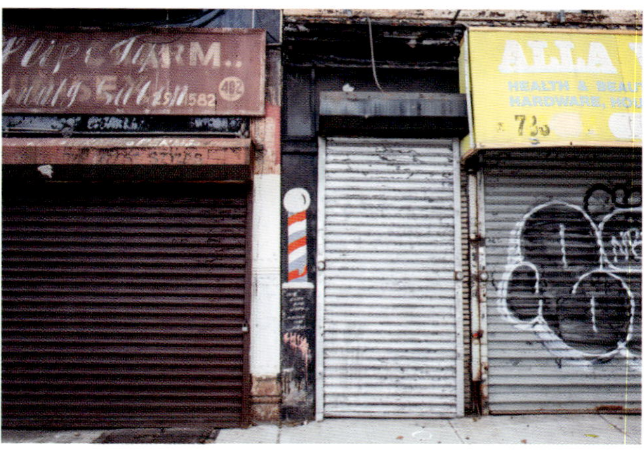

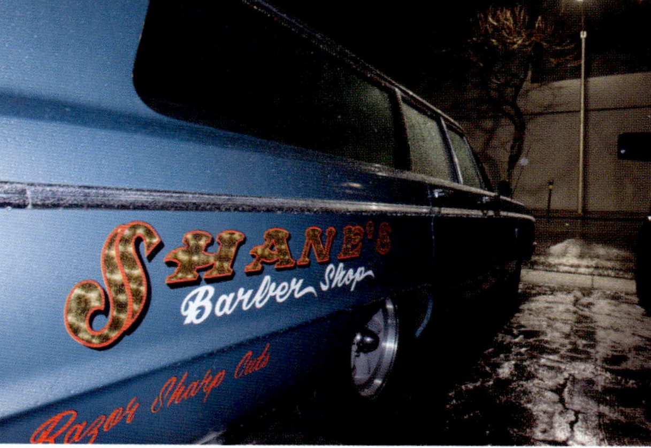
SHANE'S
Barber Shop
Razor Sharp Cuts

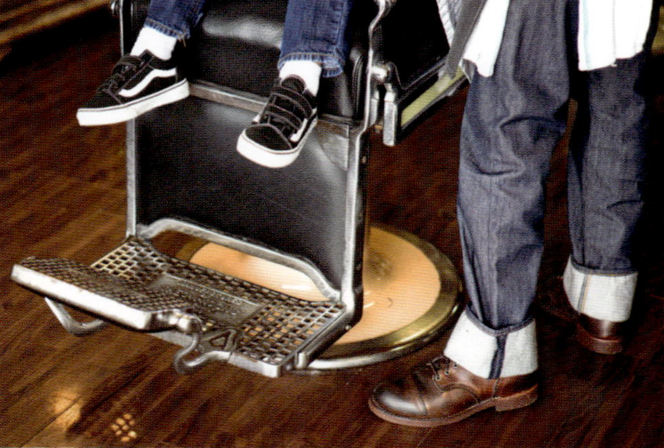

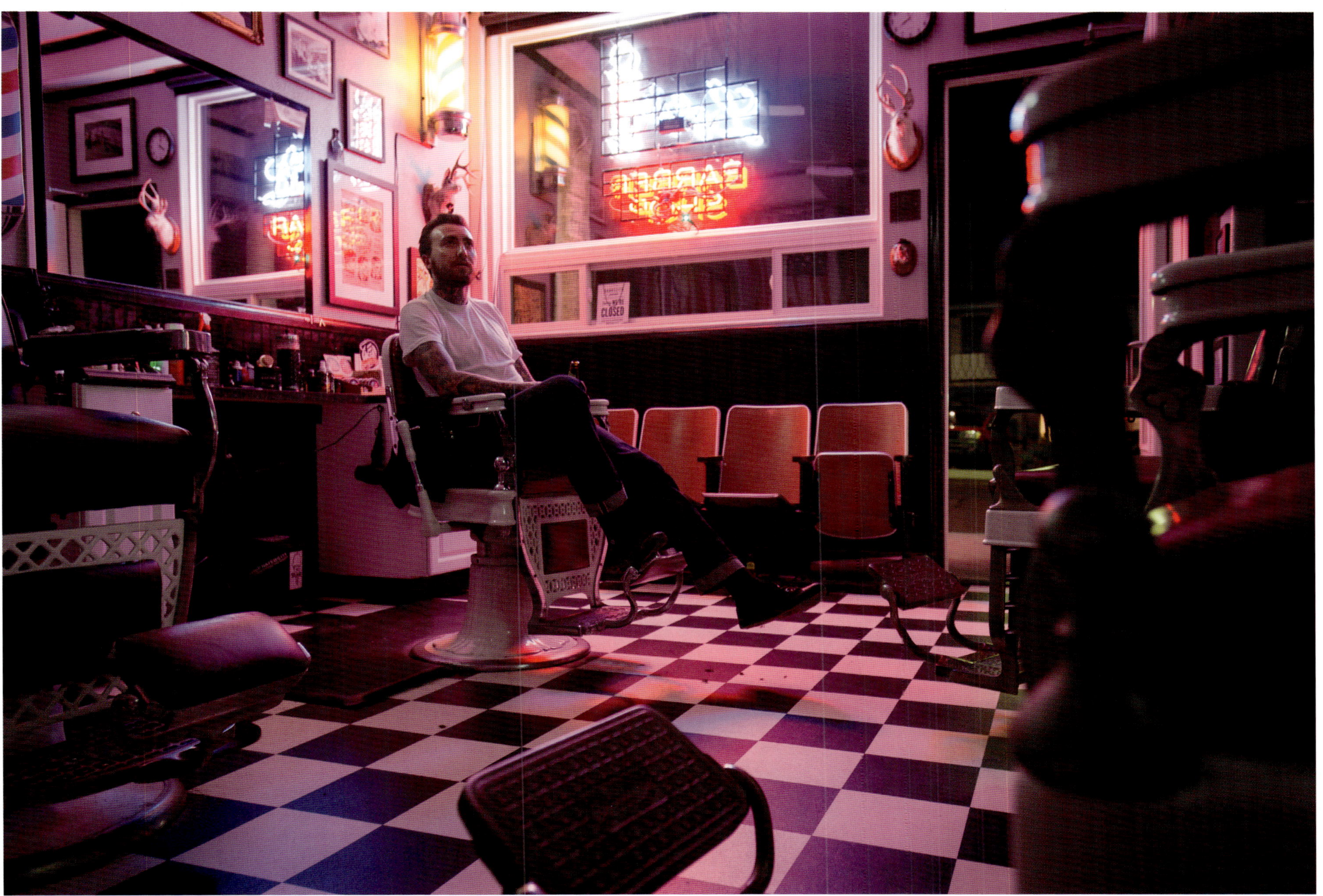

Lefty's Barbershop, San Diego, California

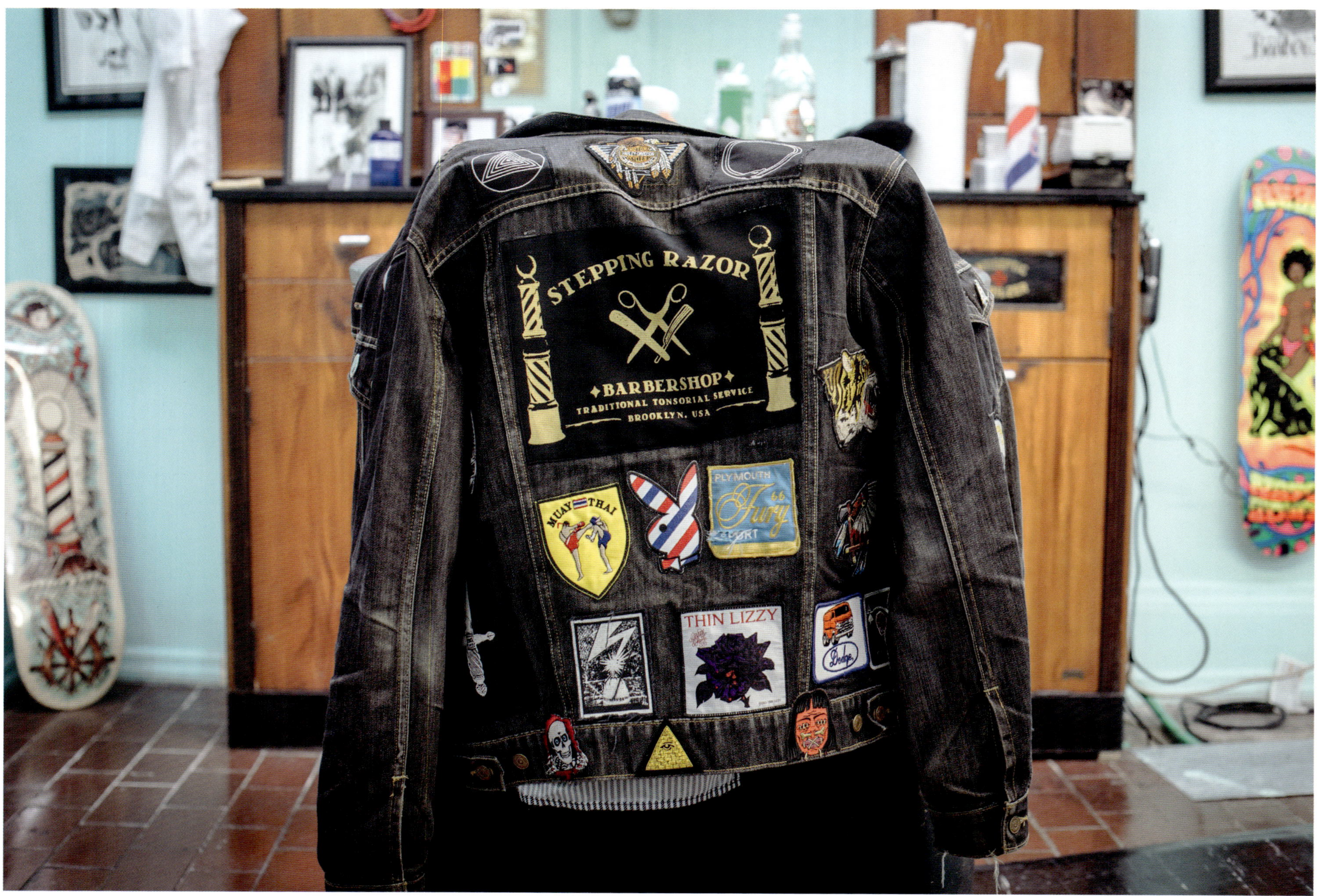

Stepping Razor Barbershop, Brooklyn, New York

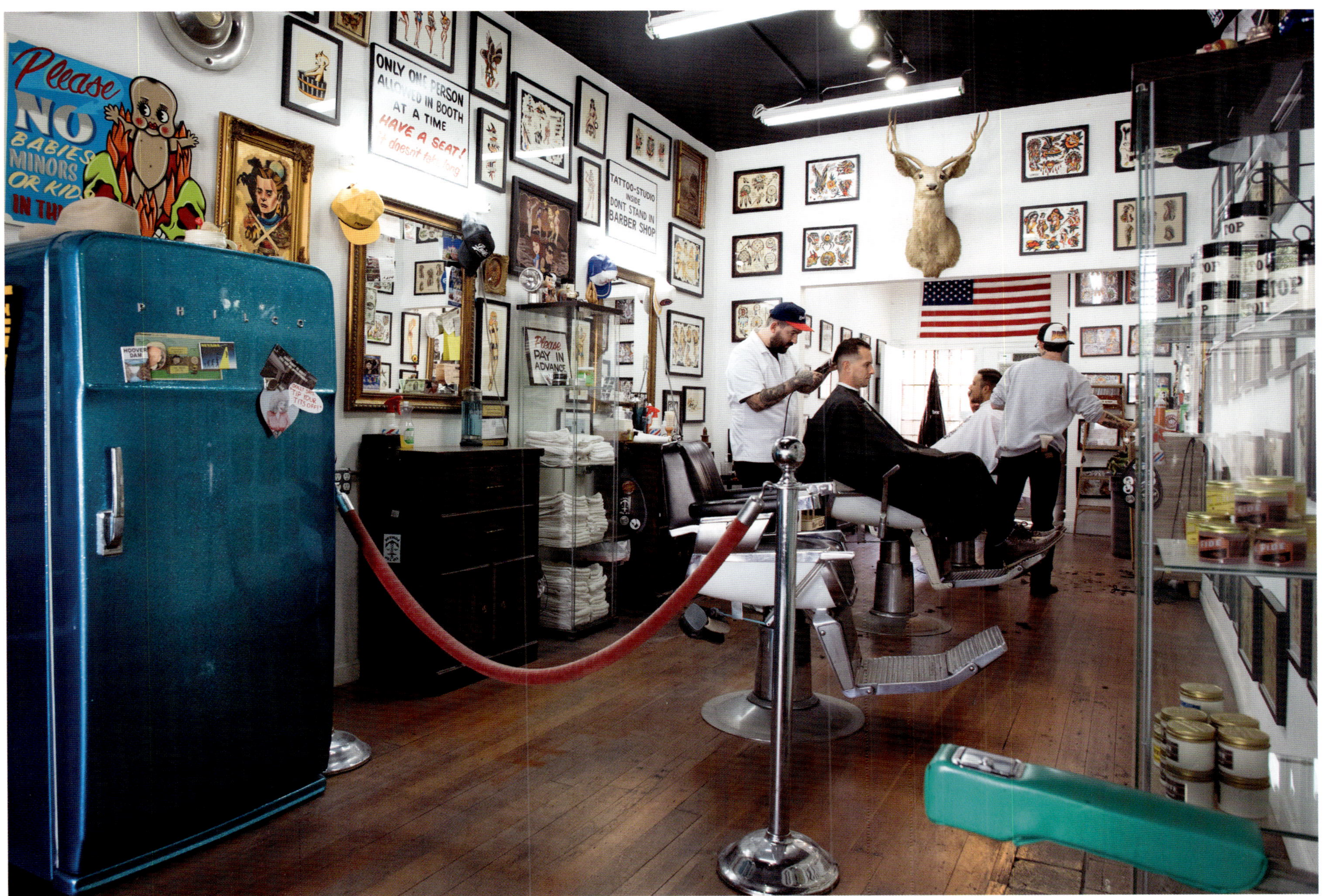

Tip Top Barbershop, Whittier, California

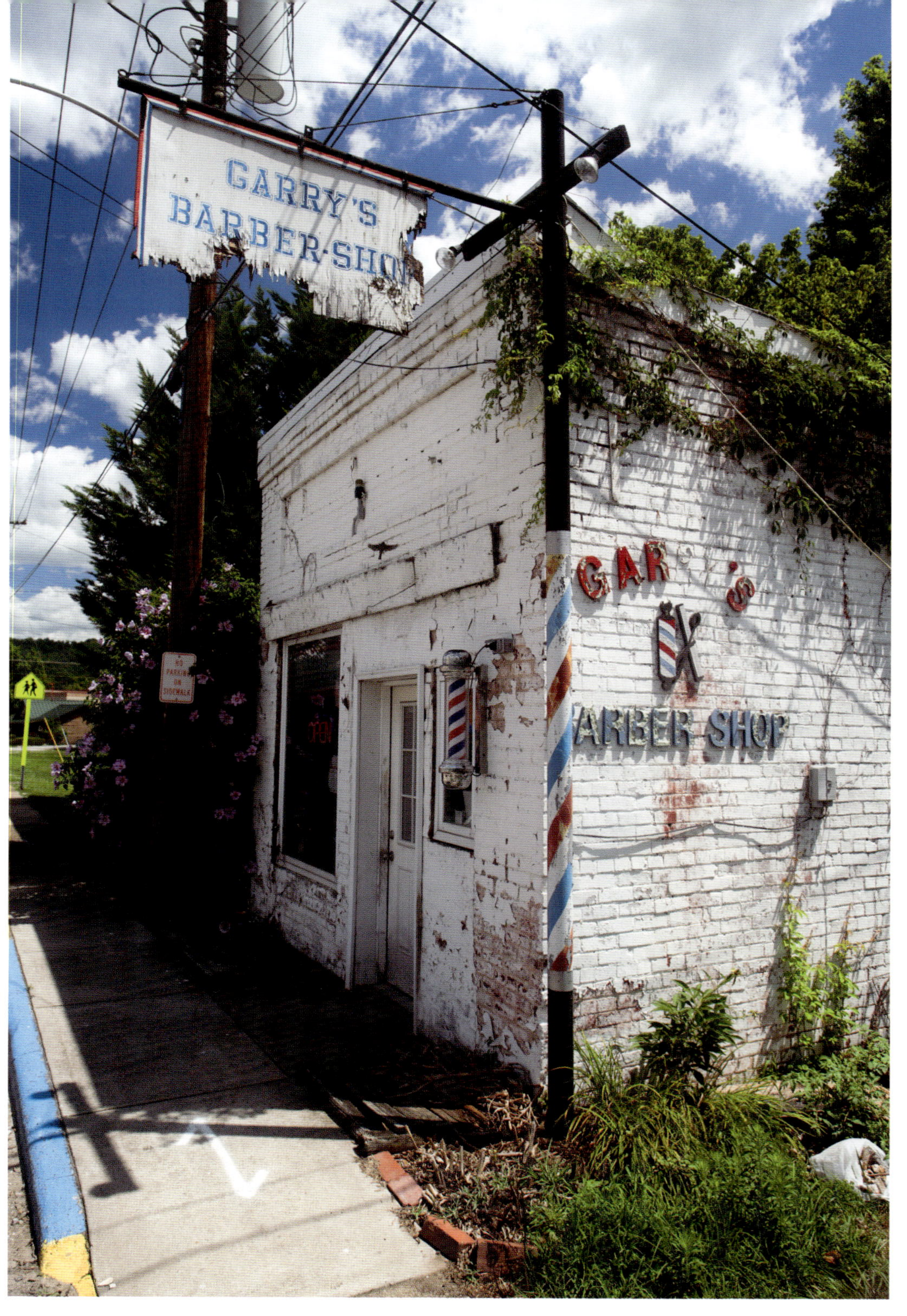

Garry's Barbershop, Poca, West Virginia

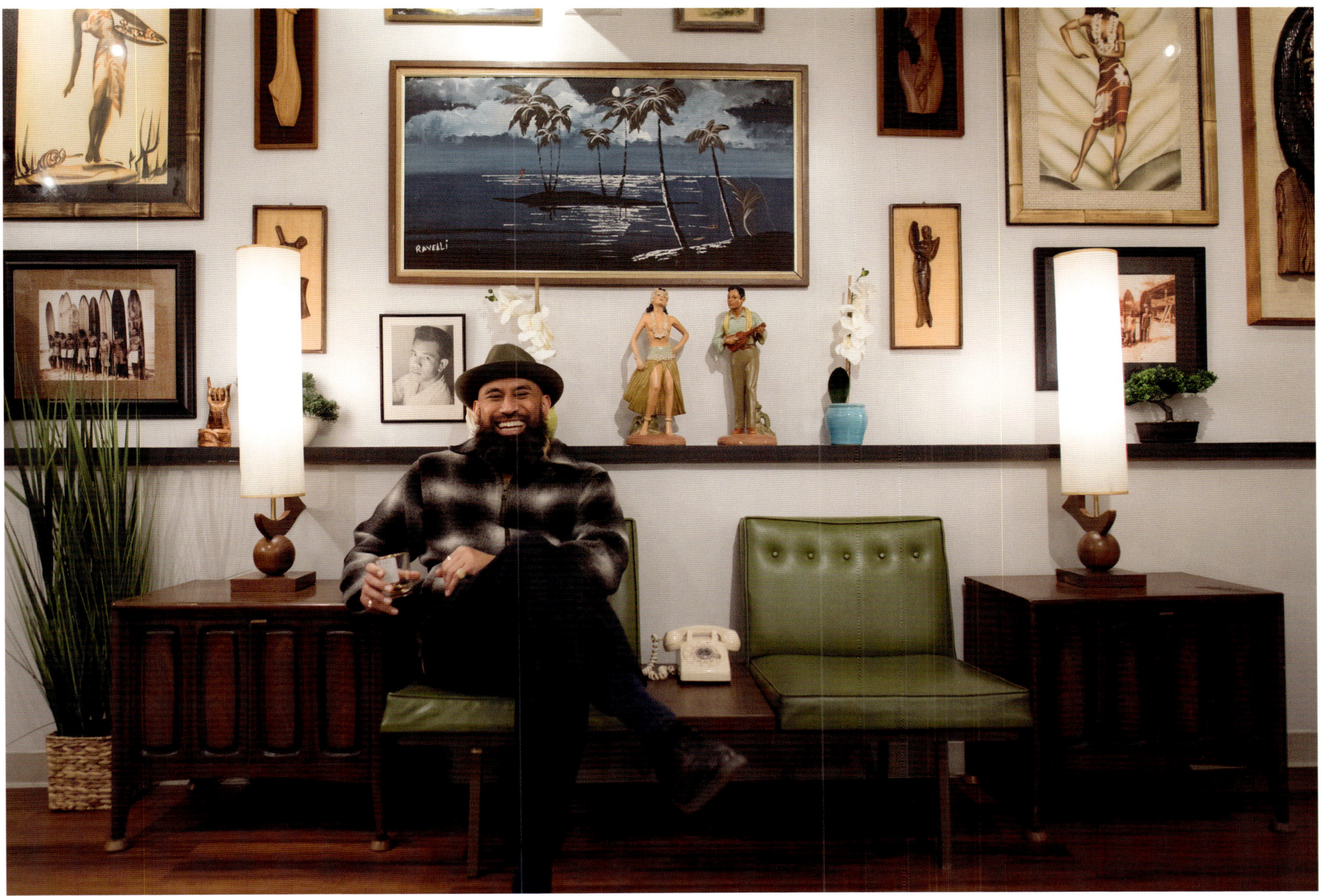

Mark-Jason Solofa Men's Grooming, Danville, California

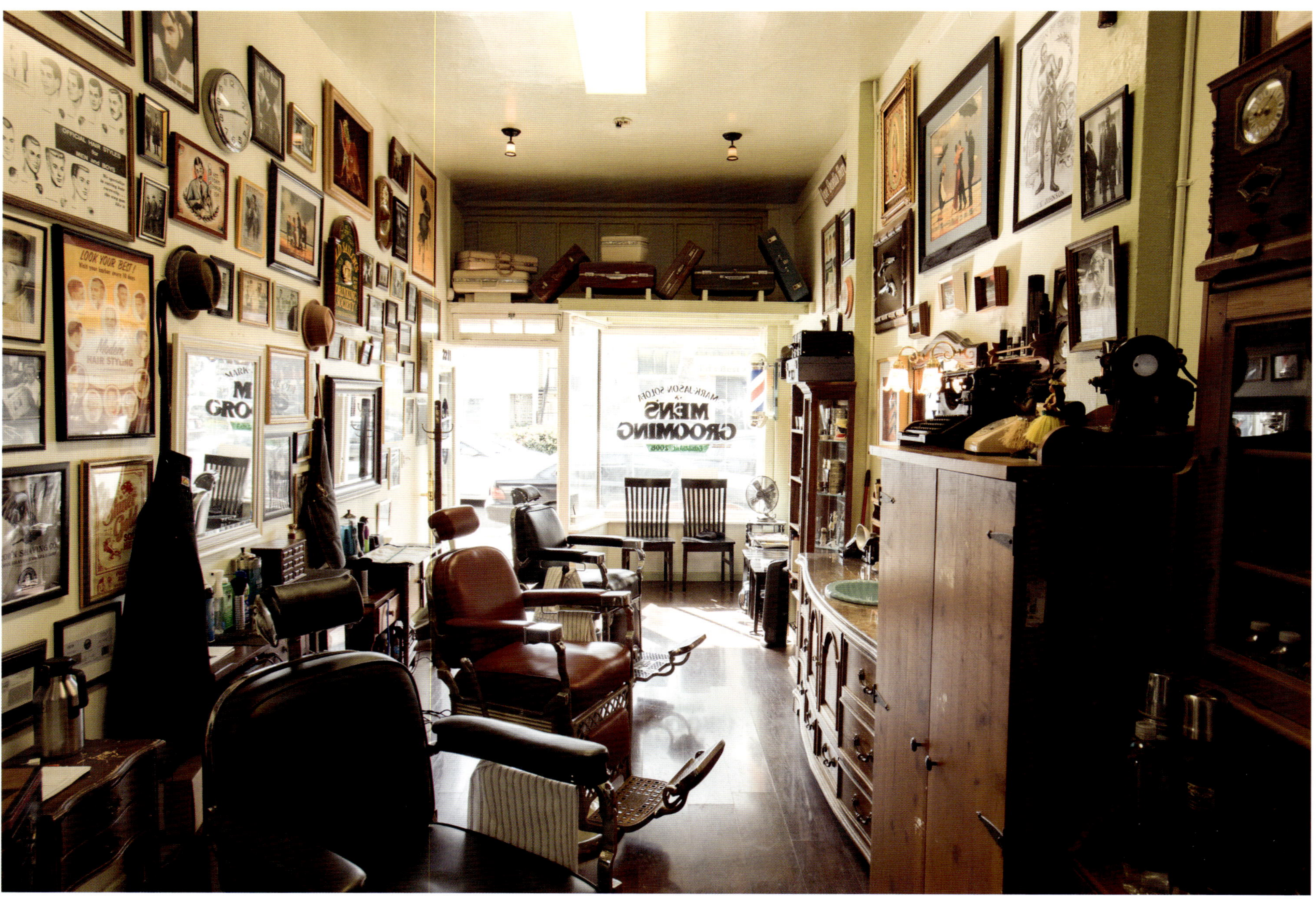

Mark-Jason Solofa Men's Grooming, Berkeley, California

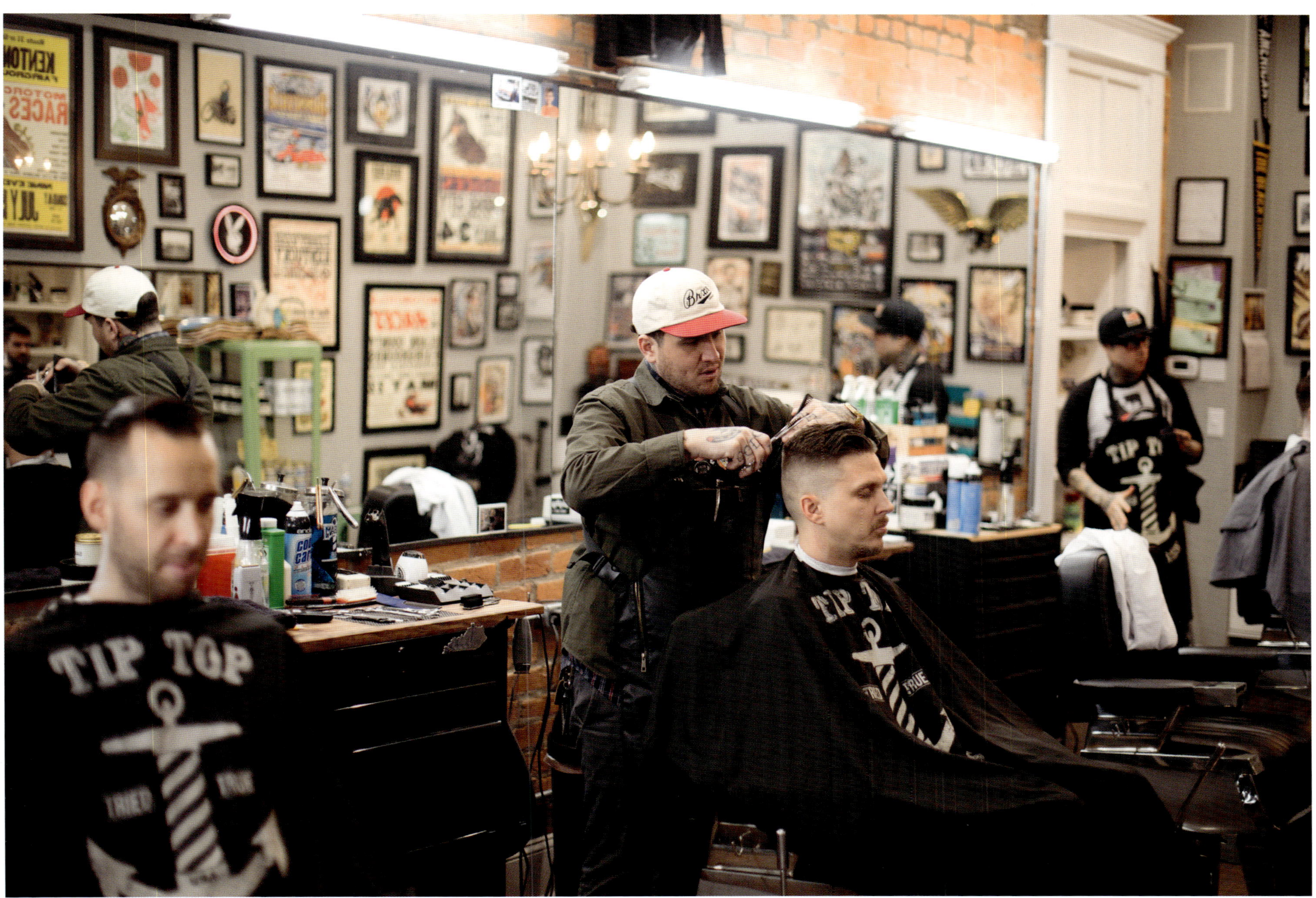

Spanky's Barbershop, Newport, Kentucky

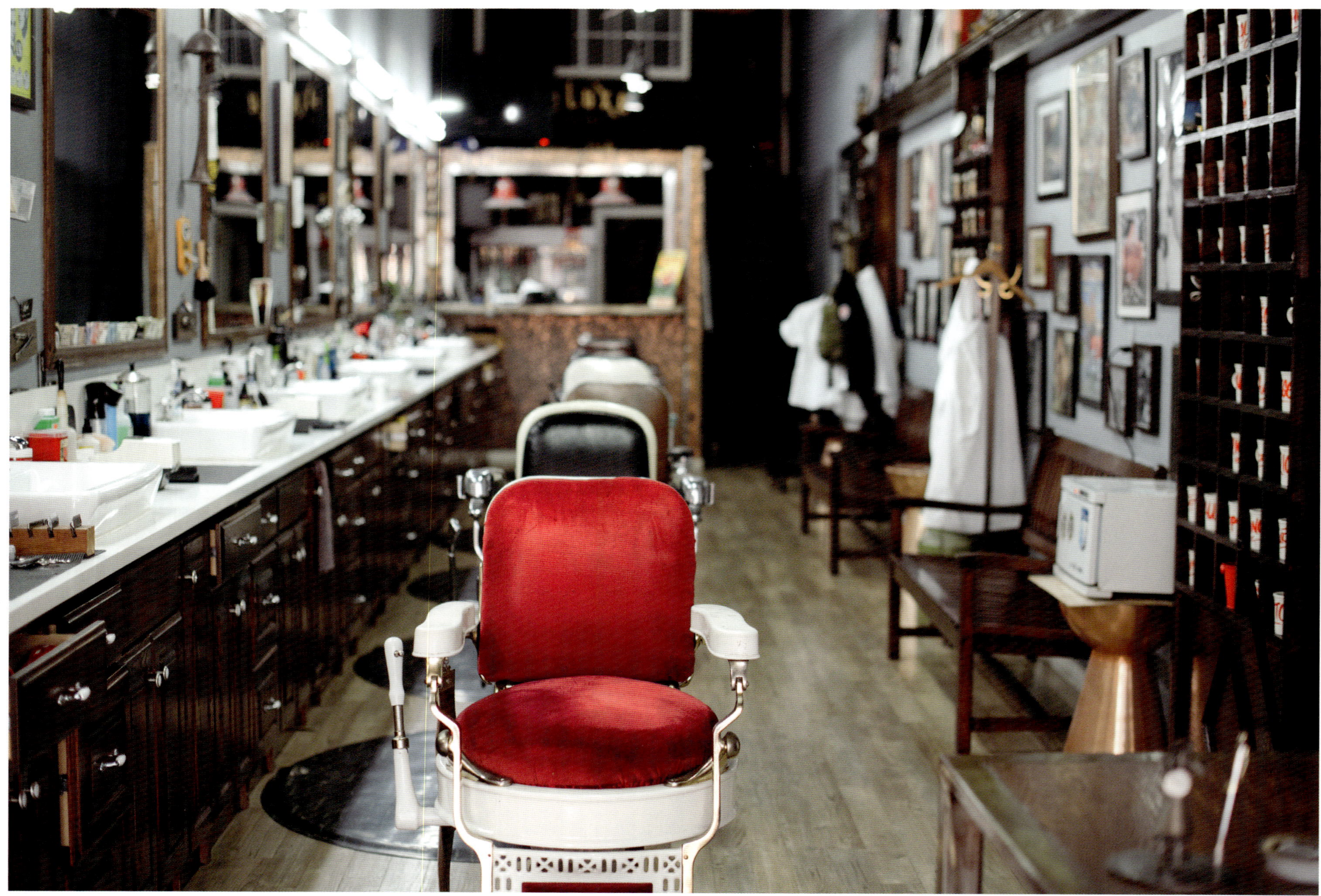

Deluxe Parlor & Shave Club, Long Beach, California

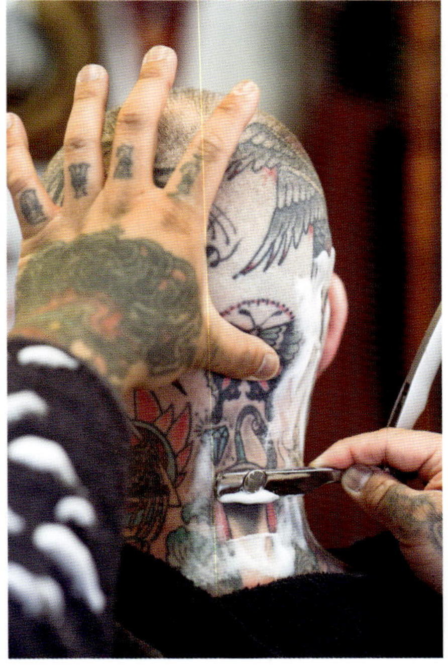

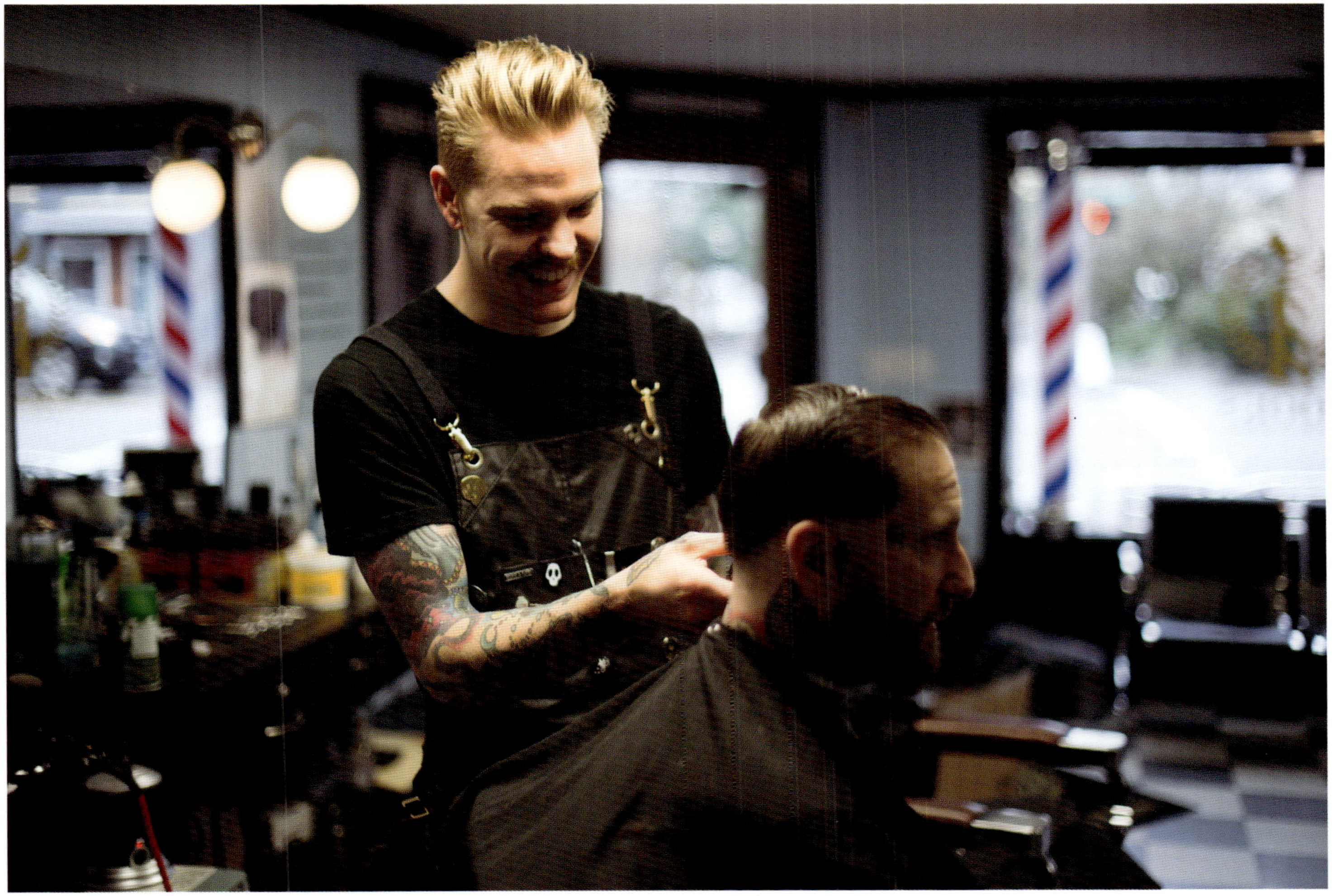

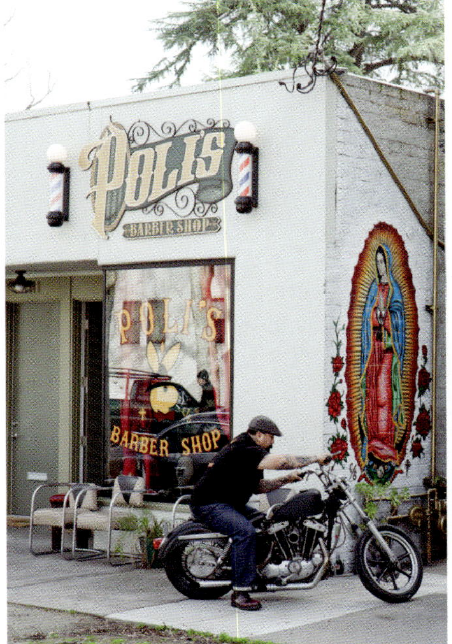
POLIS
BARBER SHOP
POLI'S
BARBER SHOP

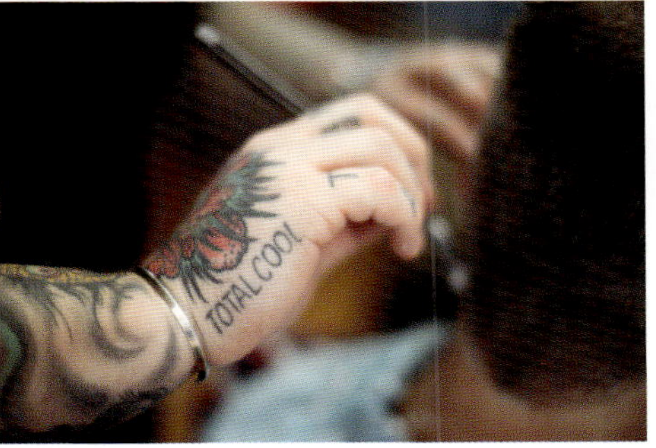
TOTAL COOL

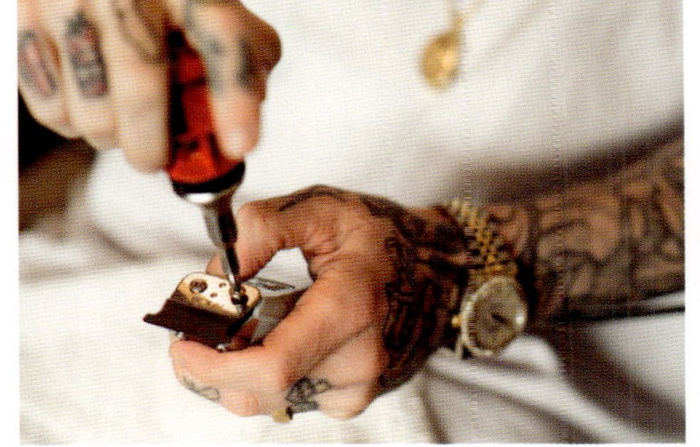

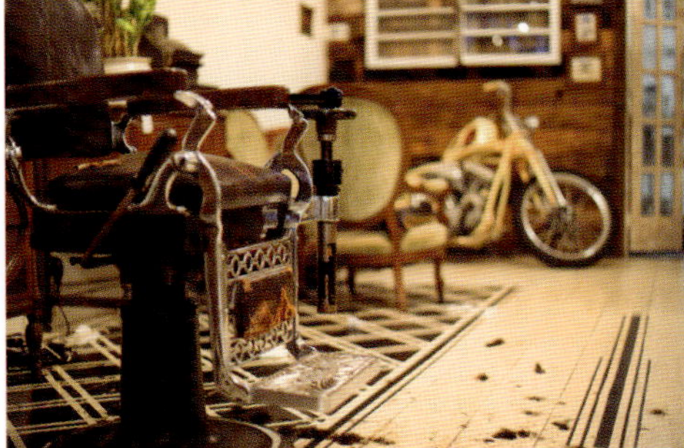

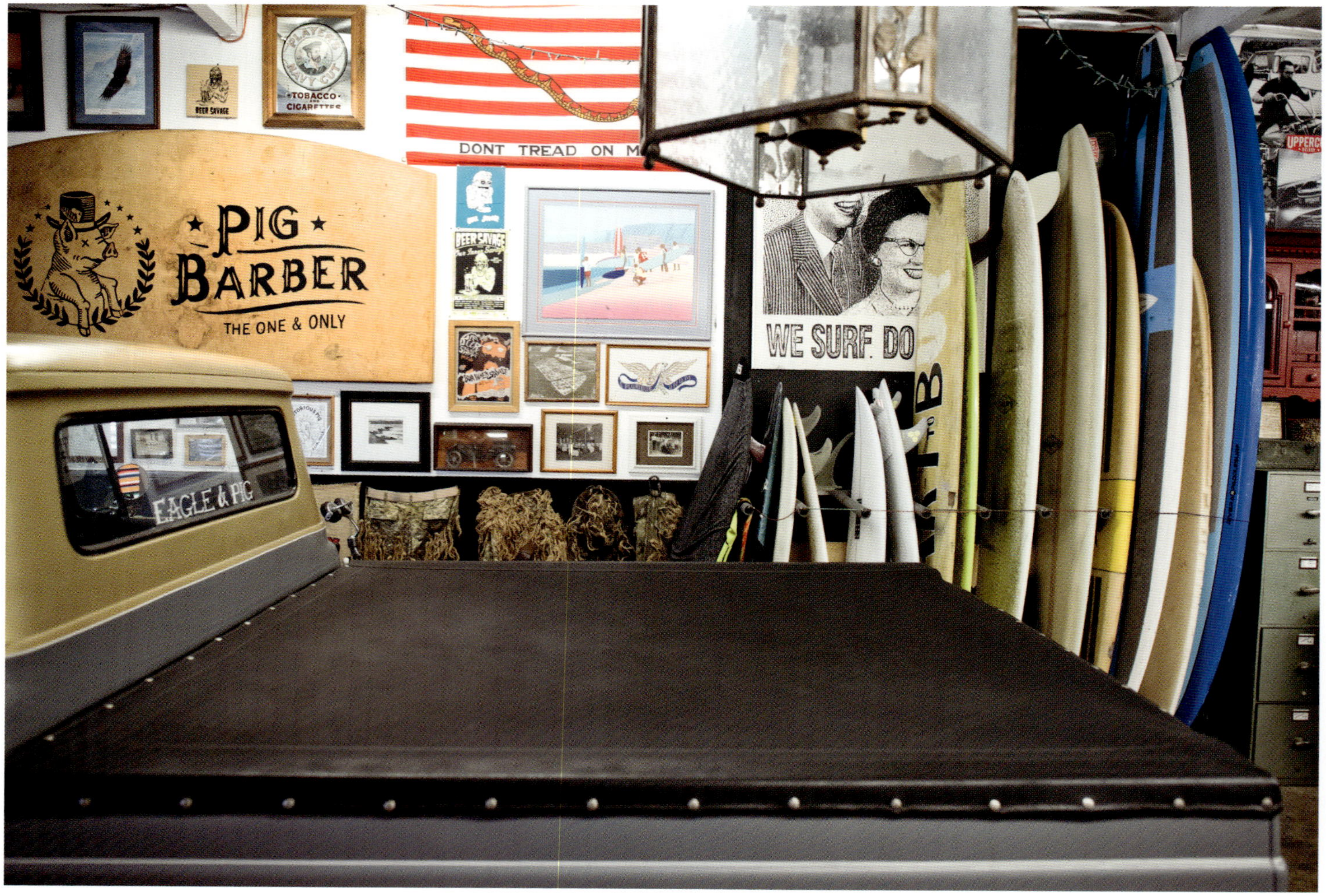

PIG
BARBER
THE ONE & ONLY
DONT TREAD ON M
WE SURF. DO
EAGLE & PIG
UPPERC

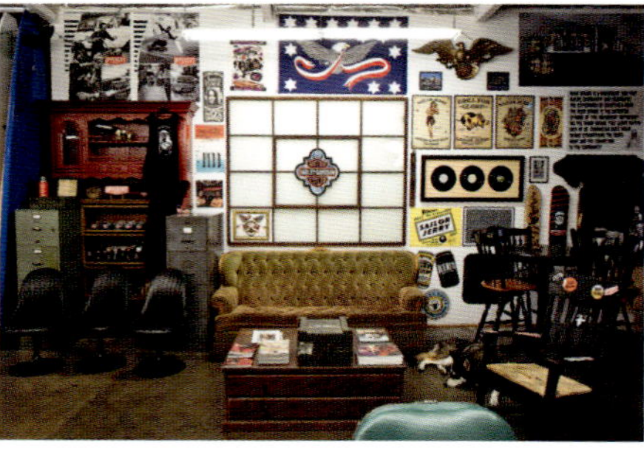

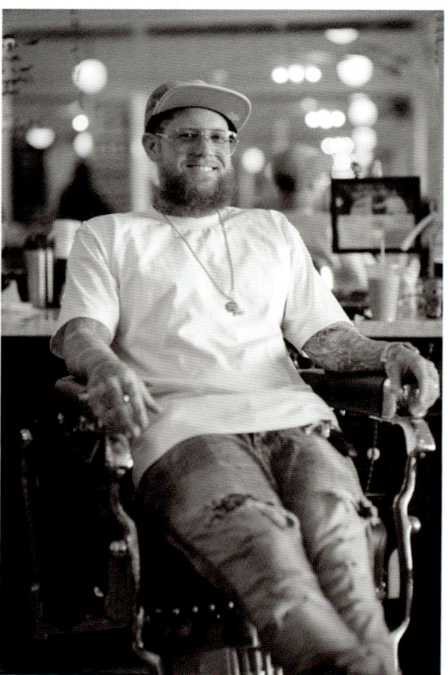

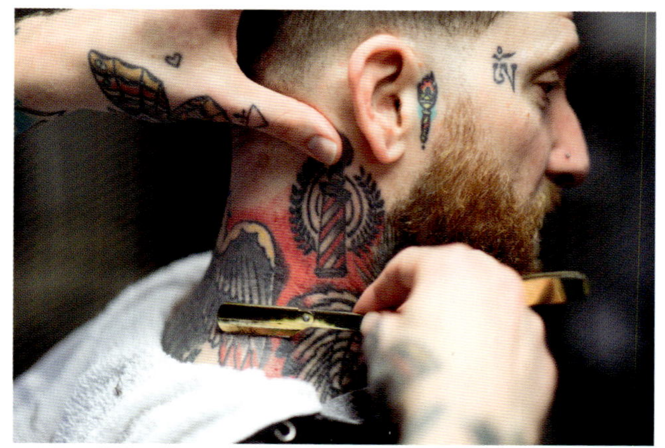

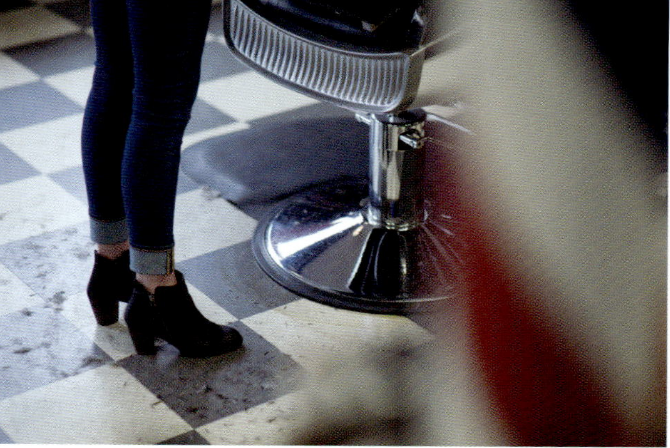

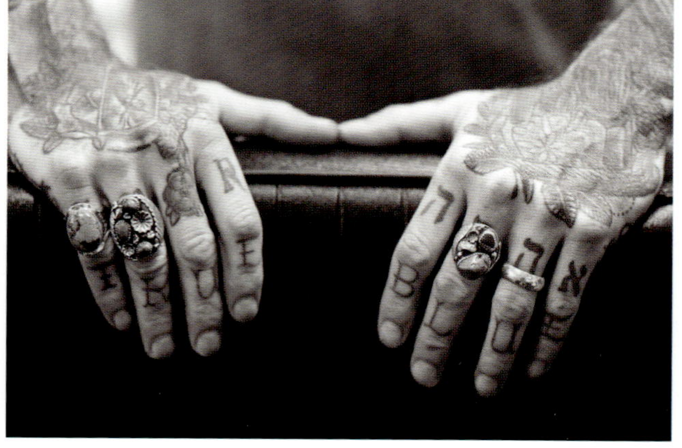

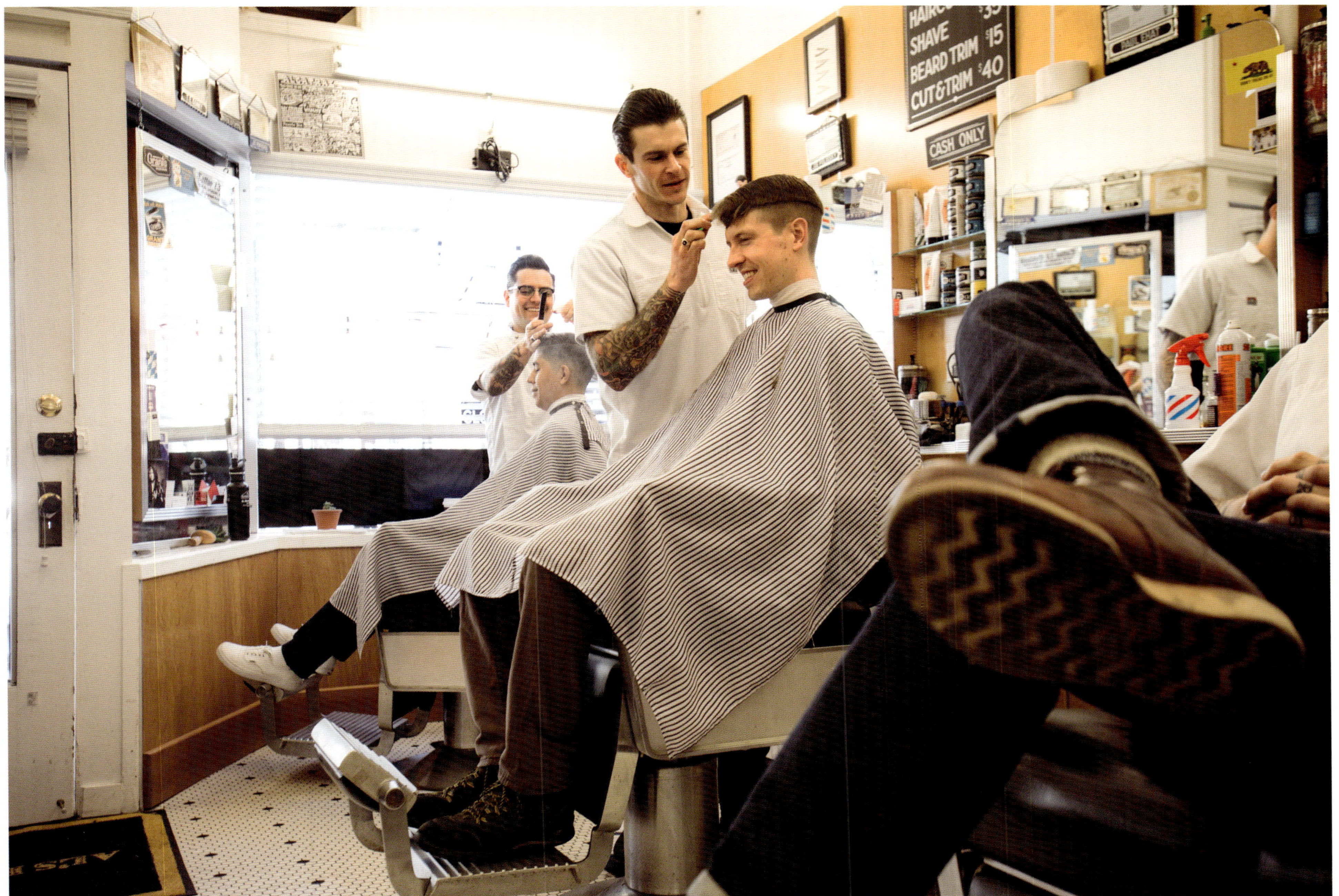

Al's Barbershop, Alameda, California

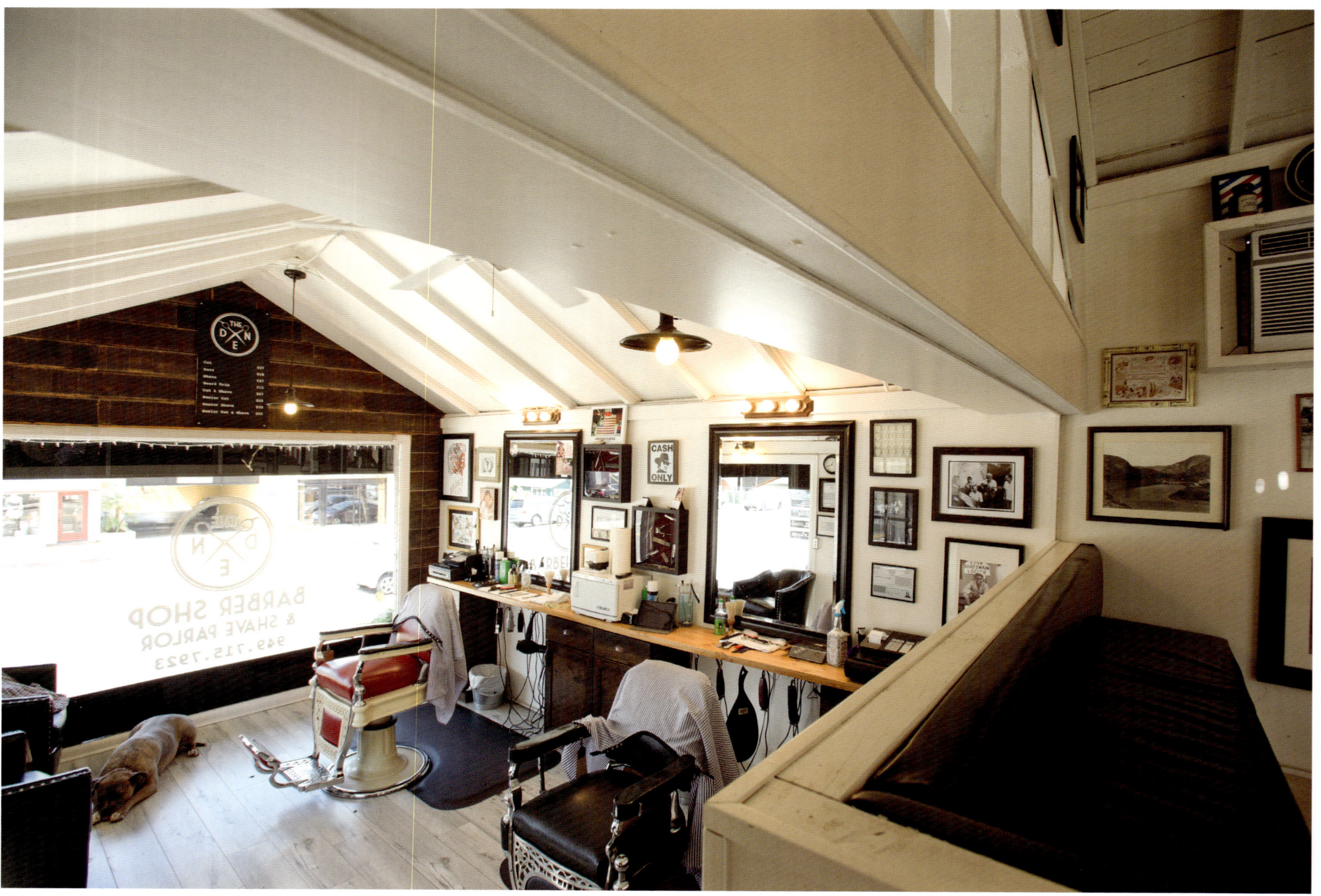

The Den Barbershop, Laguna, California

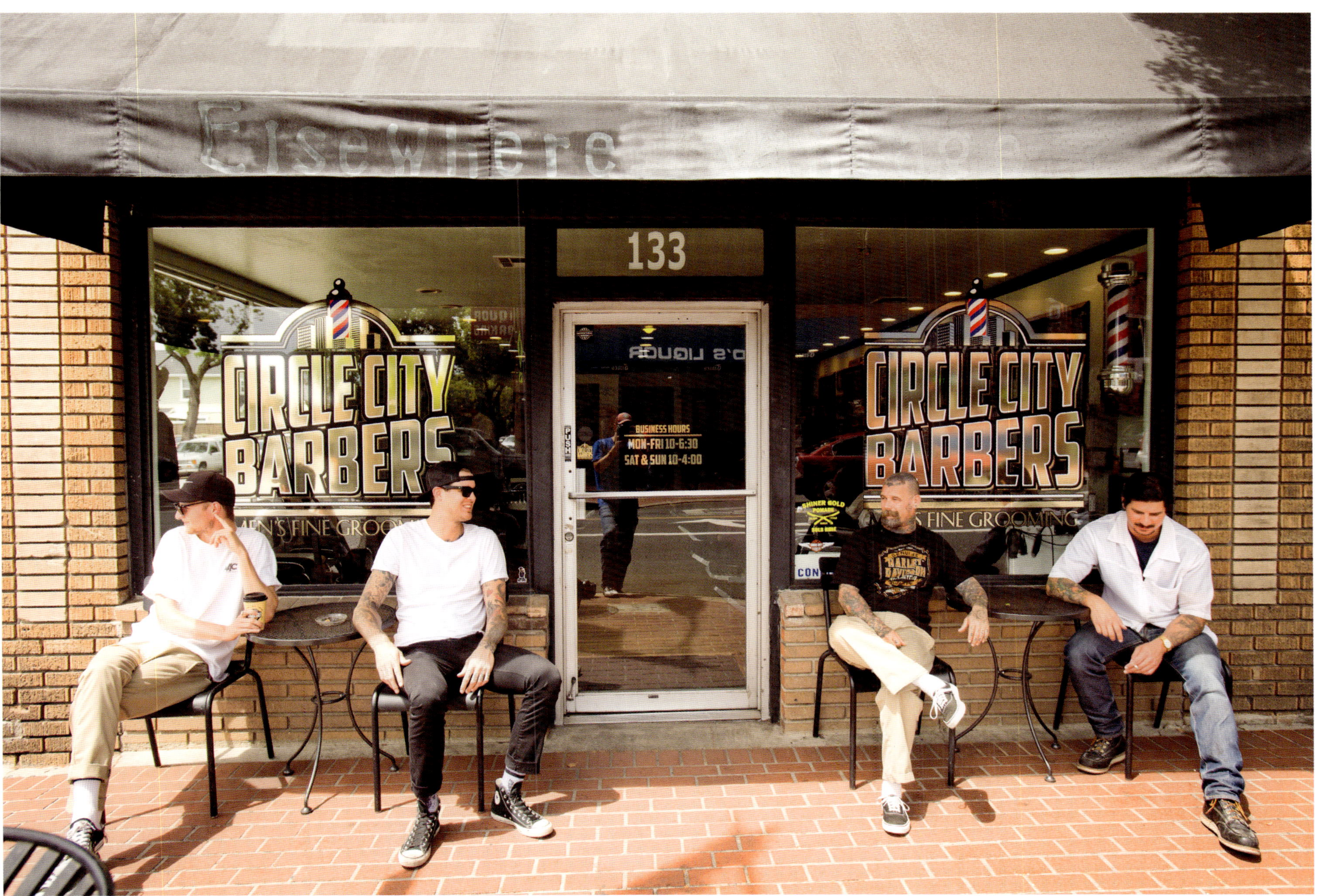

Circle City Barbers, Orange, California

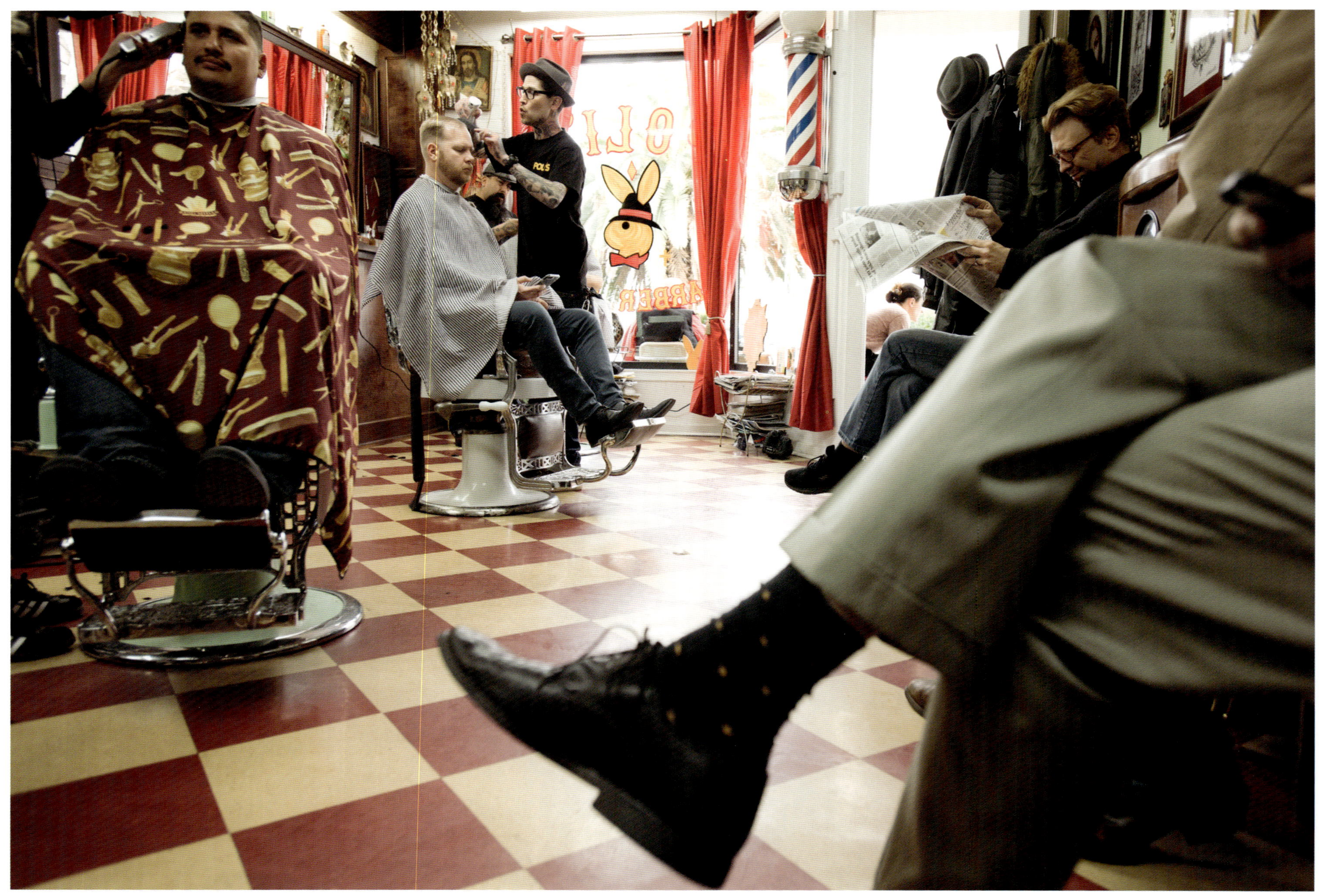

Poli's Barbershop, Sacramento, California

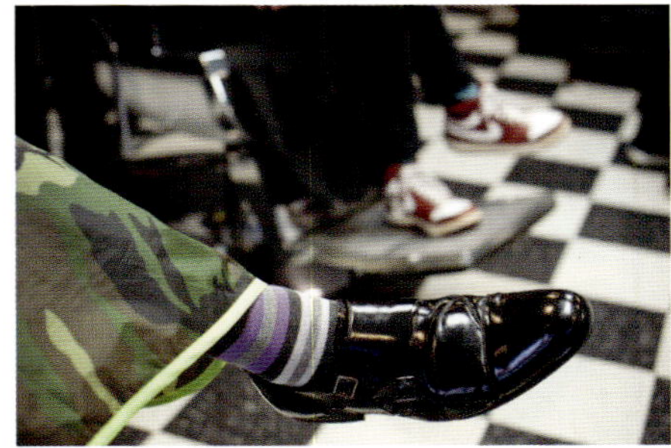

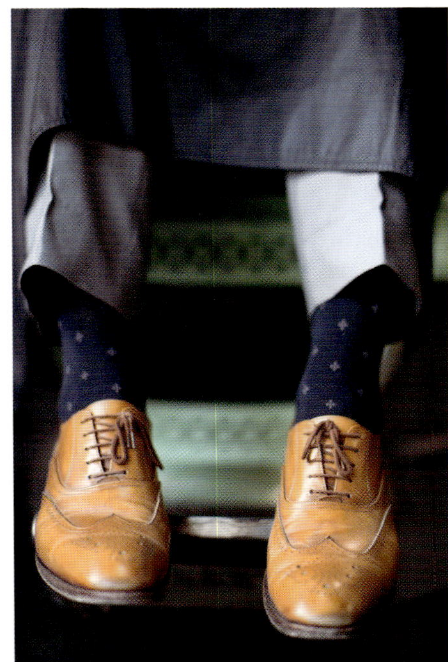

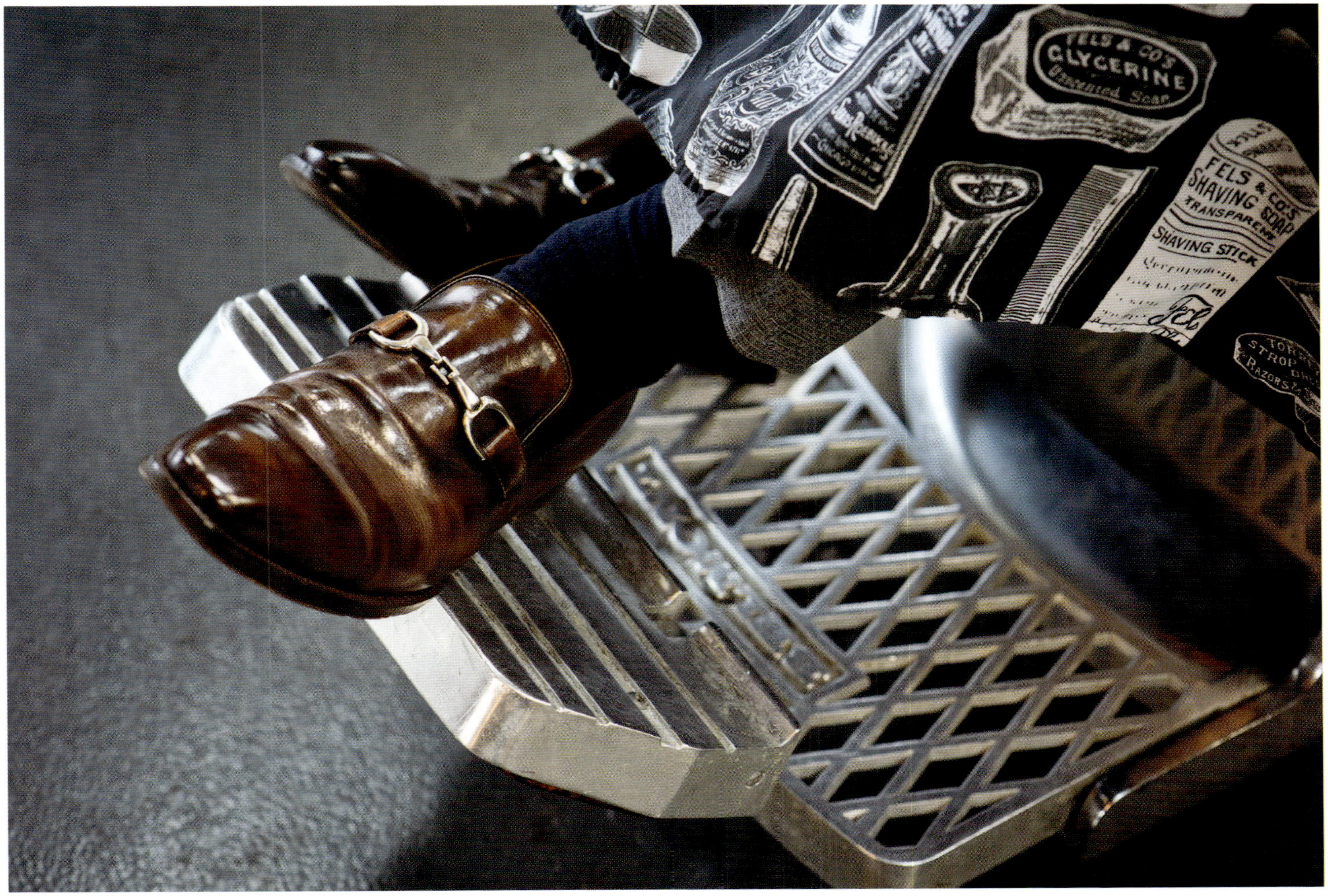

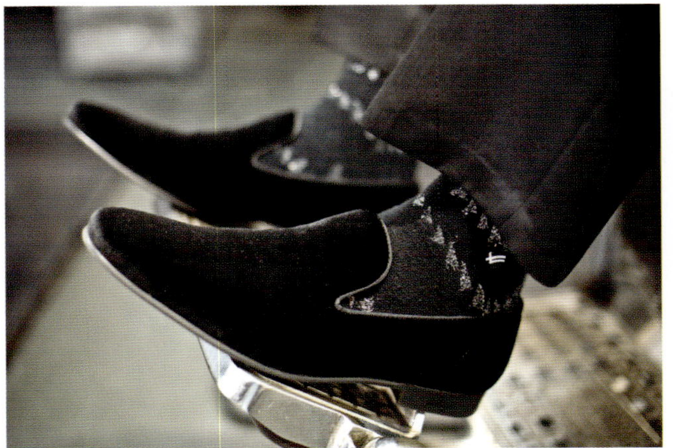

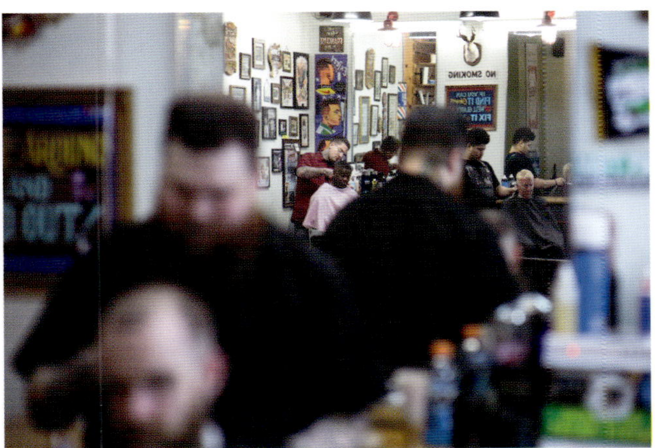

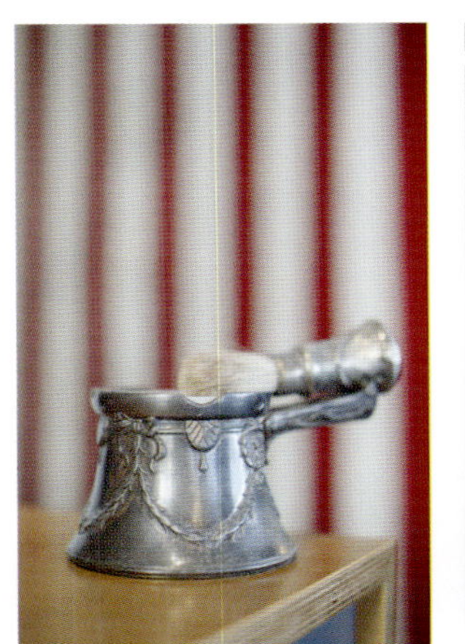

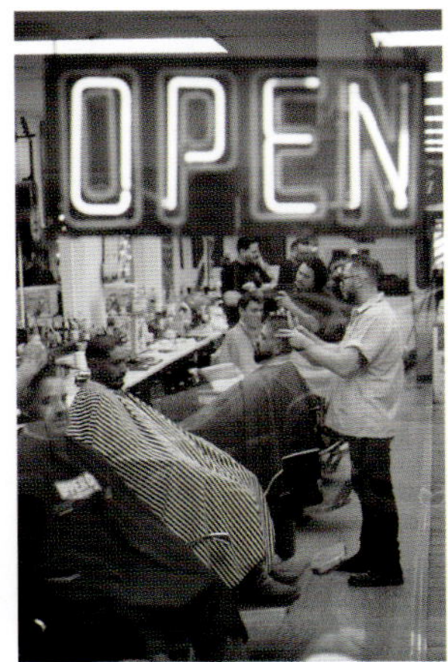
OPEN

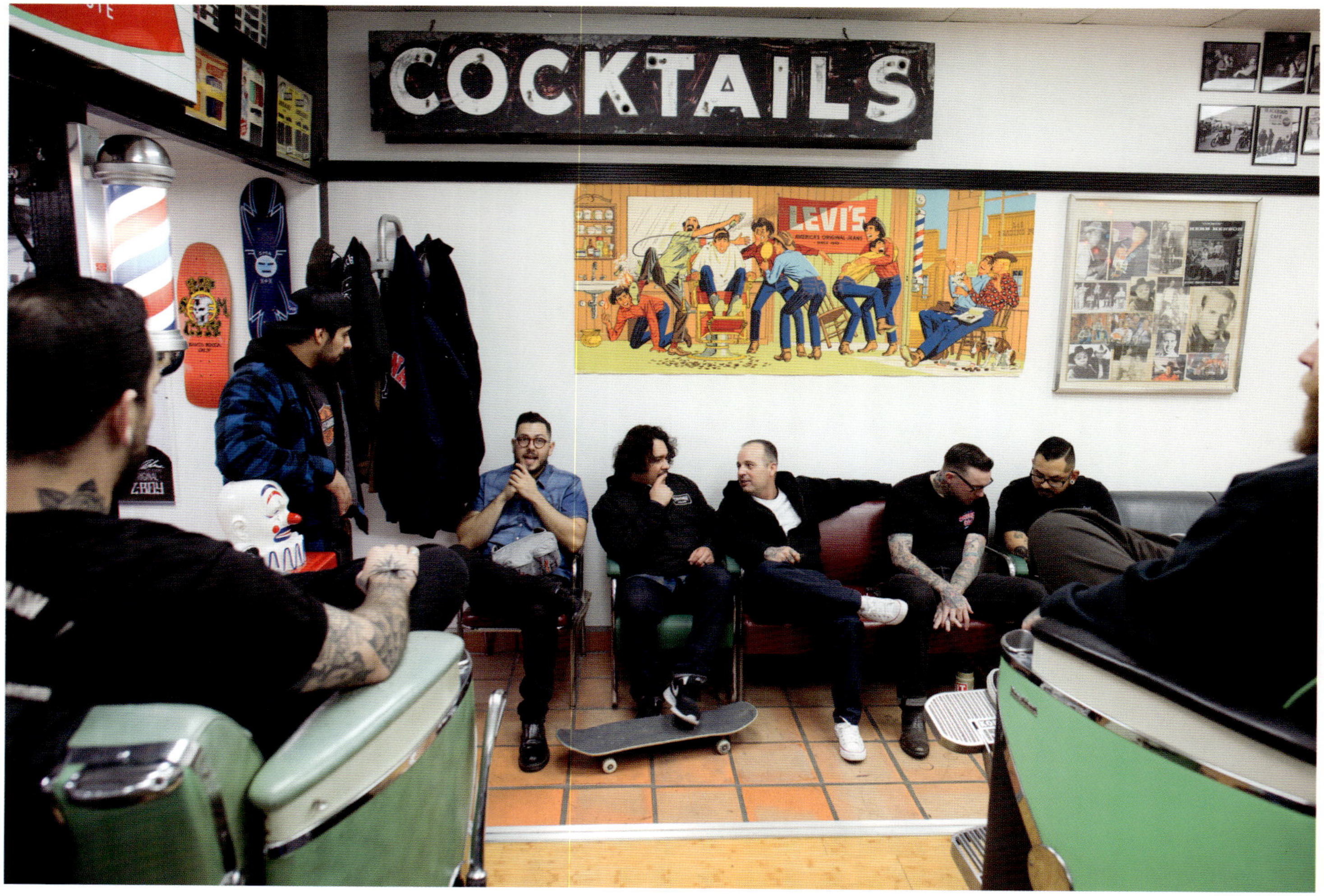

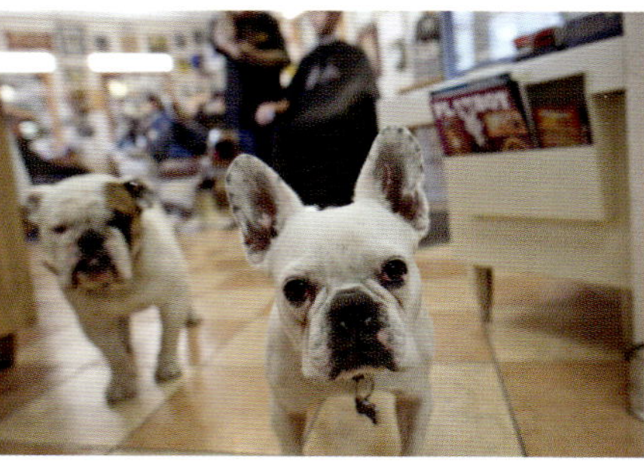

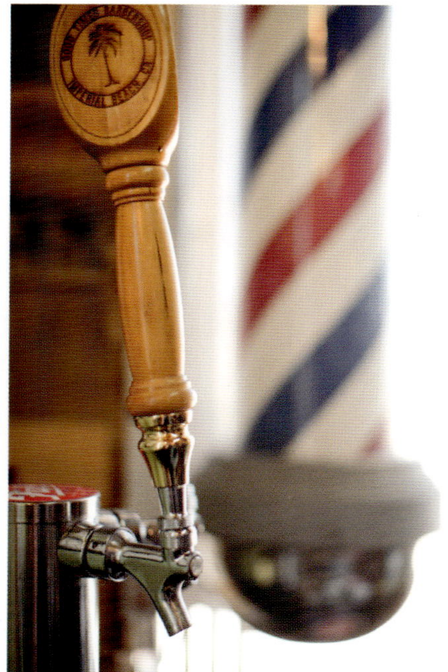

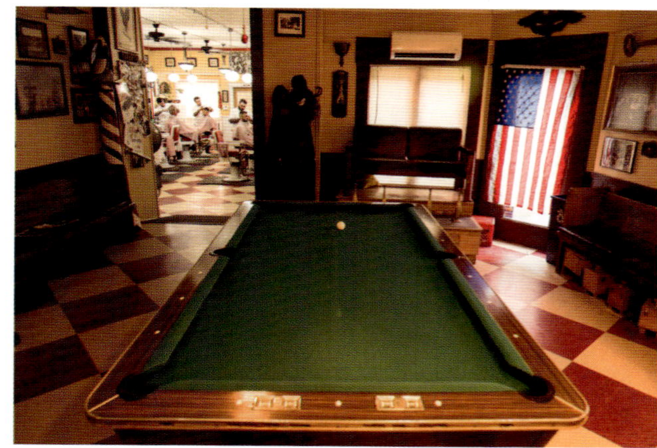

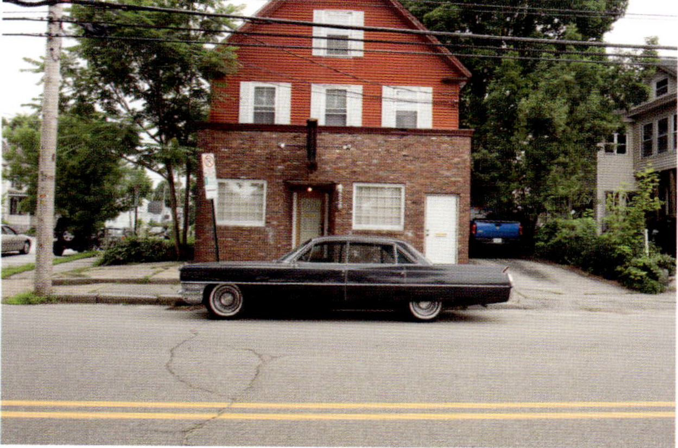

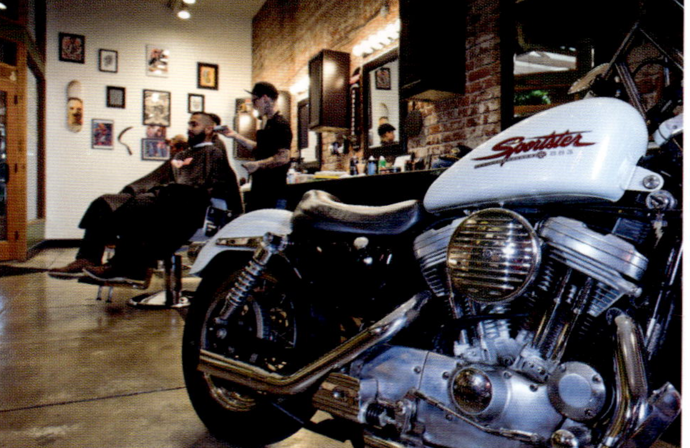
Sportster

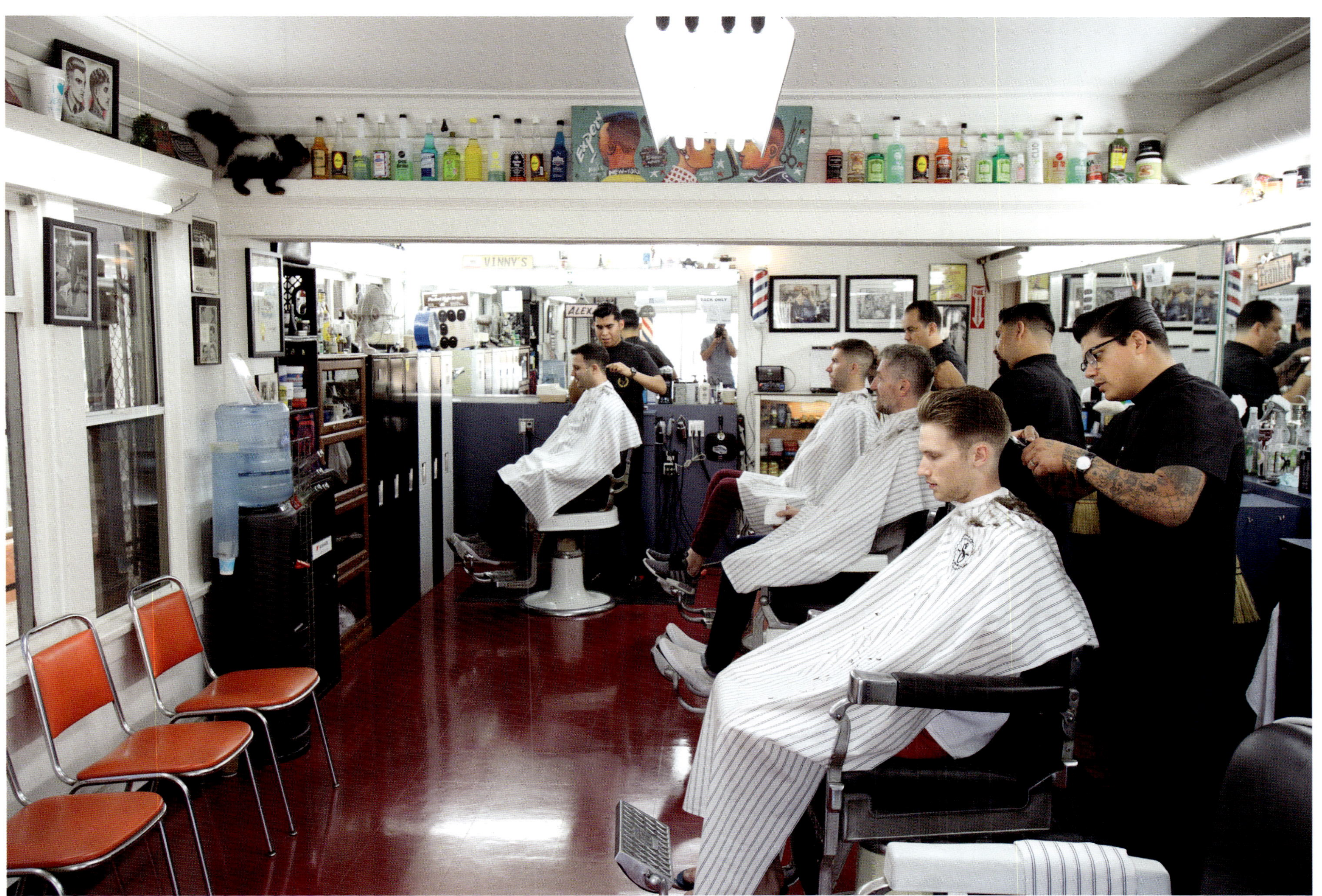

Vinnie's Barbershop, Los Angeles, California

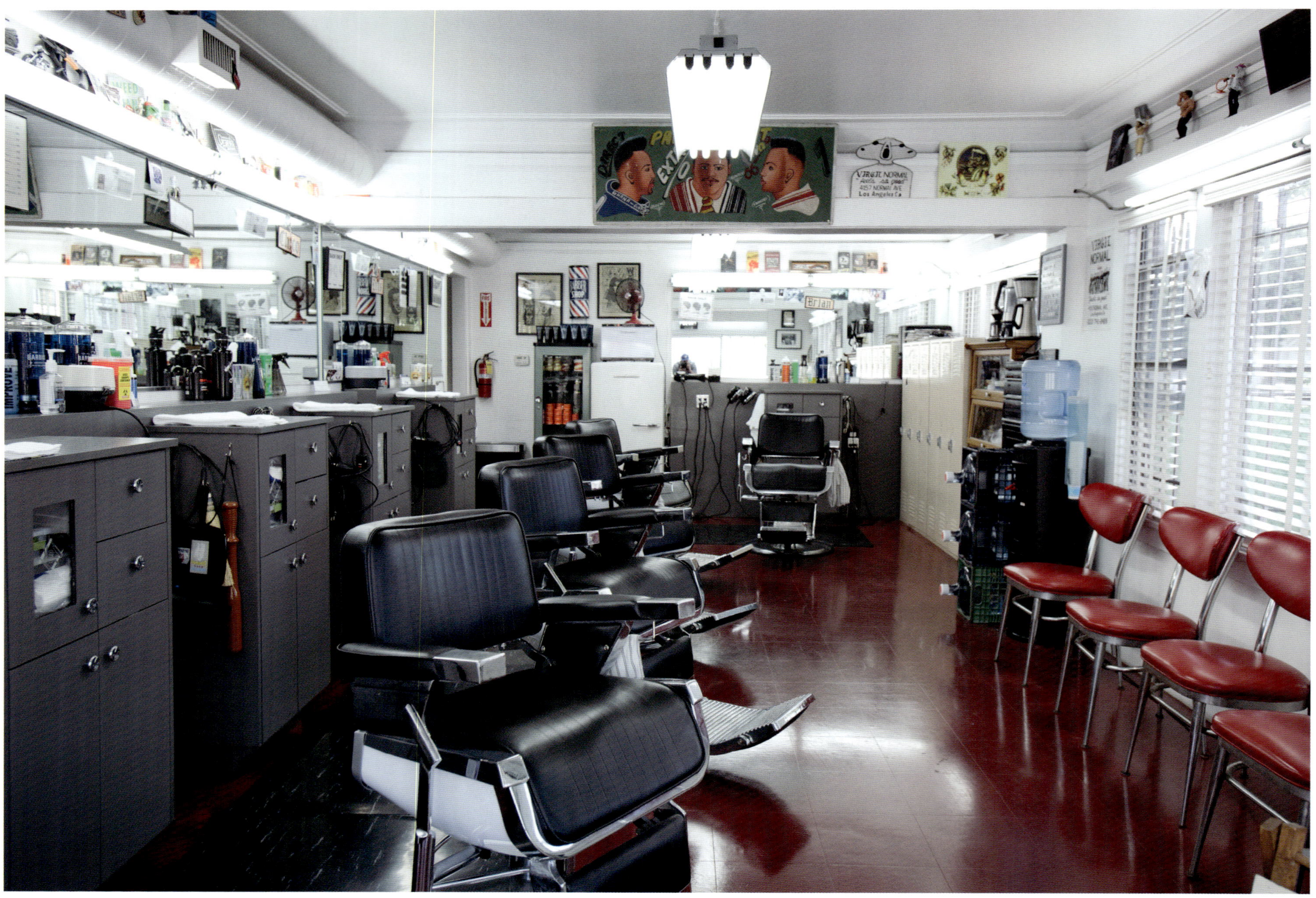

Vinnie's Barbershop, Los Angeles, California

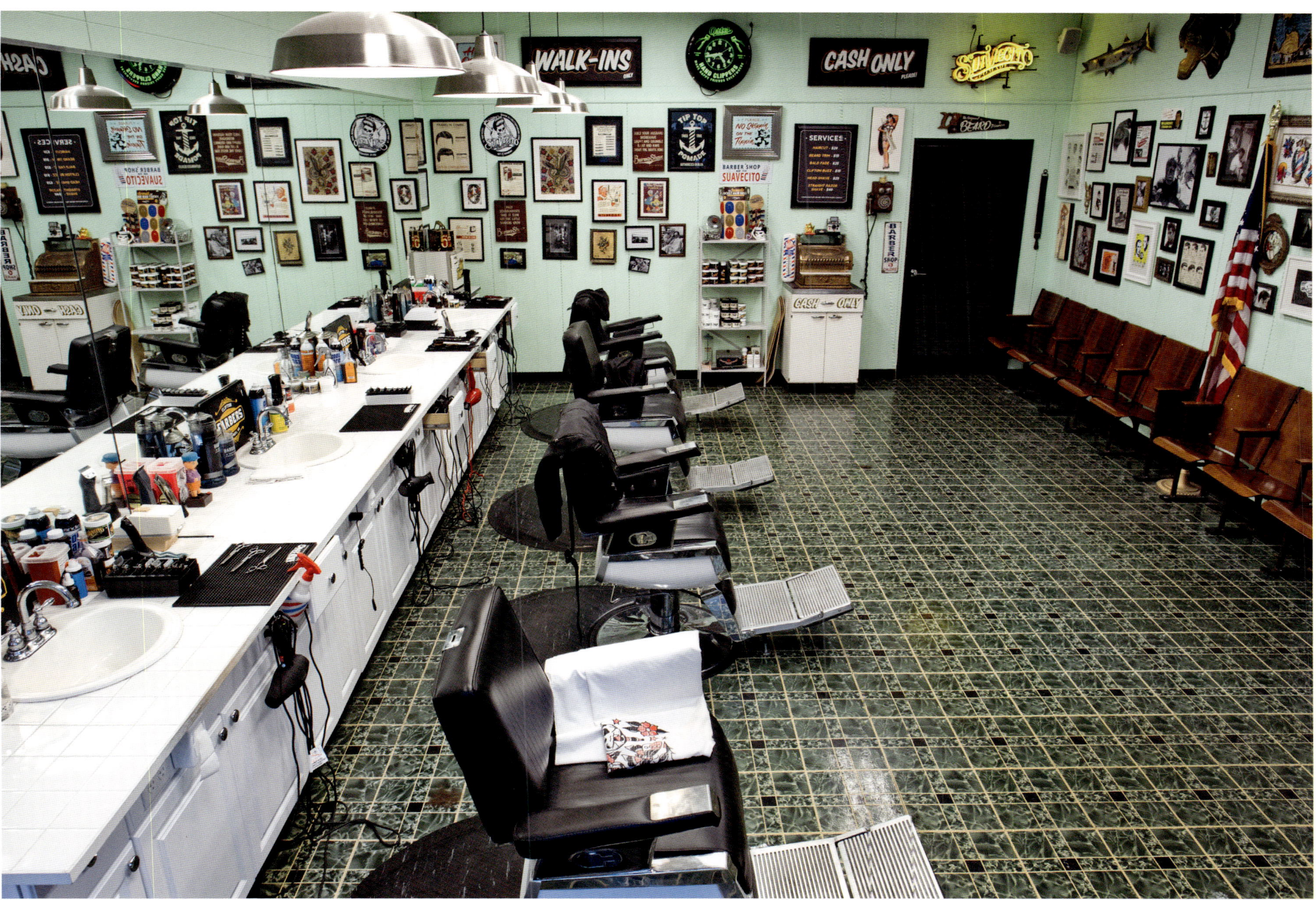

Clifton Barbershop, Cincinnati, Ohio

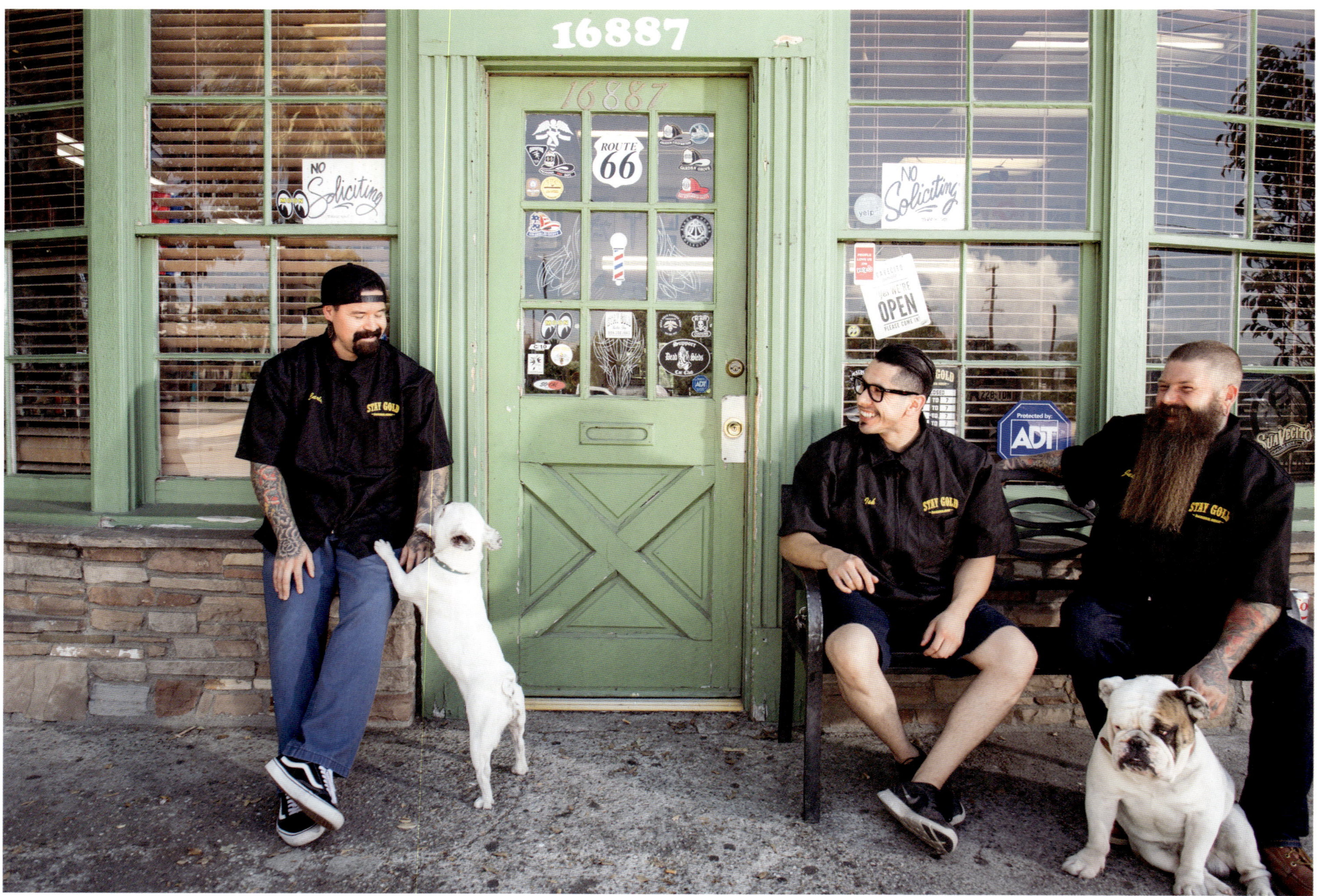

Stay Gold Barbershop, Fontana, California

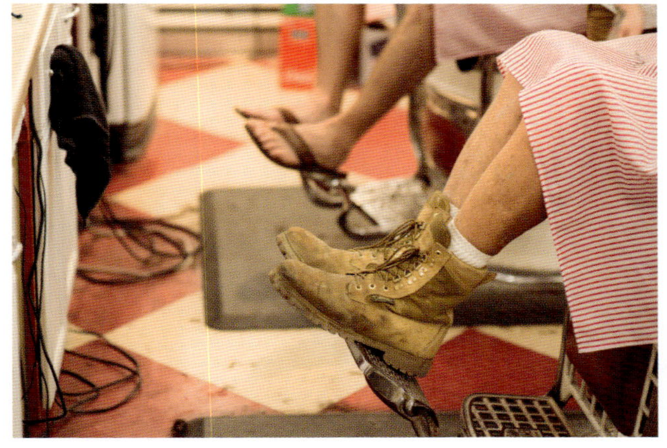
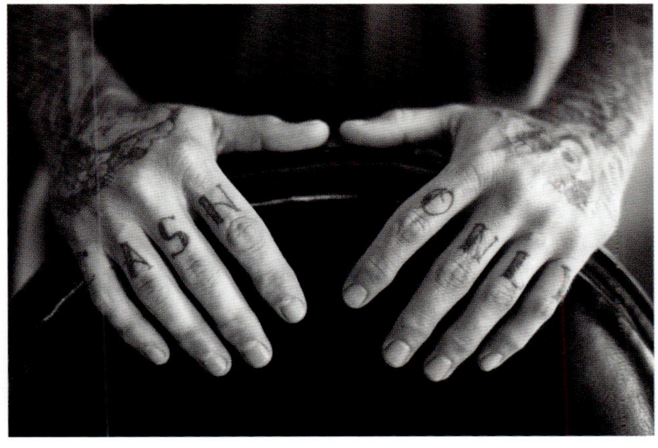
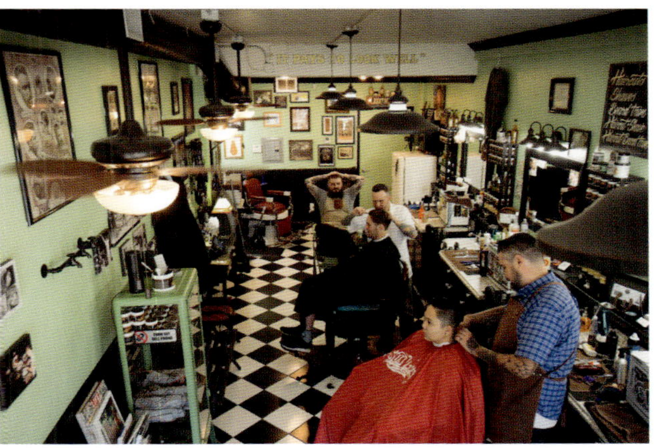
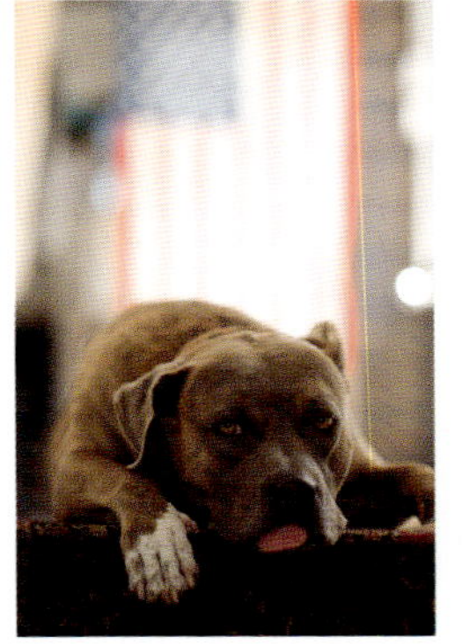
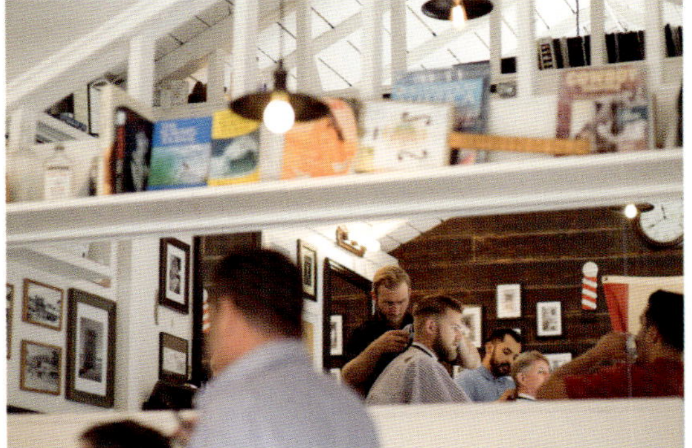
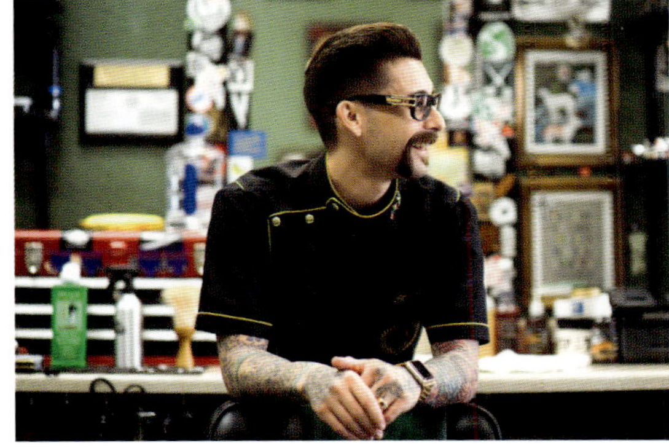
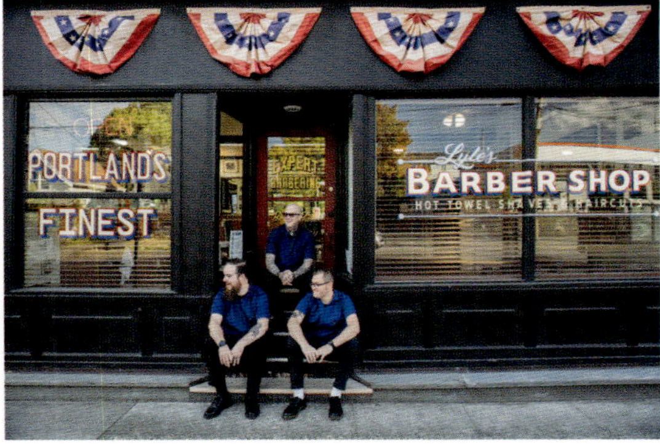
PORTLAND'S
FINEST
BARBER SHOP
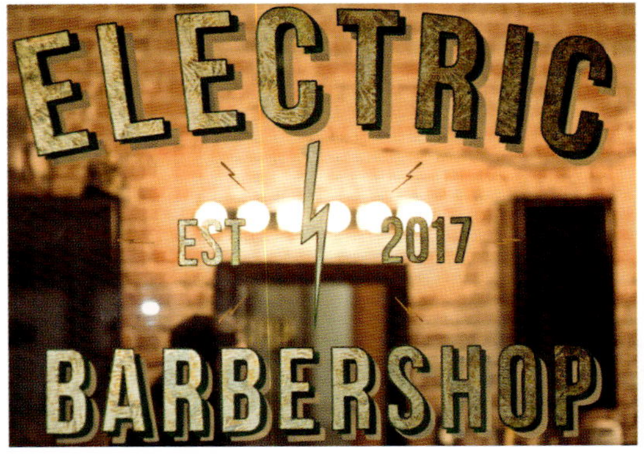
ELECTRIC
EST 2017
BARBERSHOP
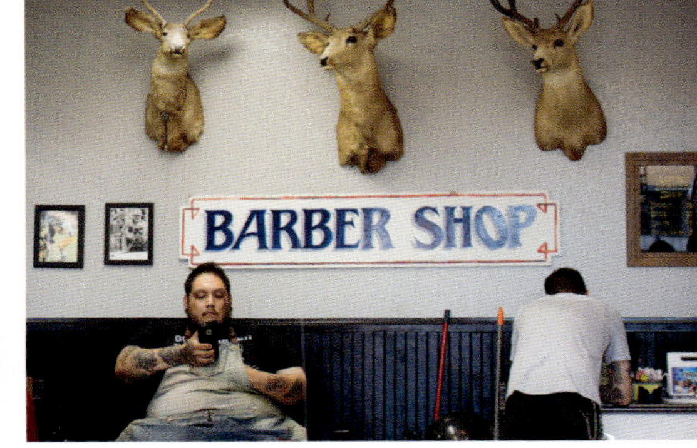
BARBER SHOP
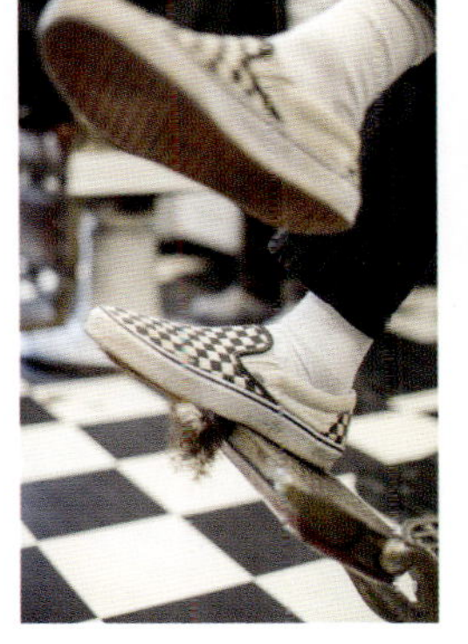
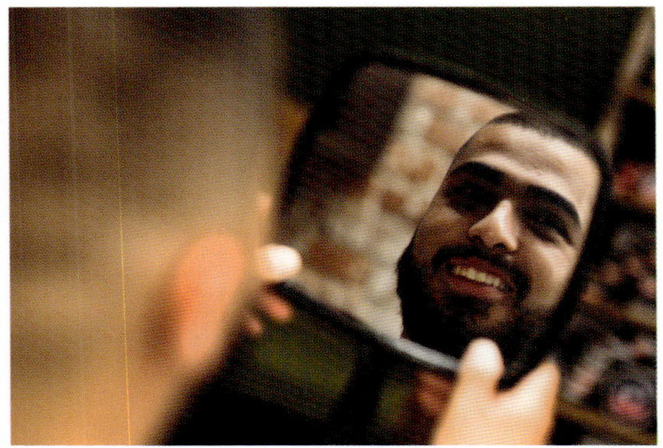

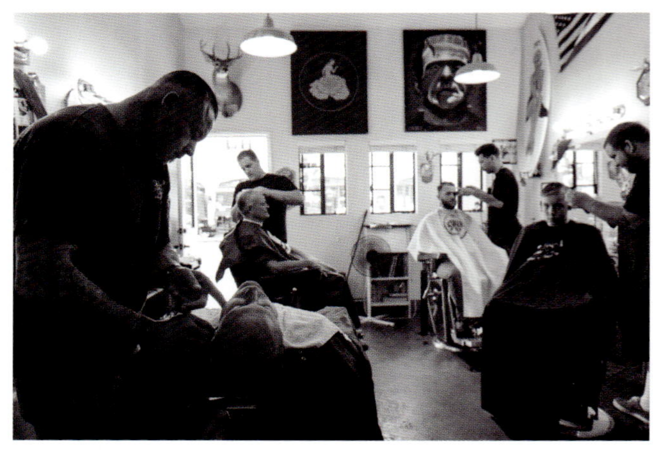

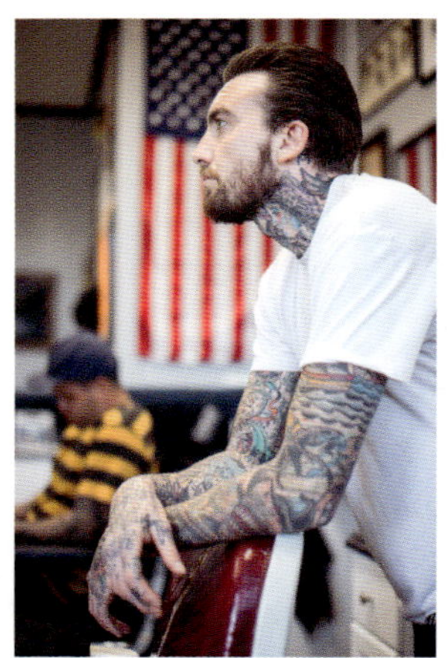

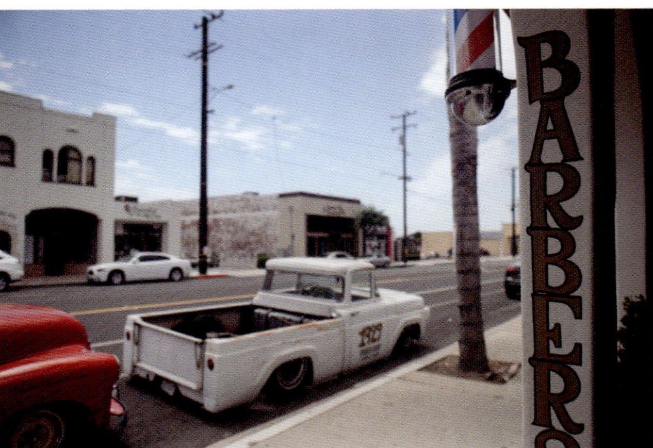
BARBER

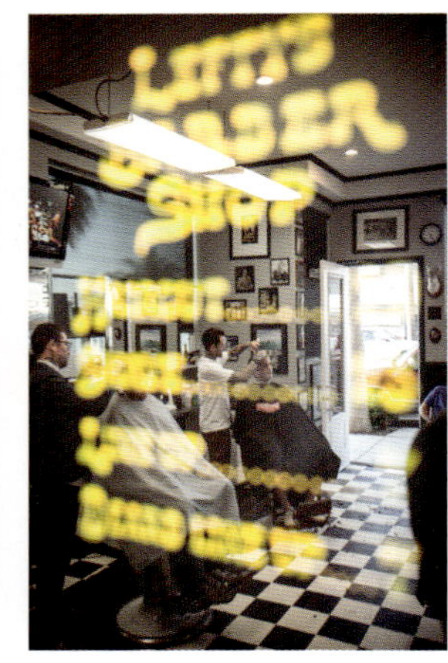

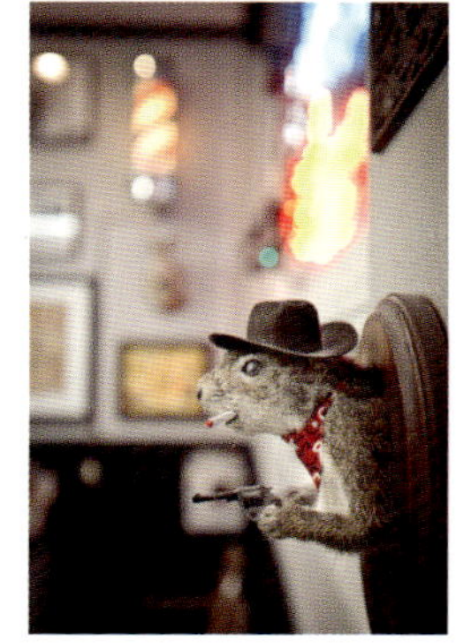

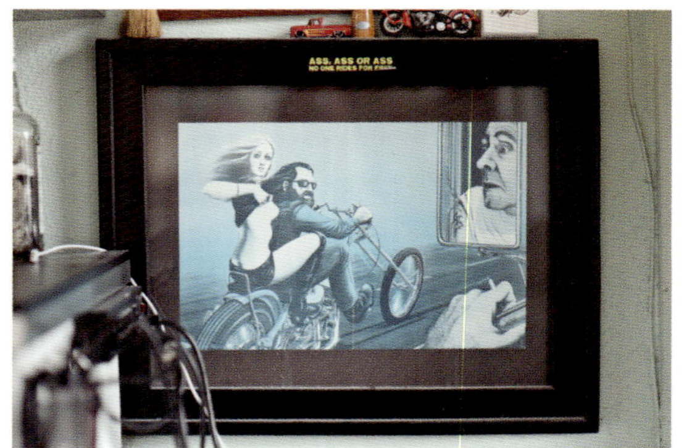
ASS, ASS OR ASS

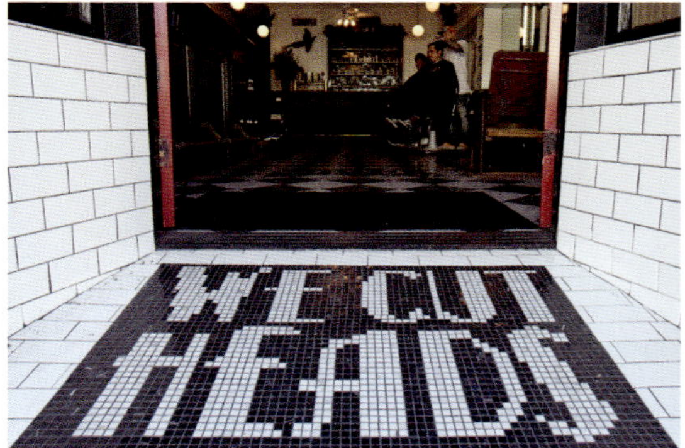
WE CUT
HEADS

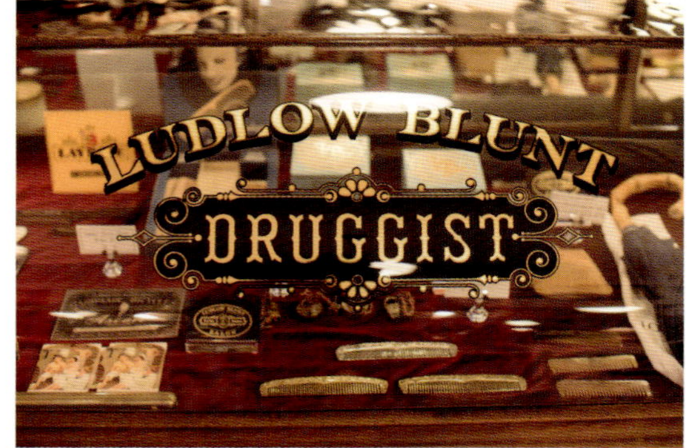
LUDLOW BLUNT
DRUGGIST

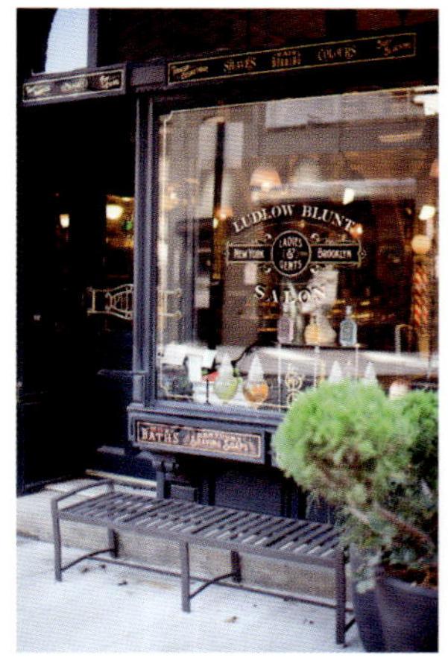
LUDLOW BLUNT

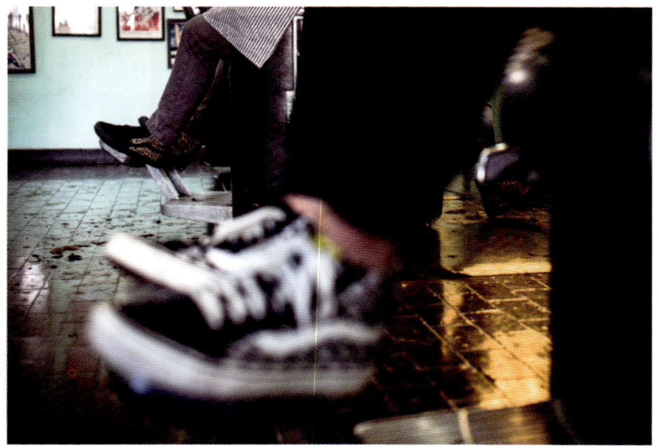

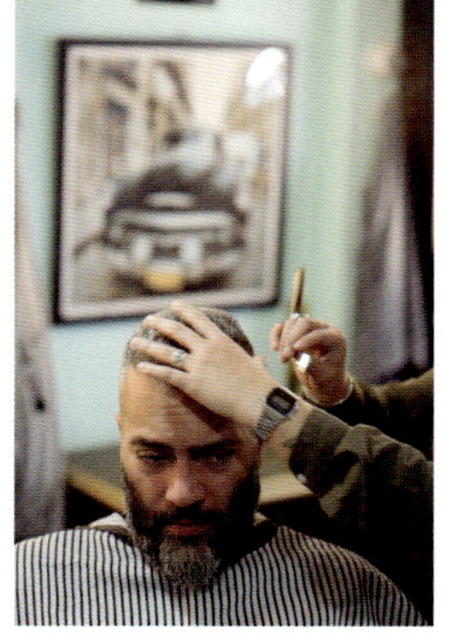

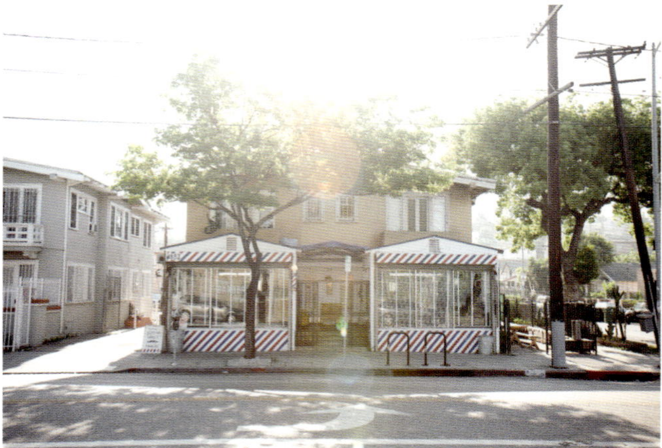

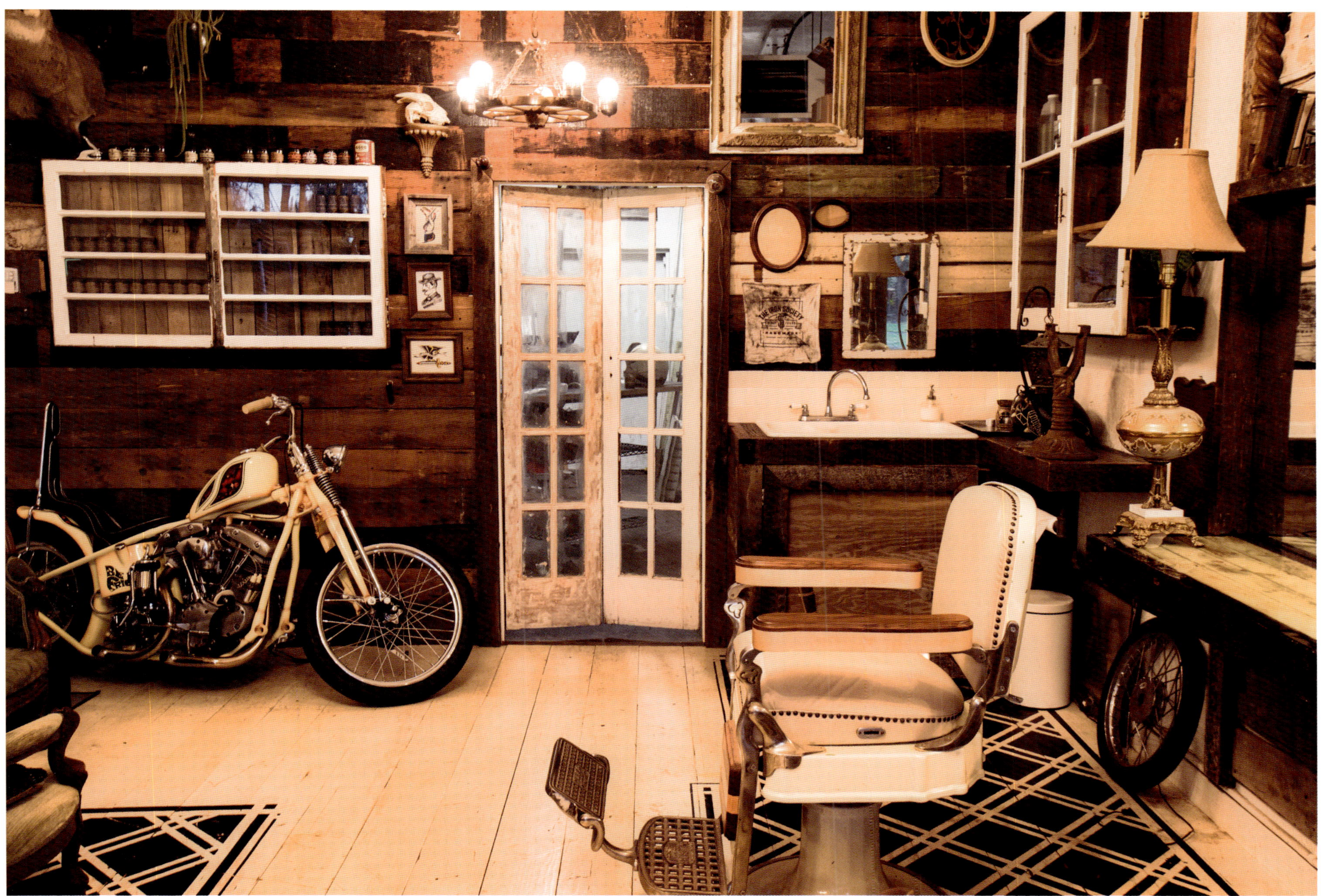

The Iron Society, Portland, Oregon

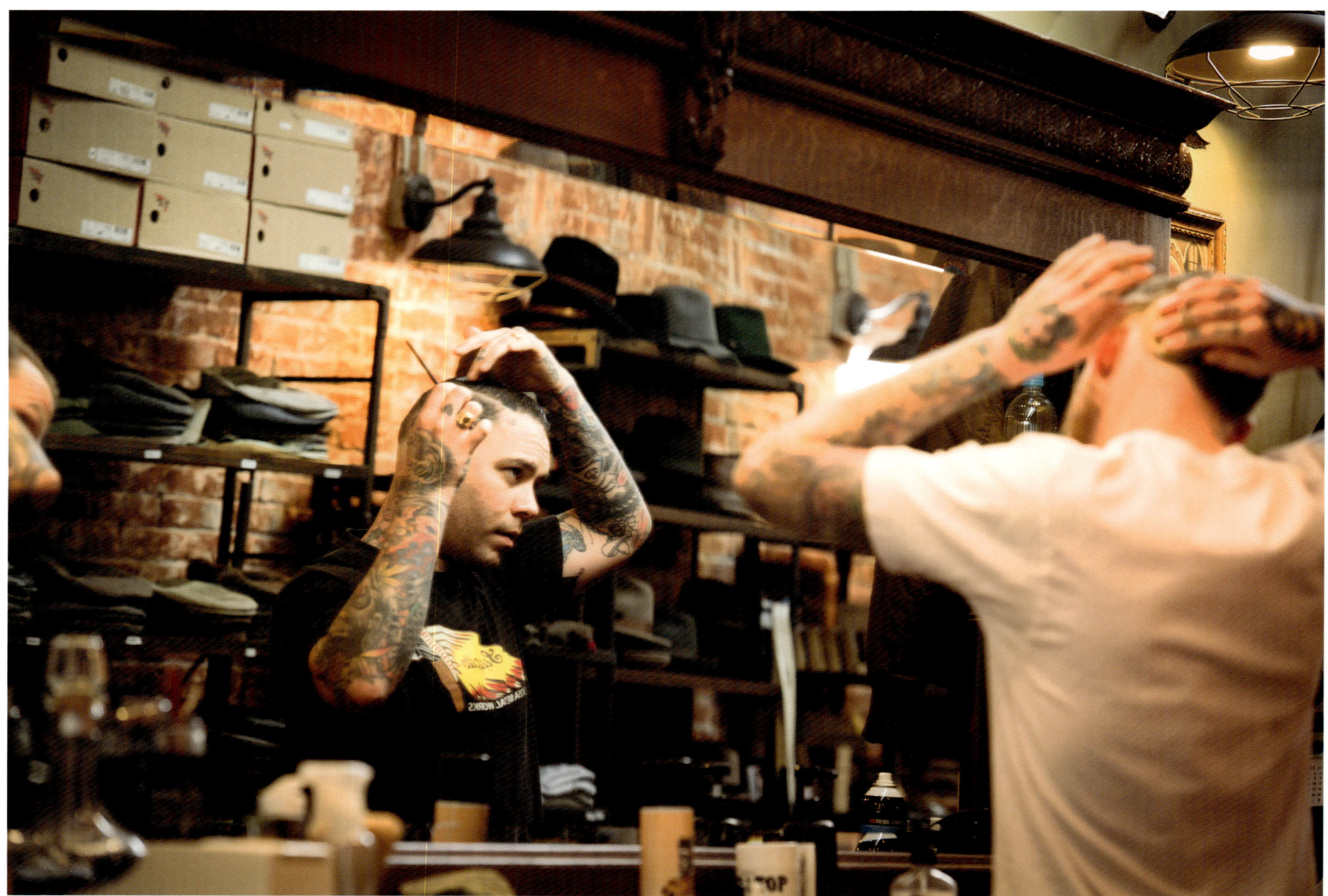

The Ritual, San Luis Obispo, California

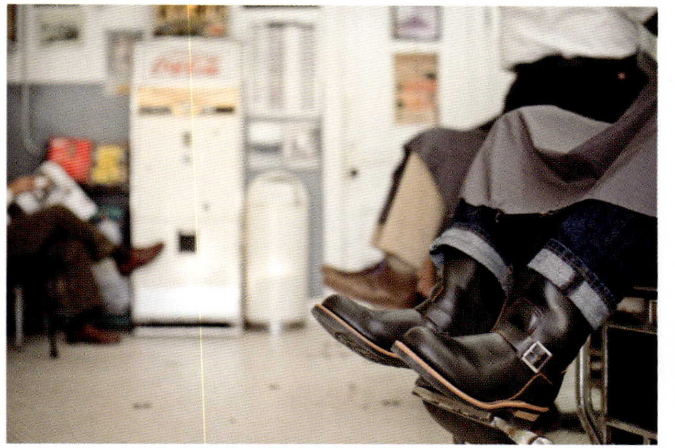

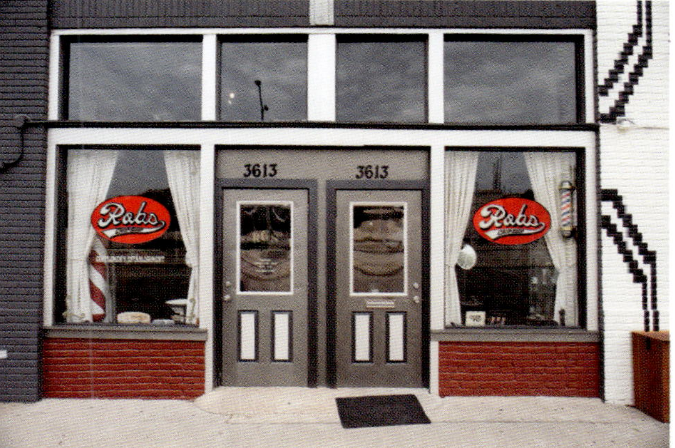

3613
3613
Rob's
Rob's

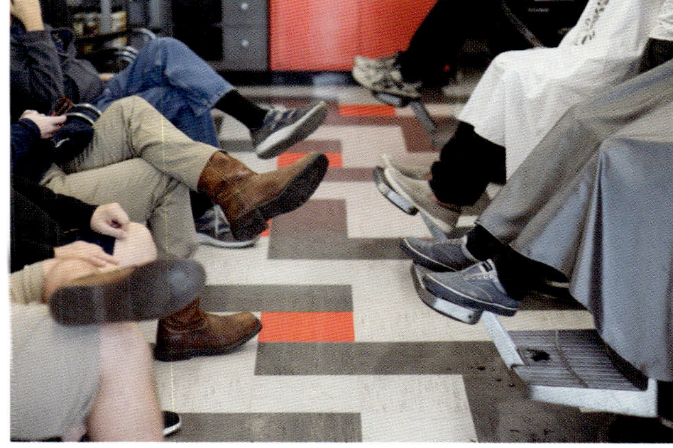

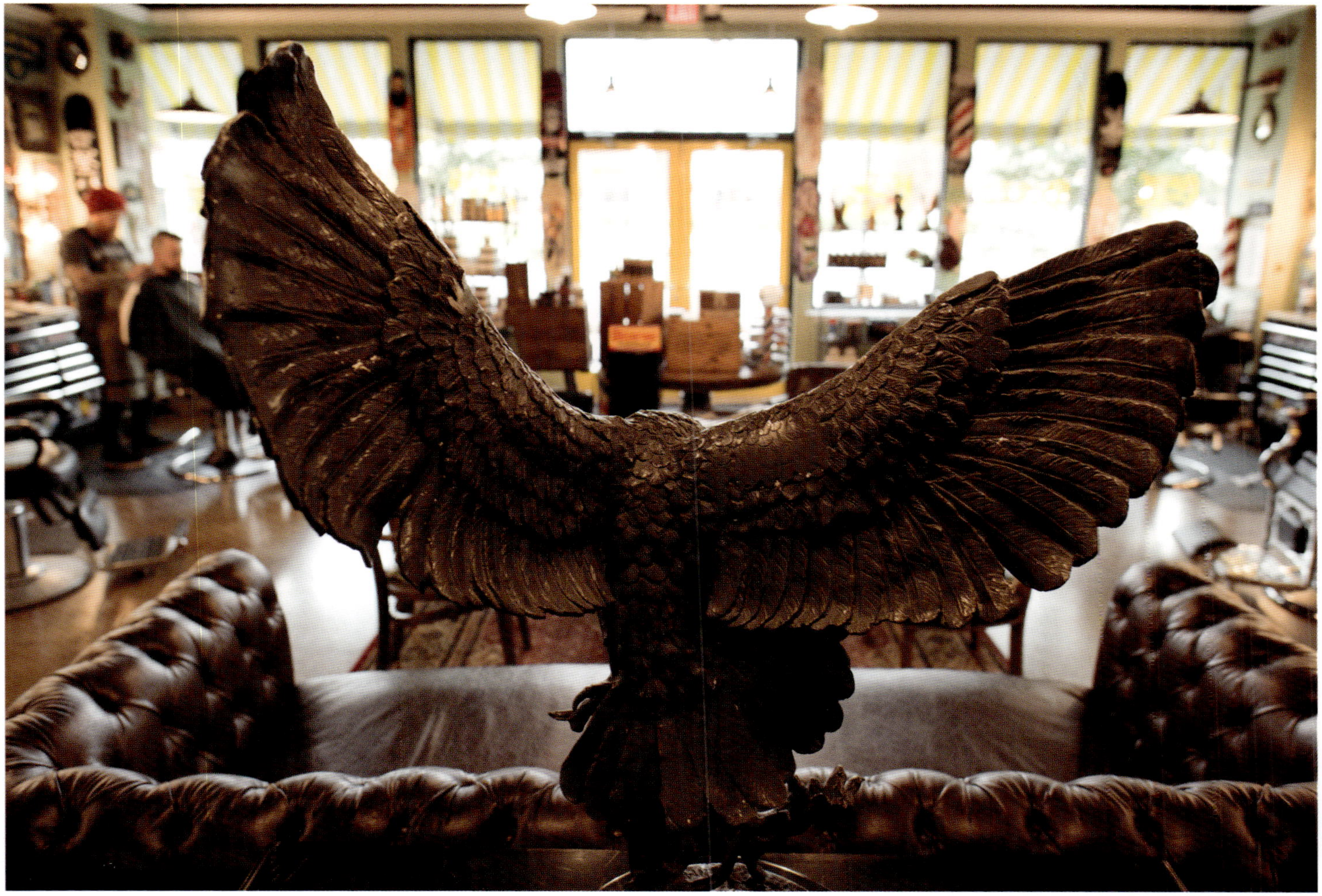

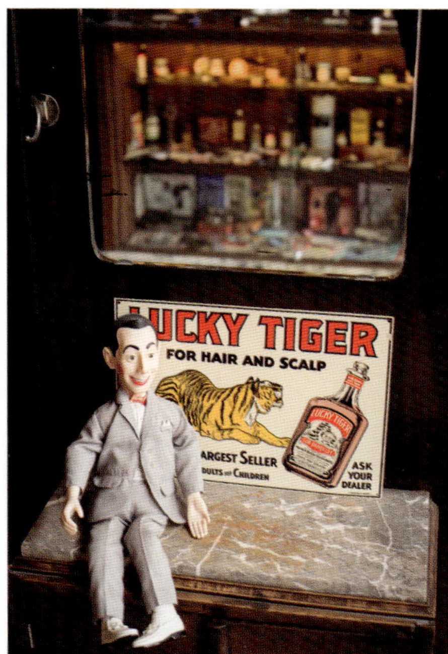

FOR HAIR AND SCALP
ASK YOUR DEALER

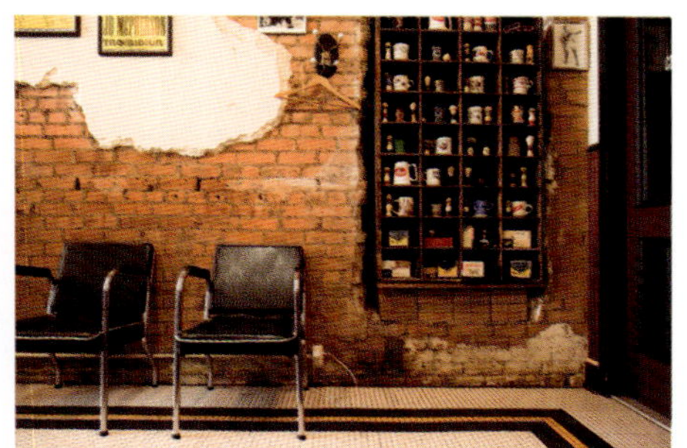

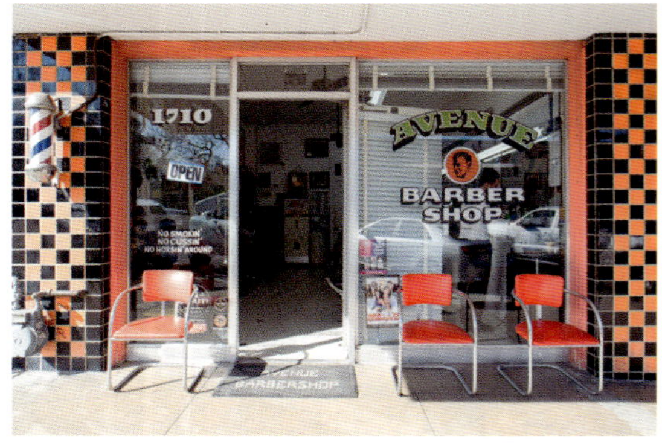
1710
AVENUE
BARBER
SHOP
OPEN

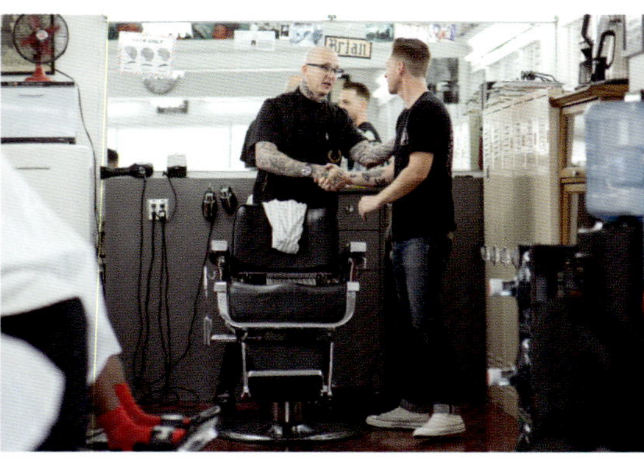
Brian

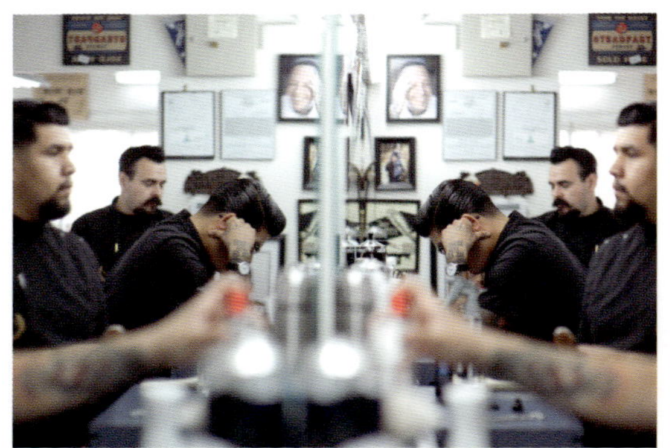

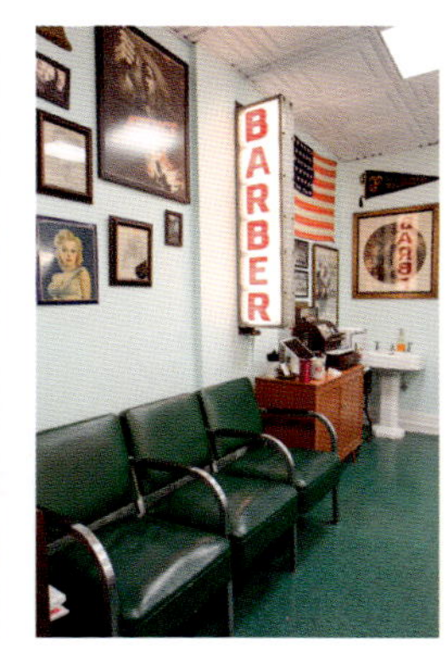
BARBER

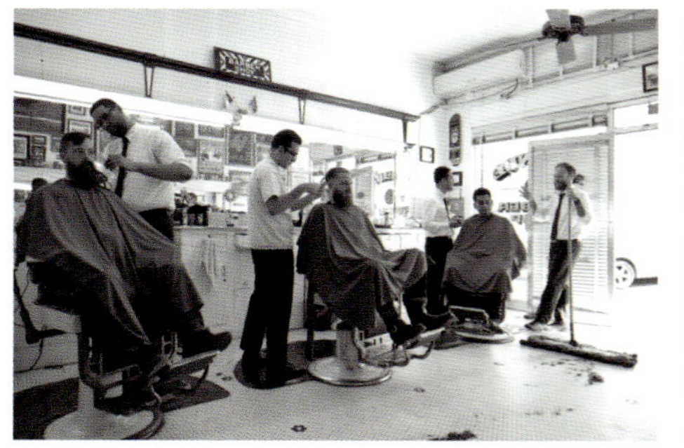

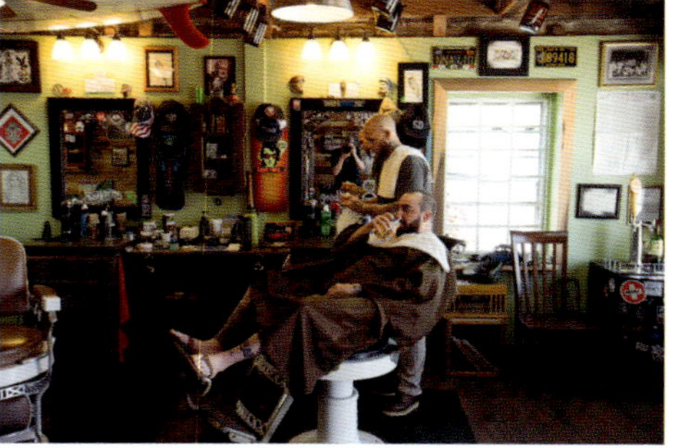

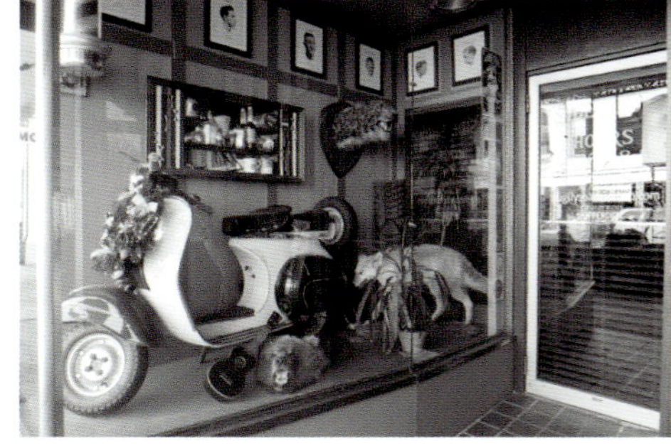

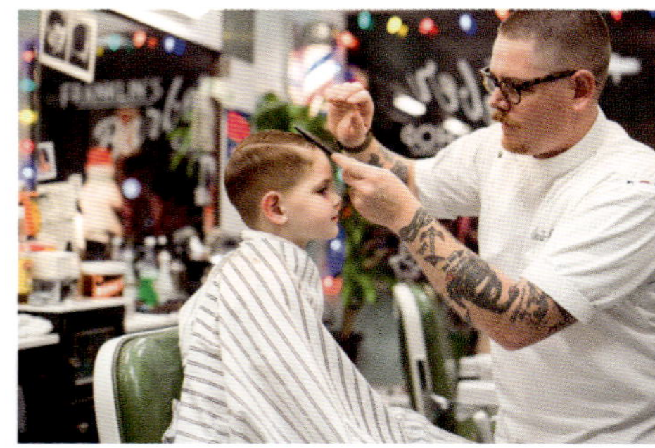

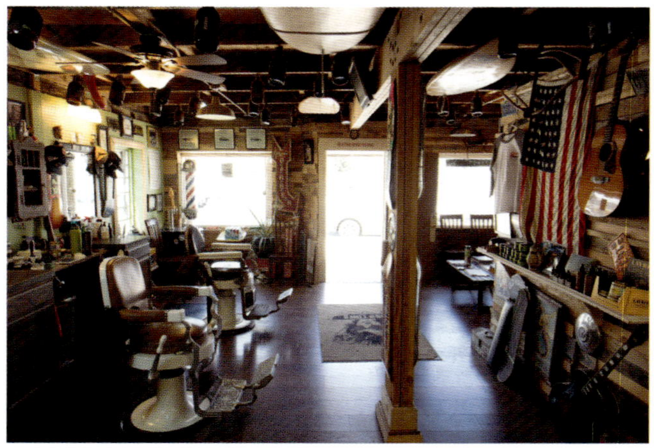

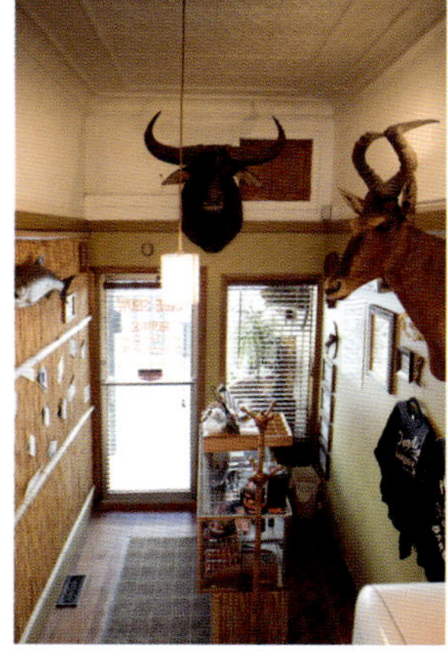

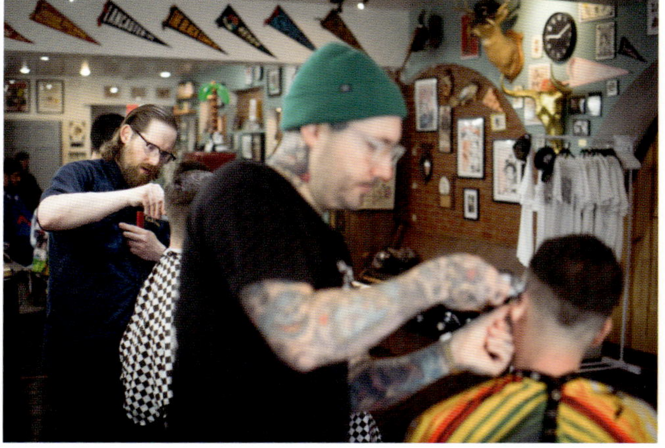

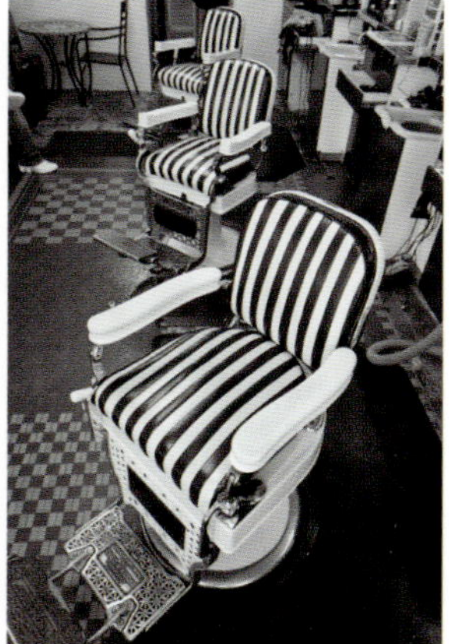

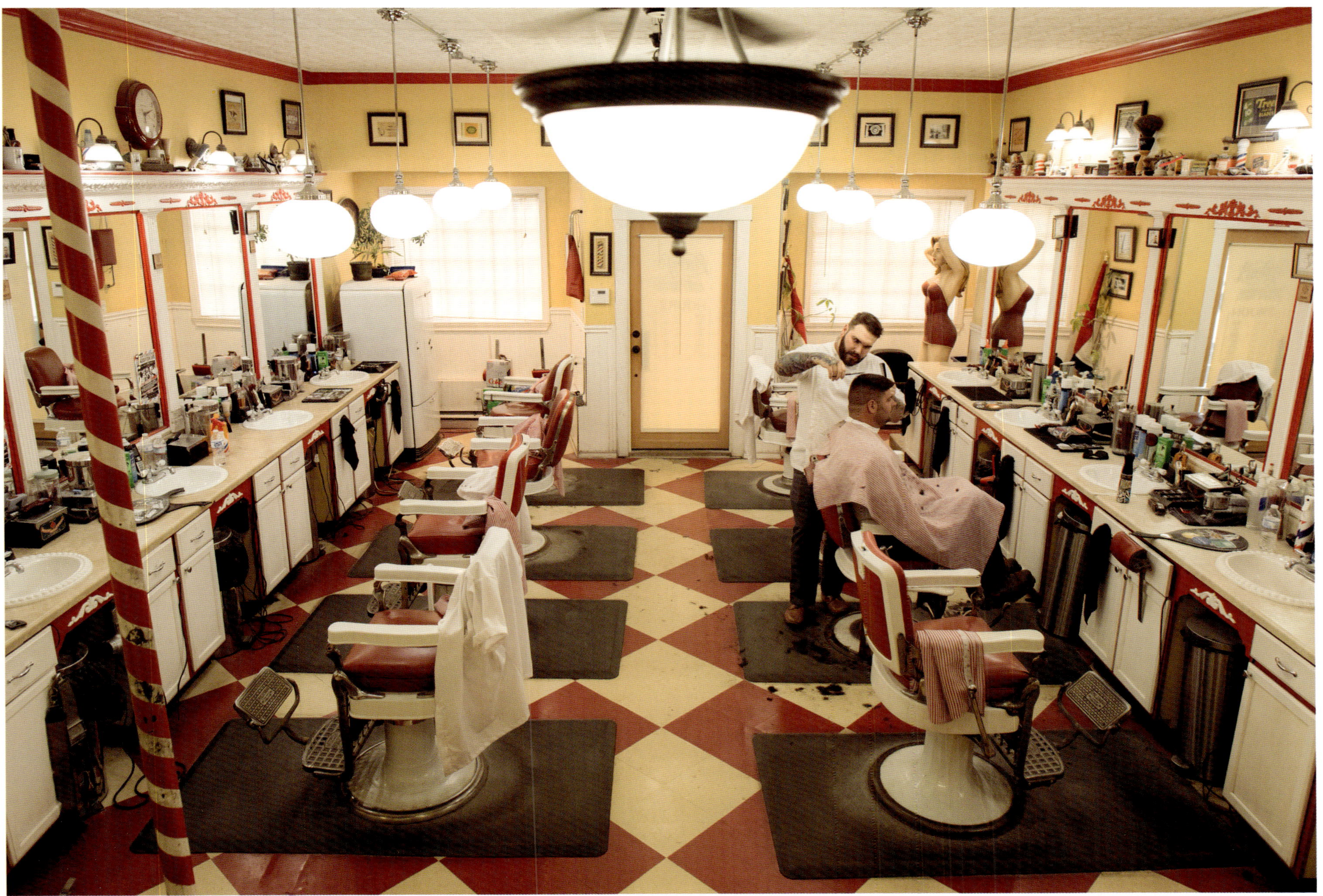

Lucky's Barbershop, Concord, New Hampshire

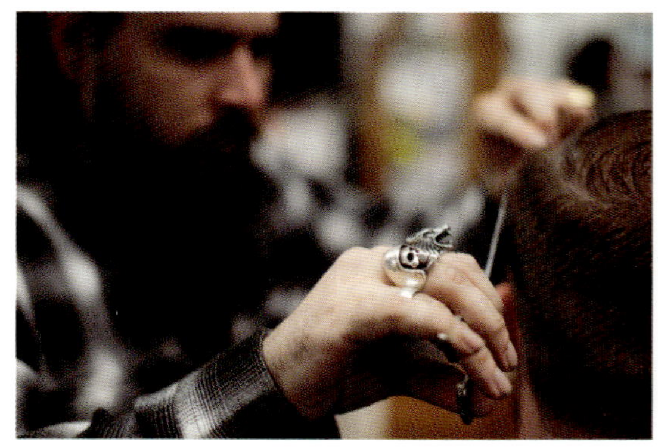

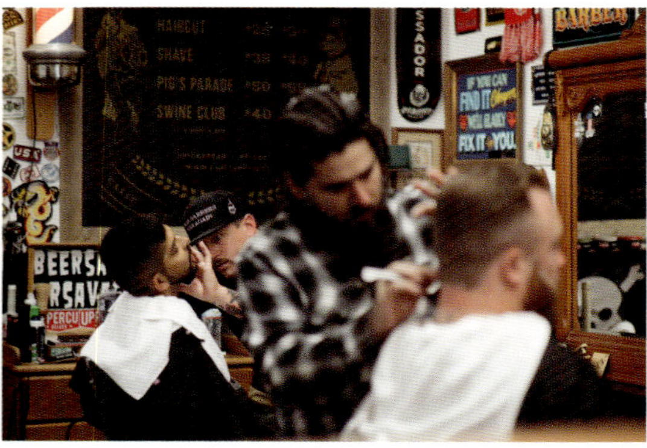

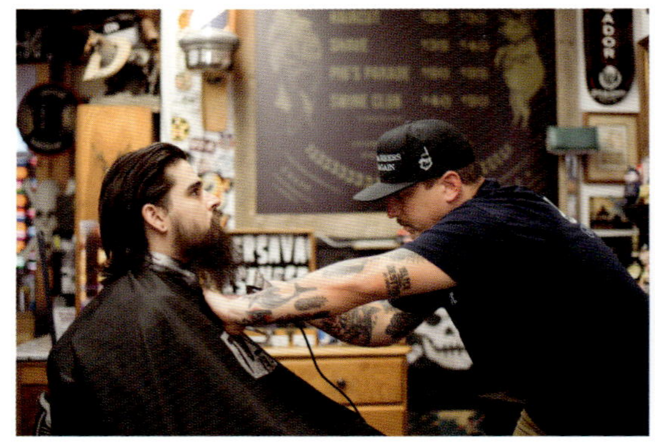

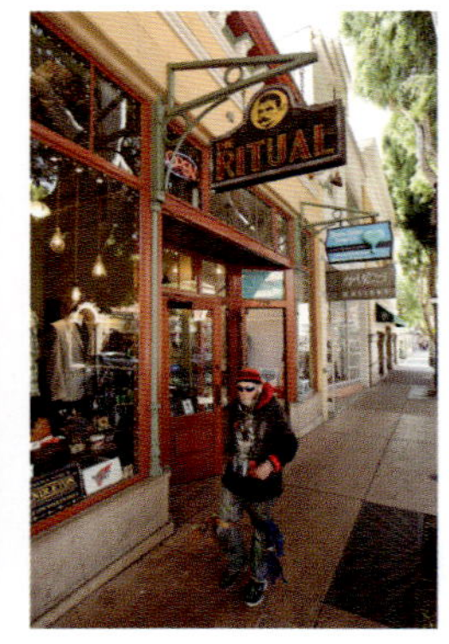
RITUAL

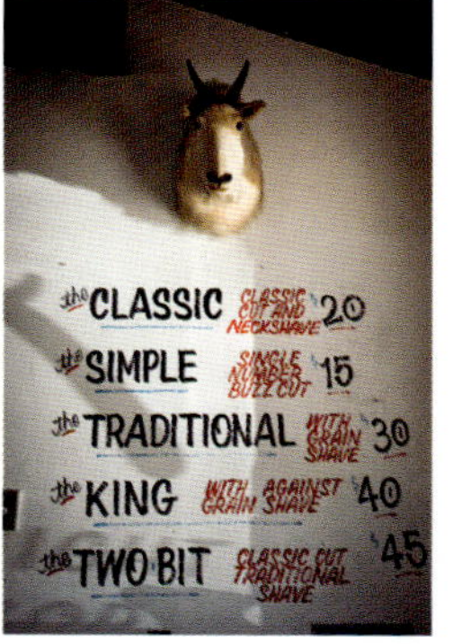
the CLASSIC 20
the SIMPLE 15
the TRADITIONAL 30
the KING 40
the TWO BIT 45

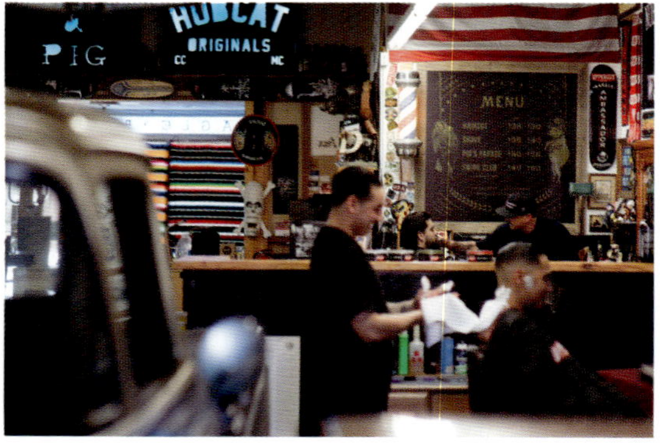
PIG
HUBCAT
ORIGINALS
MENU

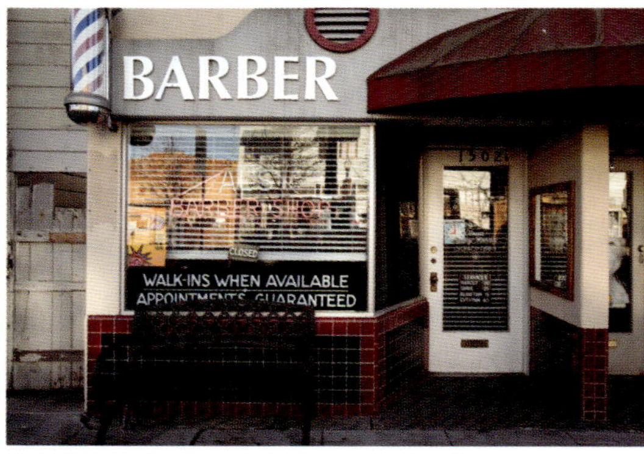
BARBER
WALK-INS WHEN AVAILABLE
APPOINTMENTS GUARANTEED

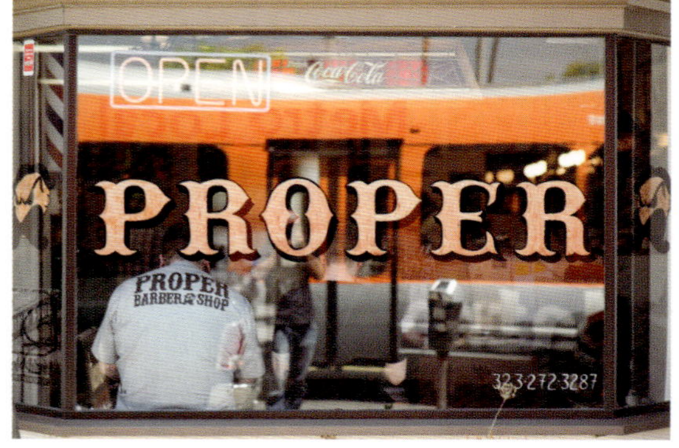
OPEN
PROPER
PROPER BARBER SHOP
323 272 3287

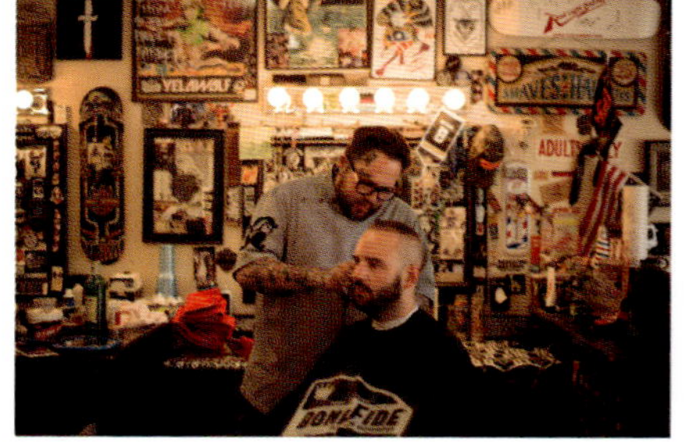

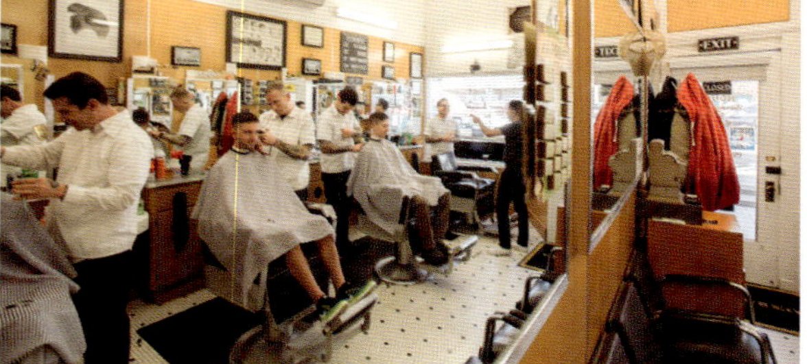

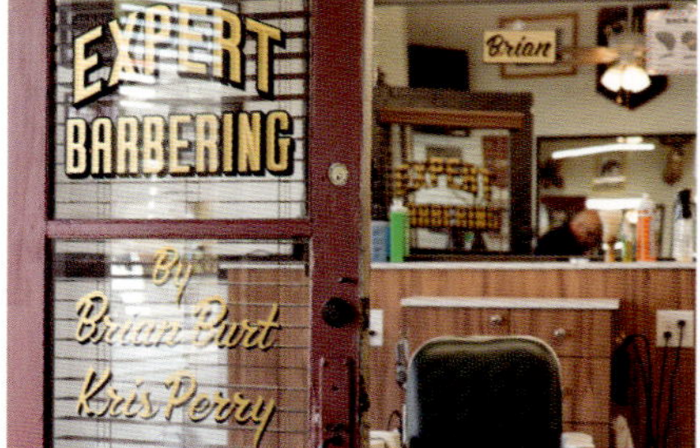
EXPERT
BARBERING
By
Brian Burt
Kris Perry
Brian

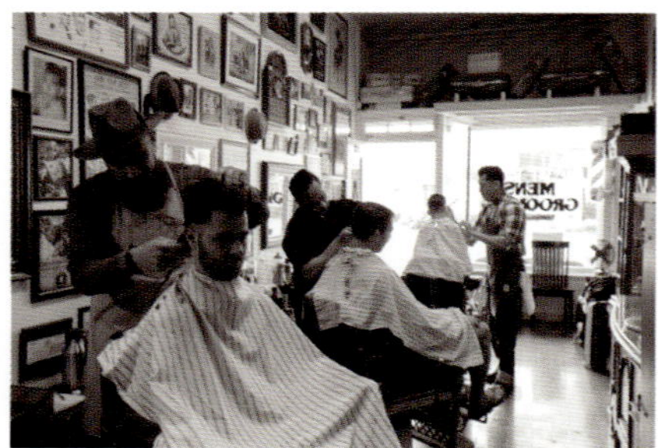

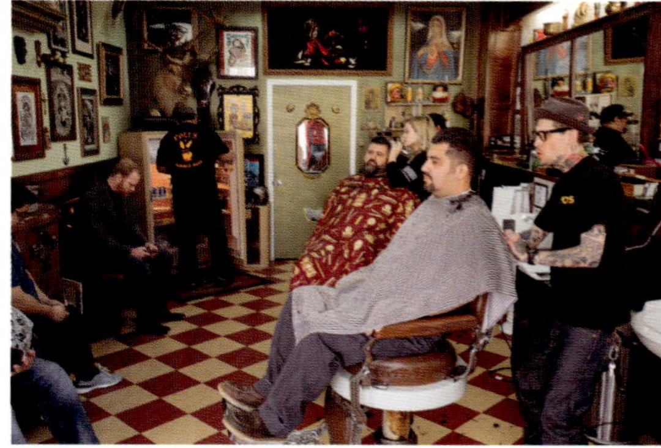

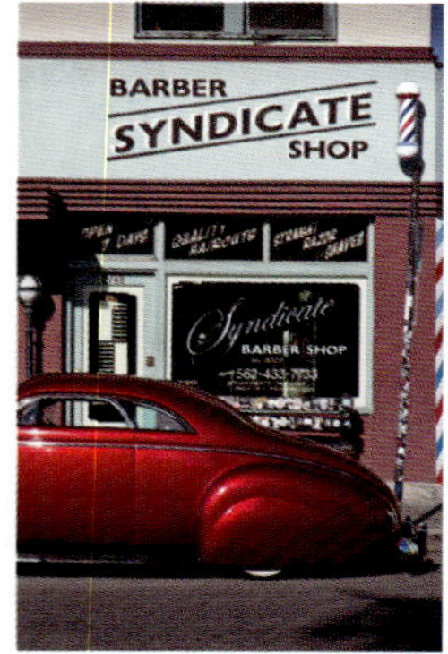
BARBER
SYNDICATE
SHOP
Syndicate
BARBER SHOP

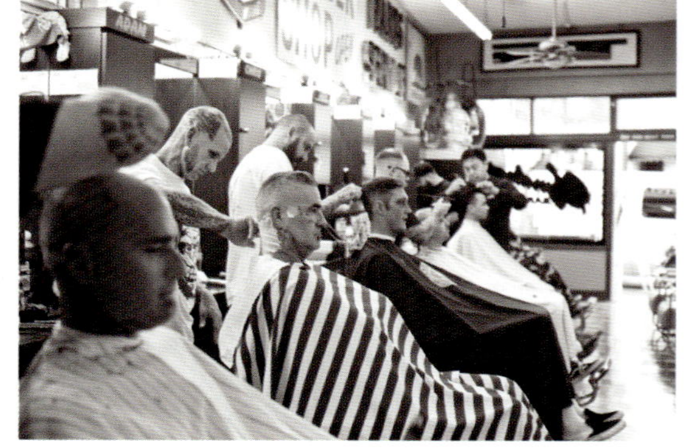

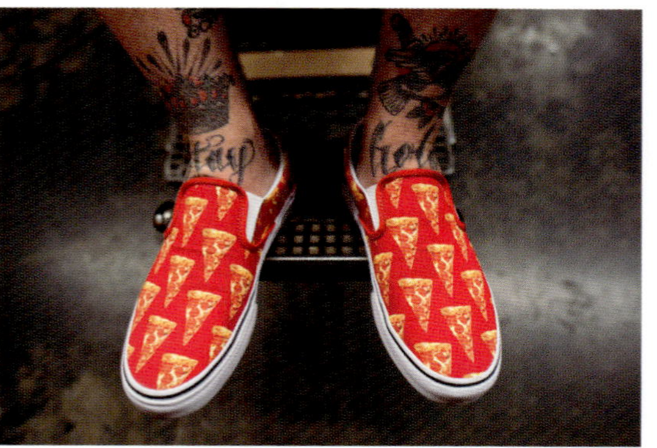

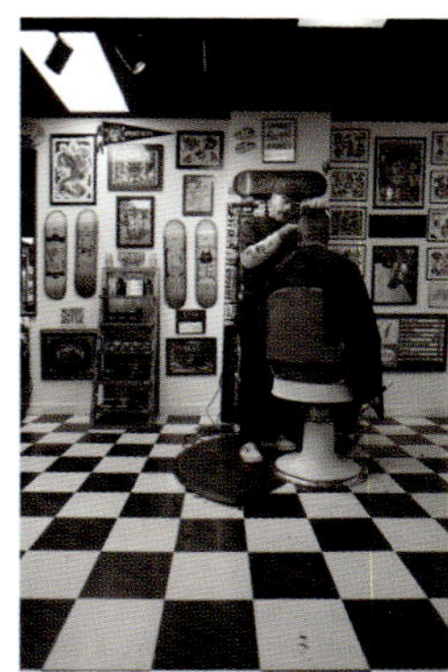
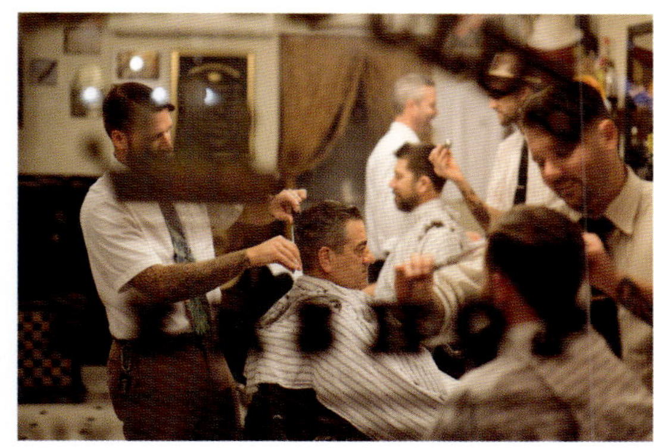
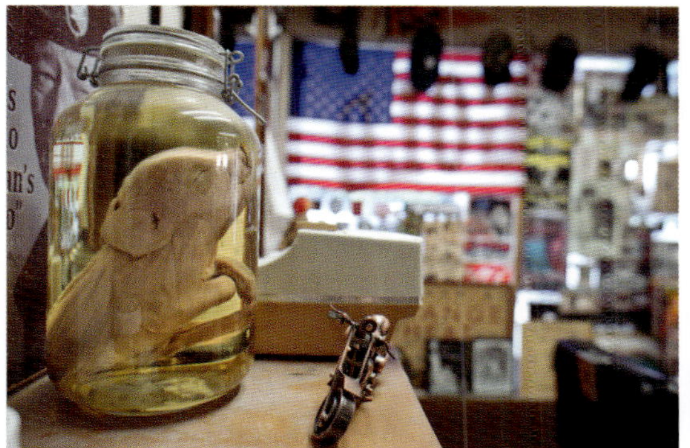
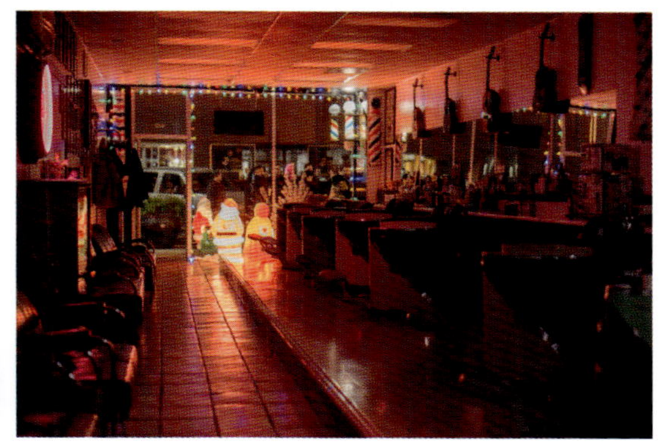
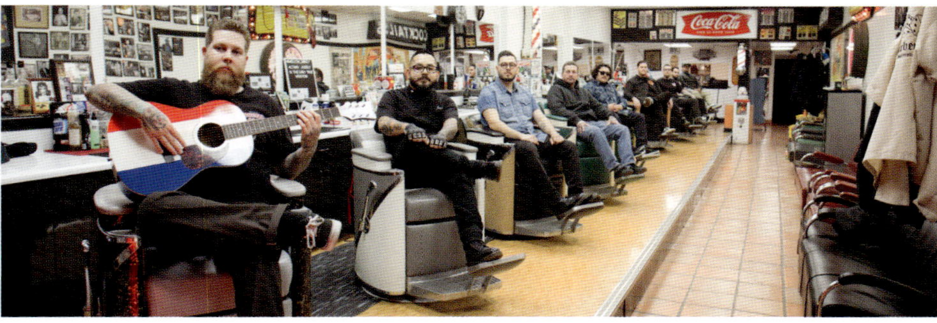
Coca-Cola
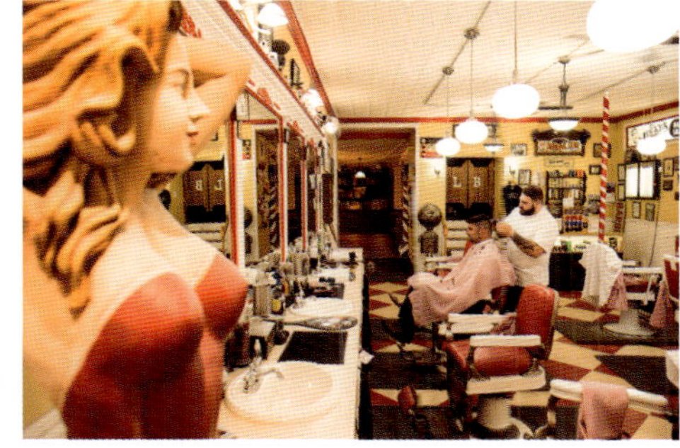
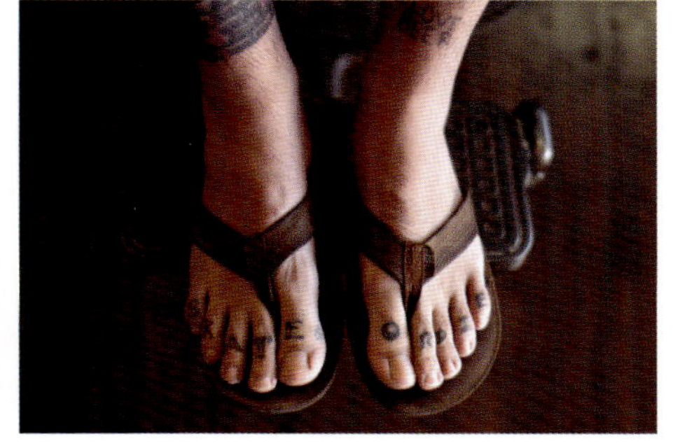
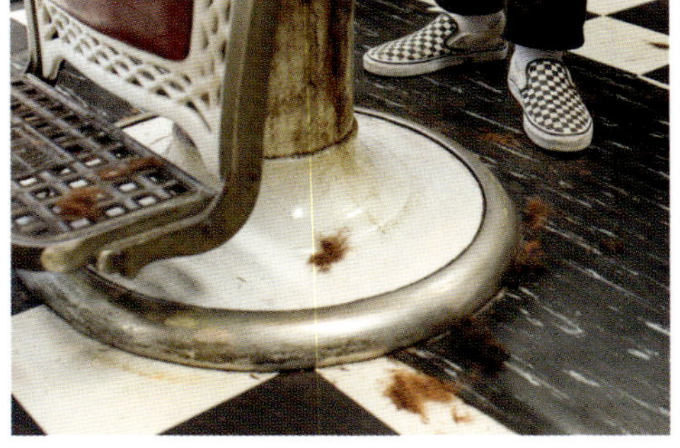
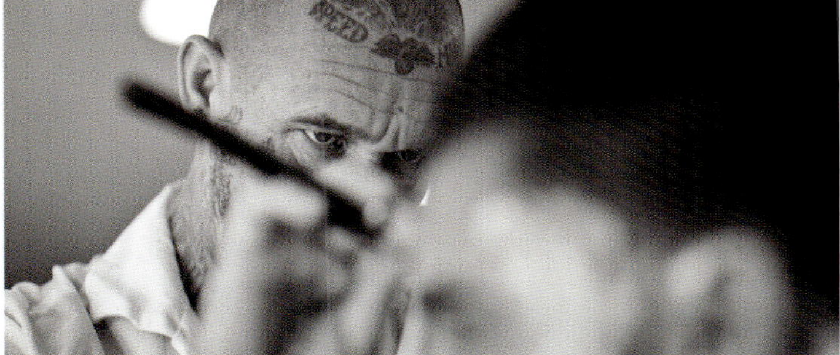
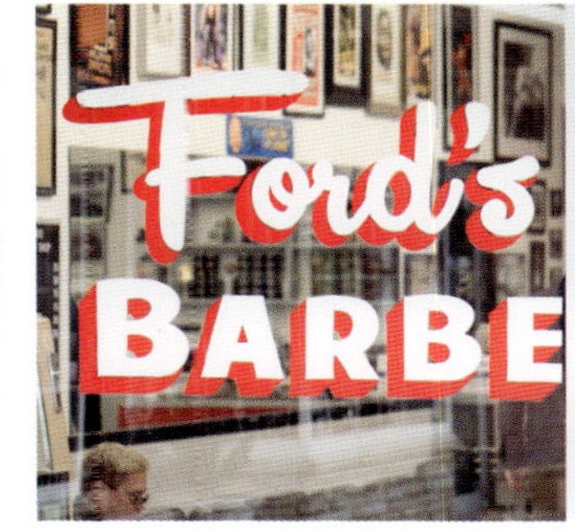
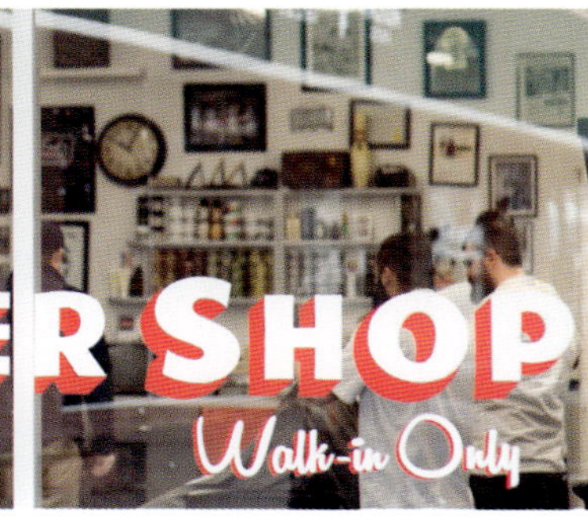
Ford's
BARBER SHOP
Walk-in Only
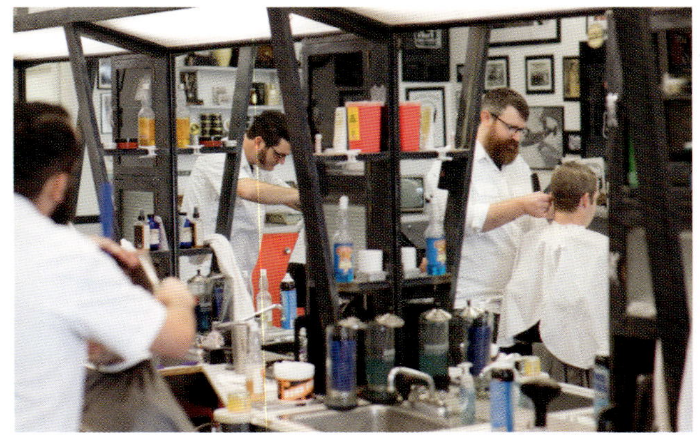
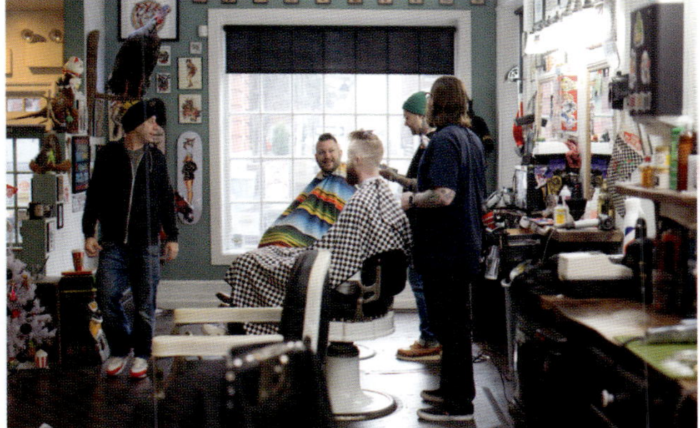
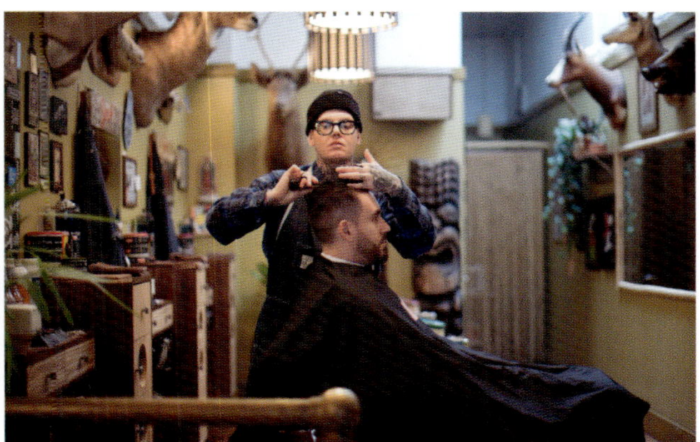

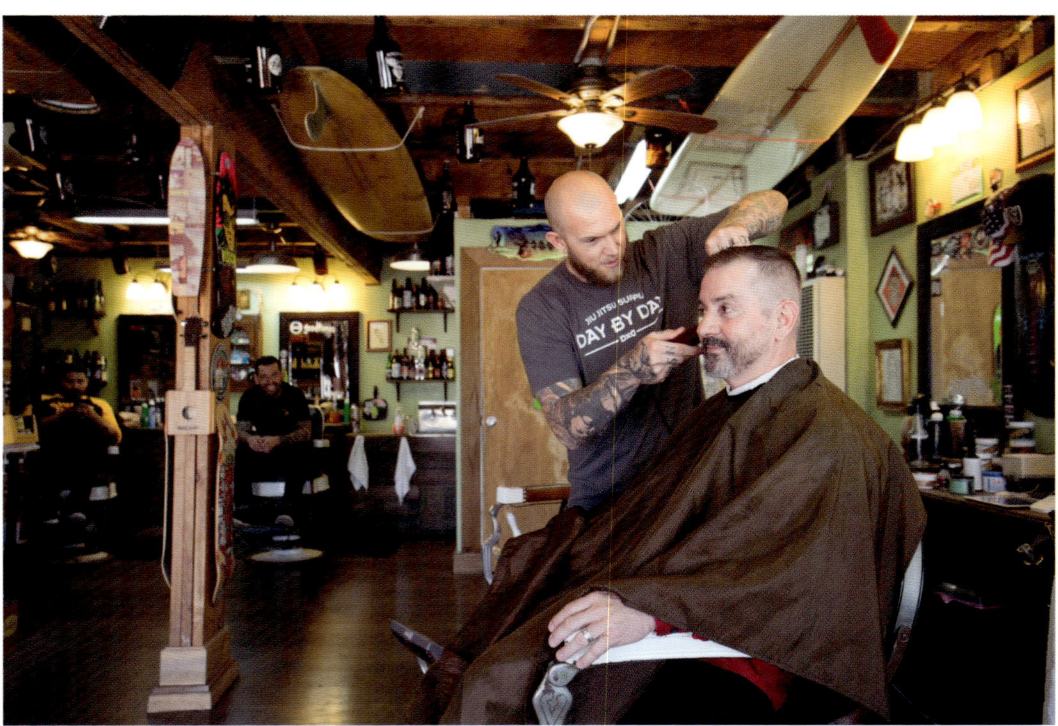

Good Times Barbershop, Imperial Beach, California

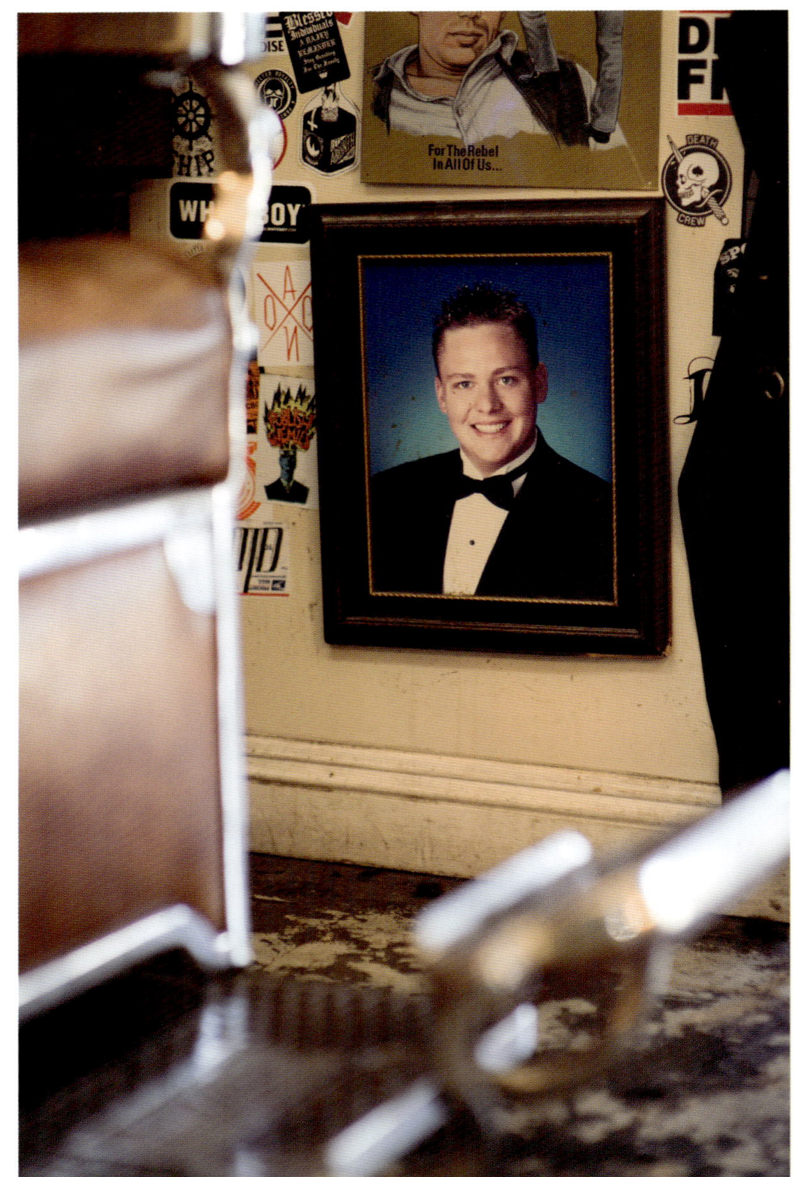

The Proper Barbershop, Los Angeles, California

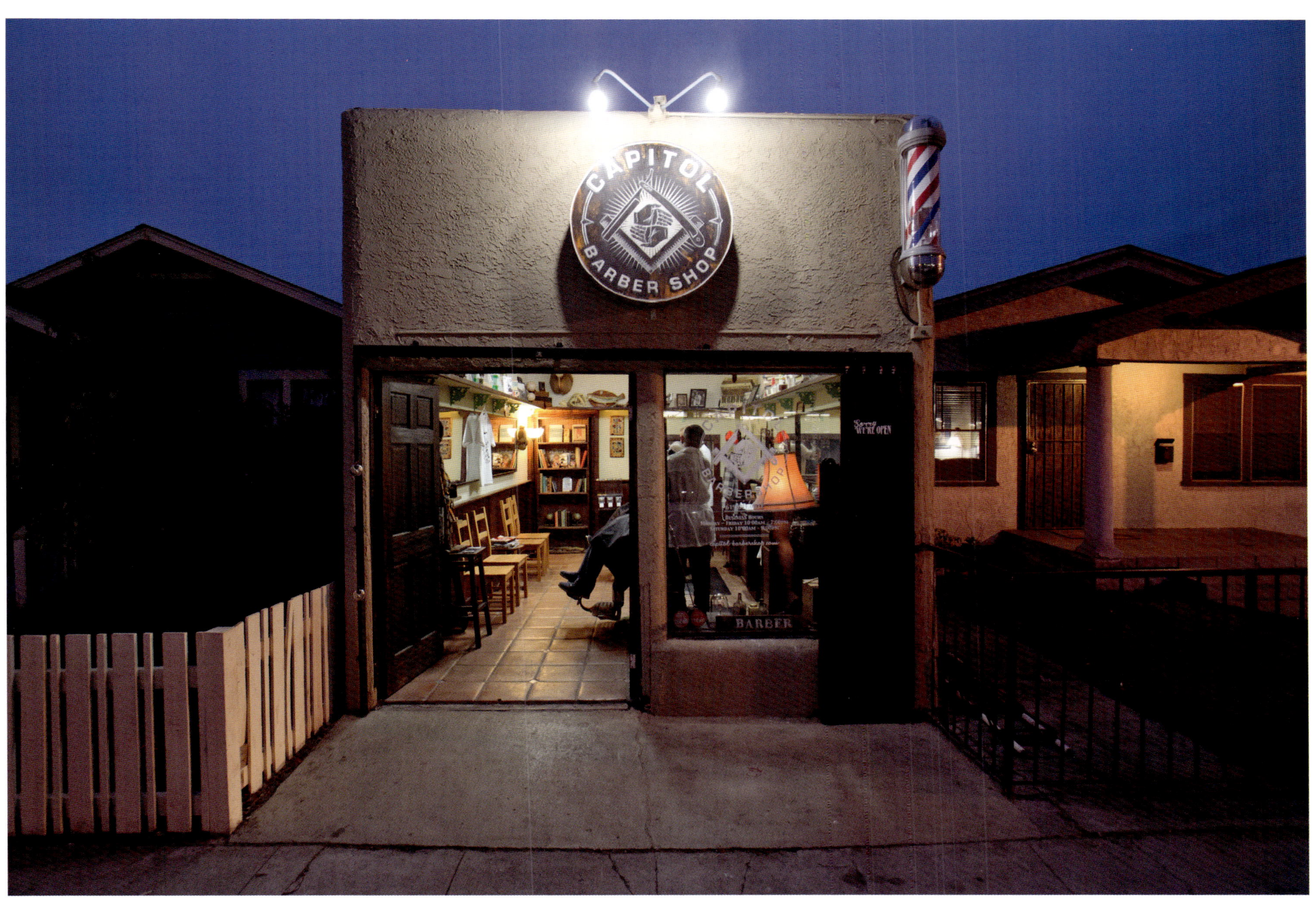

Capitol Barbershop, San Diego, California

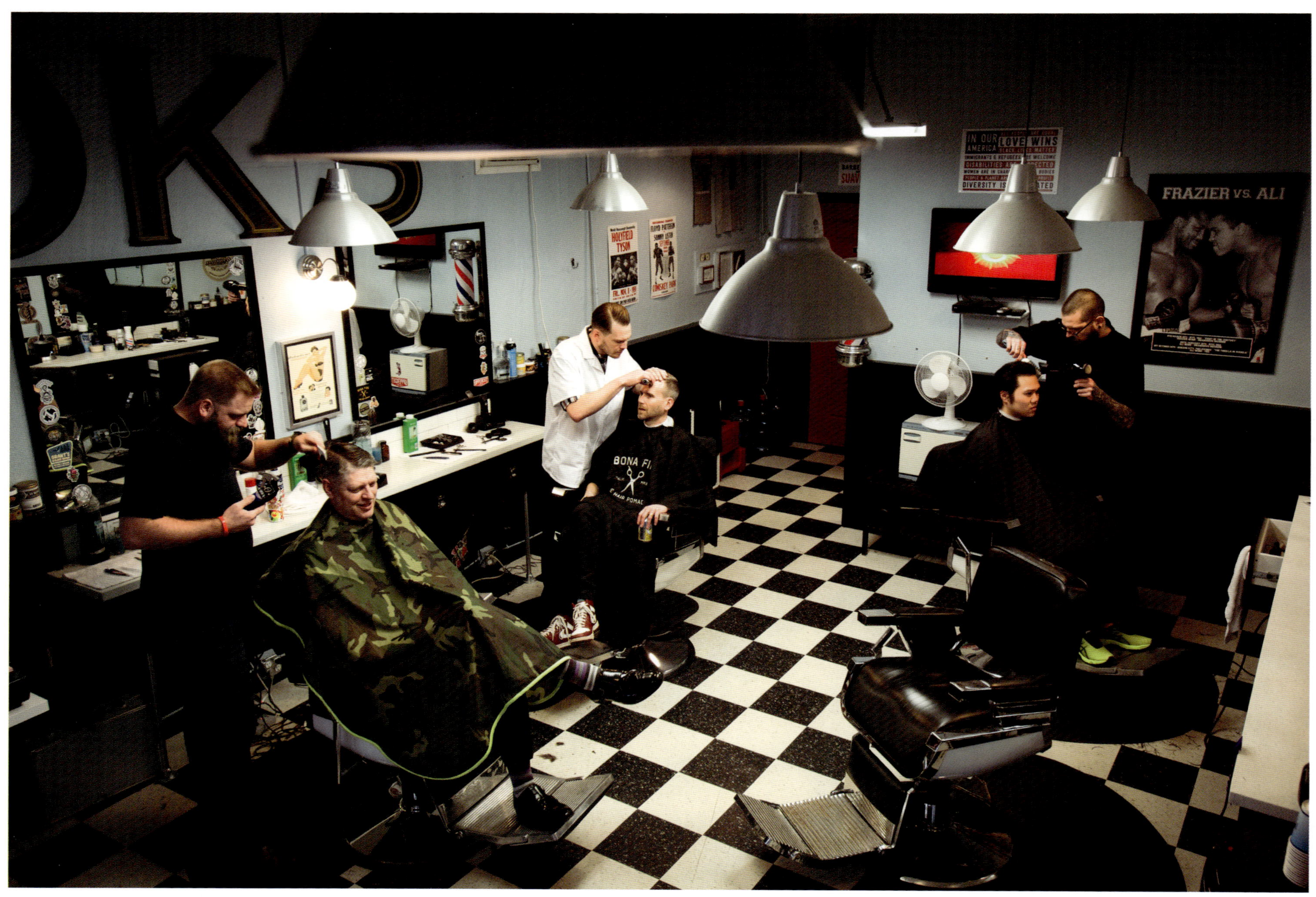

Rooks Barbershop, Portland, Oregon

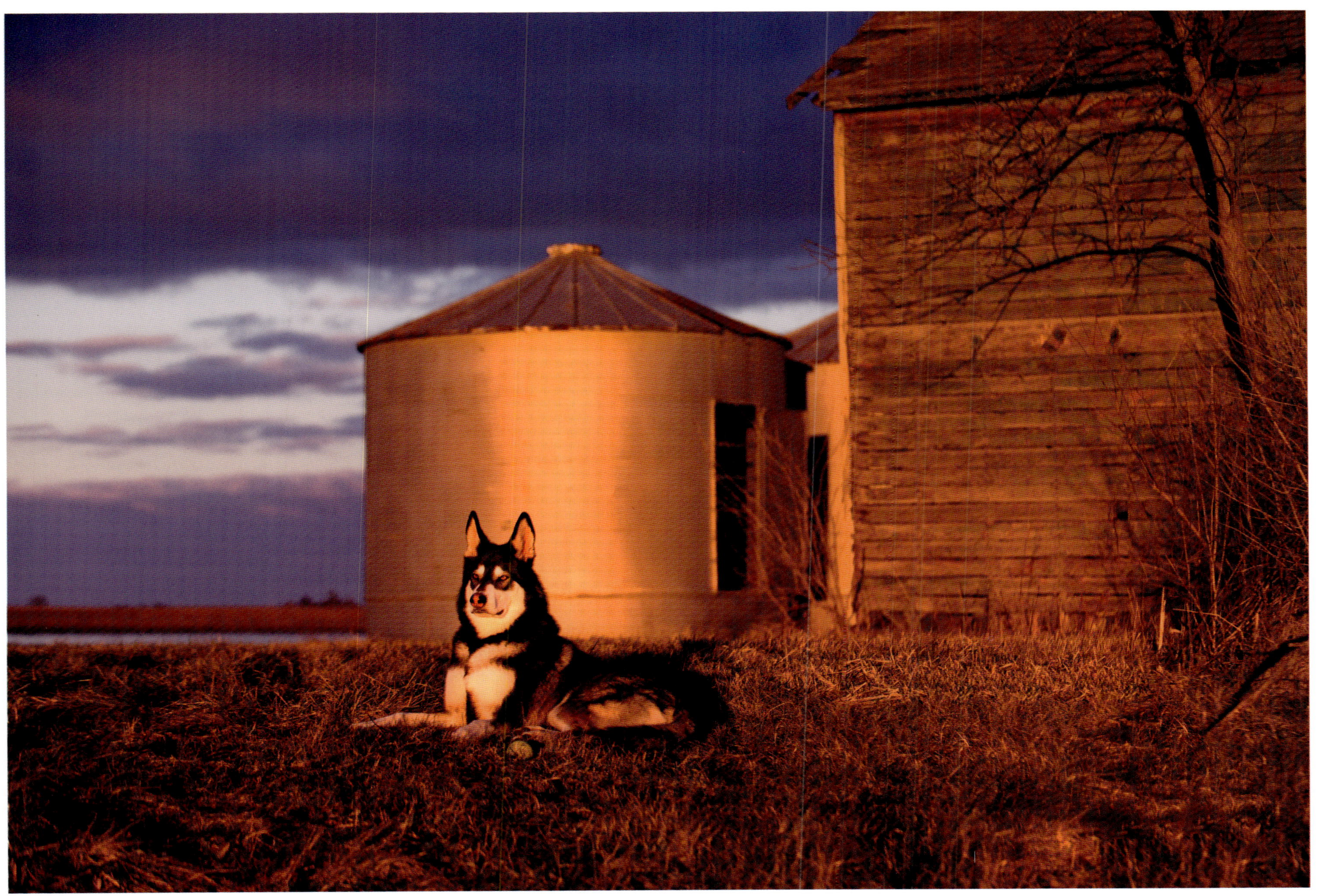

Mojo—my co-pilot on this journey. Since 2012 we've traveled more than 200,000 miles together.

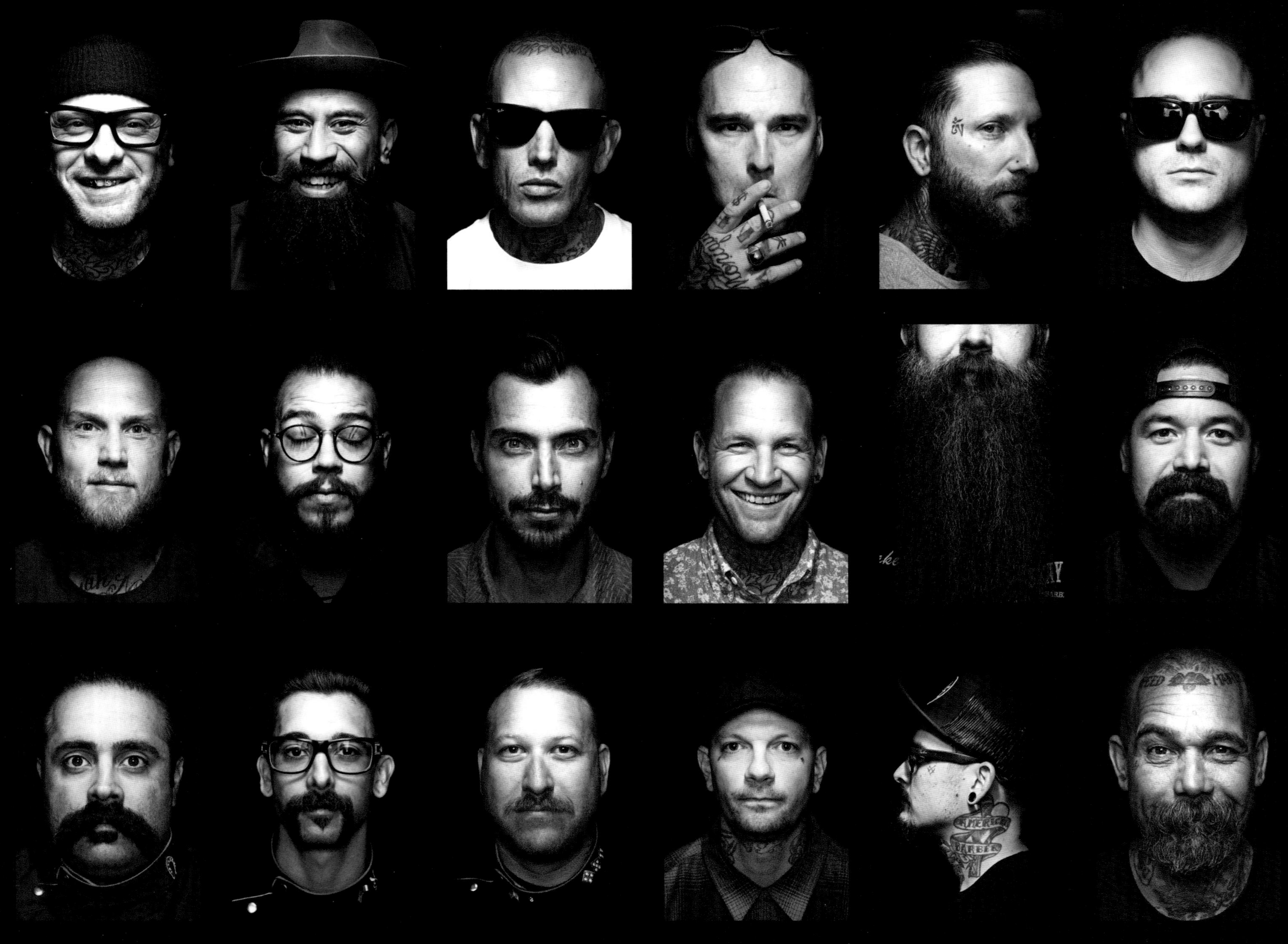
BARBER

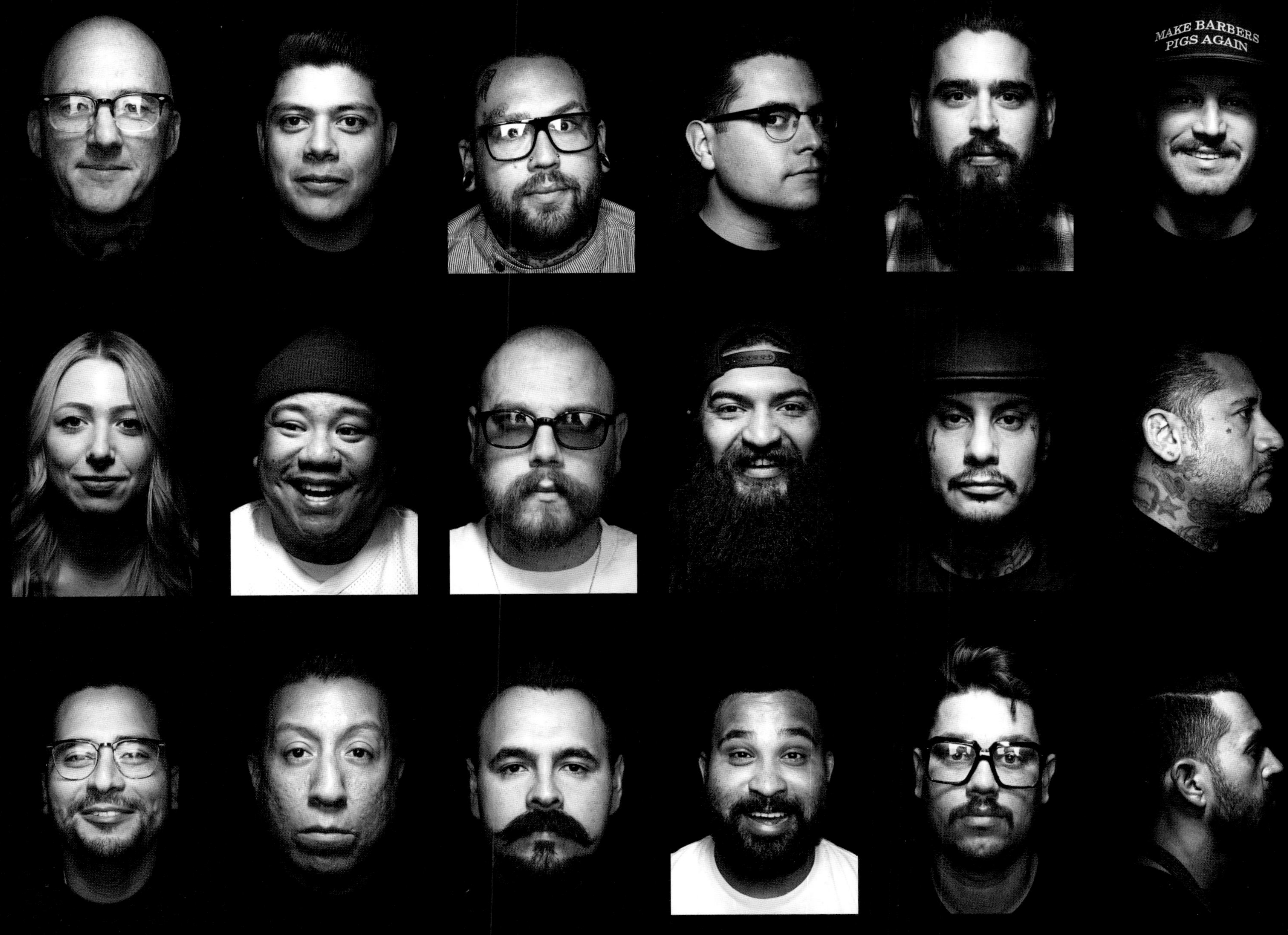
MAKE BARBERS
PIGS AGAIN

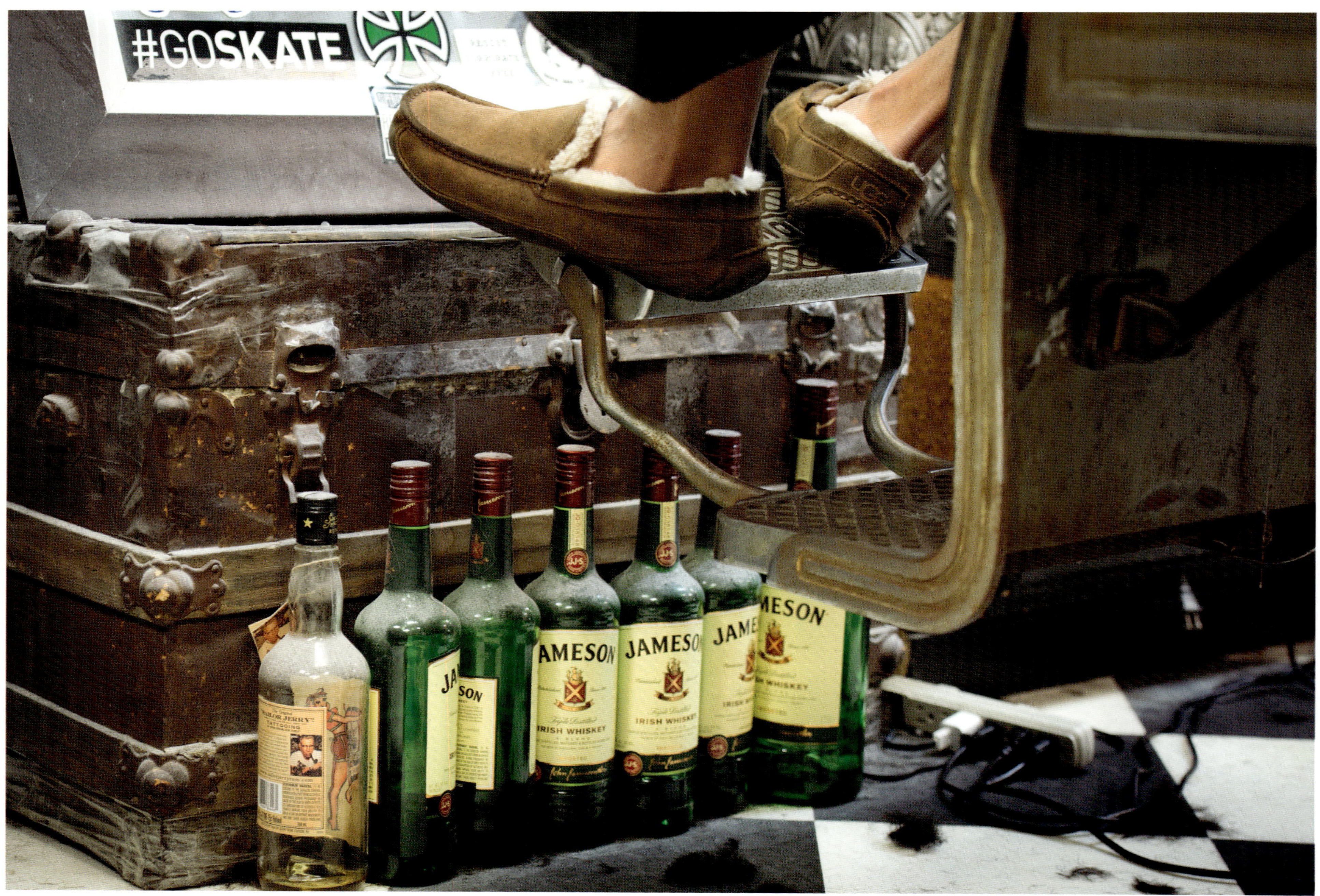

The Chop Shop, San Luis Obispo, California

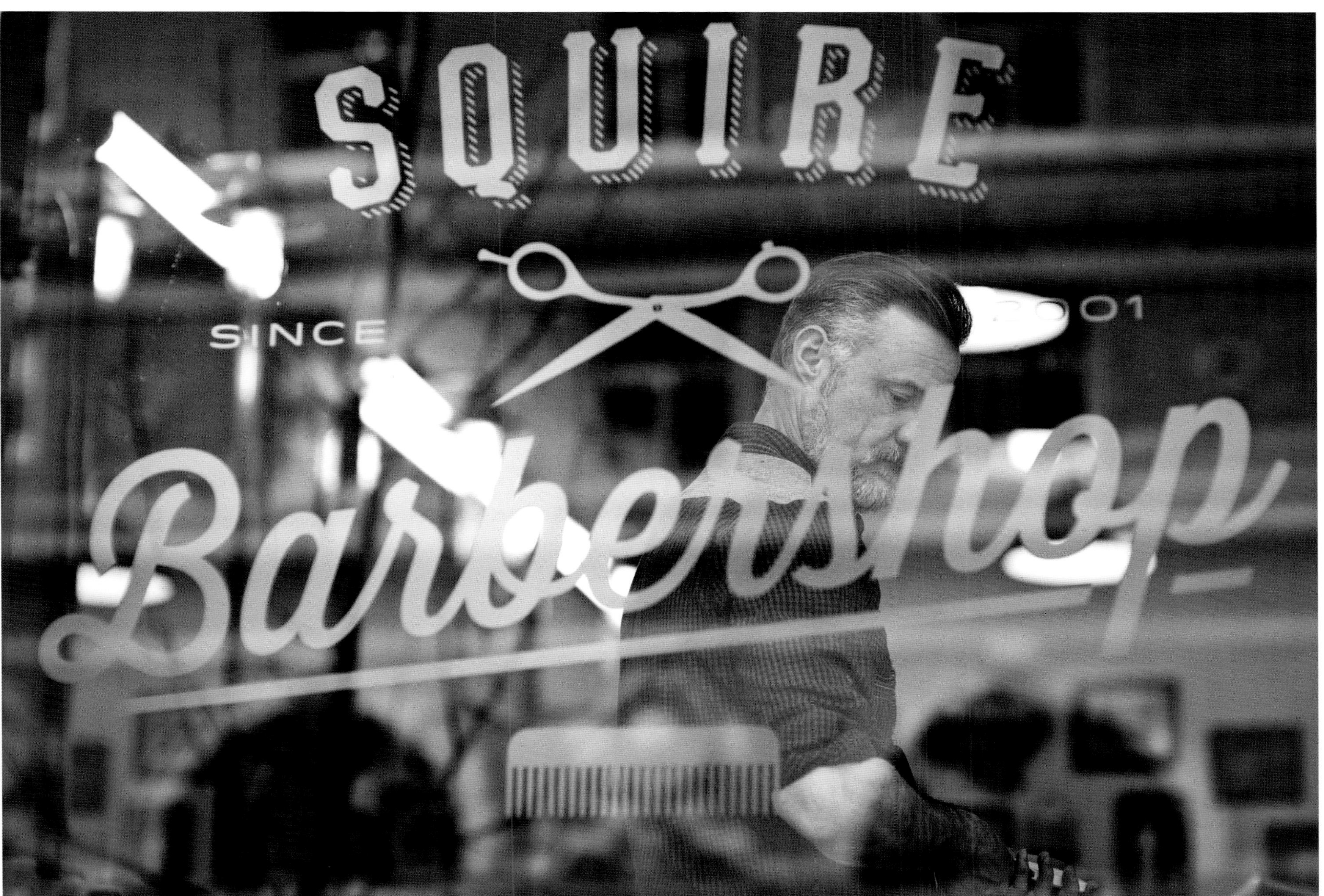

Squire Barbershop, Seattle, Washington

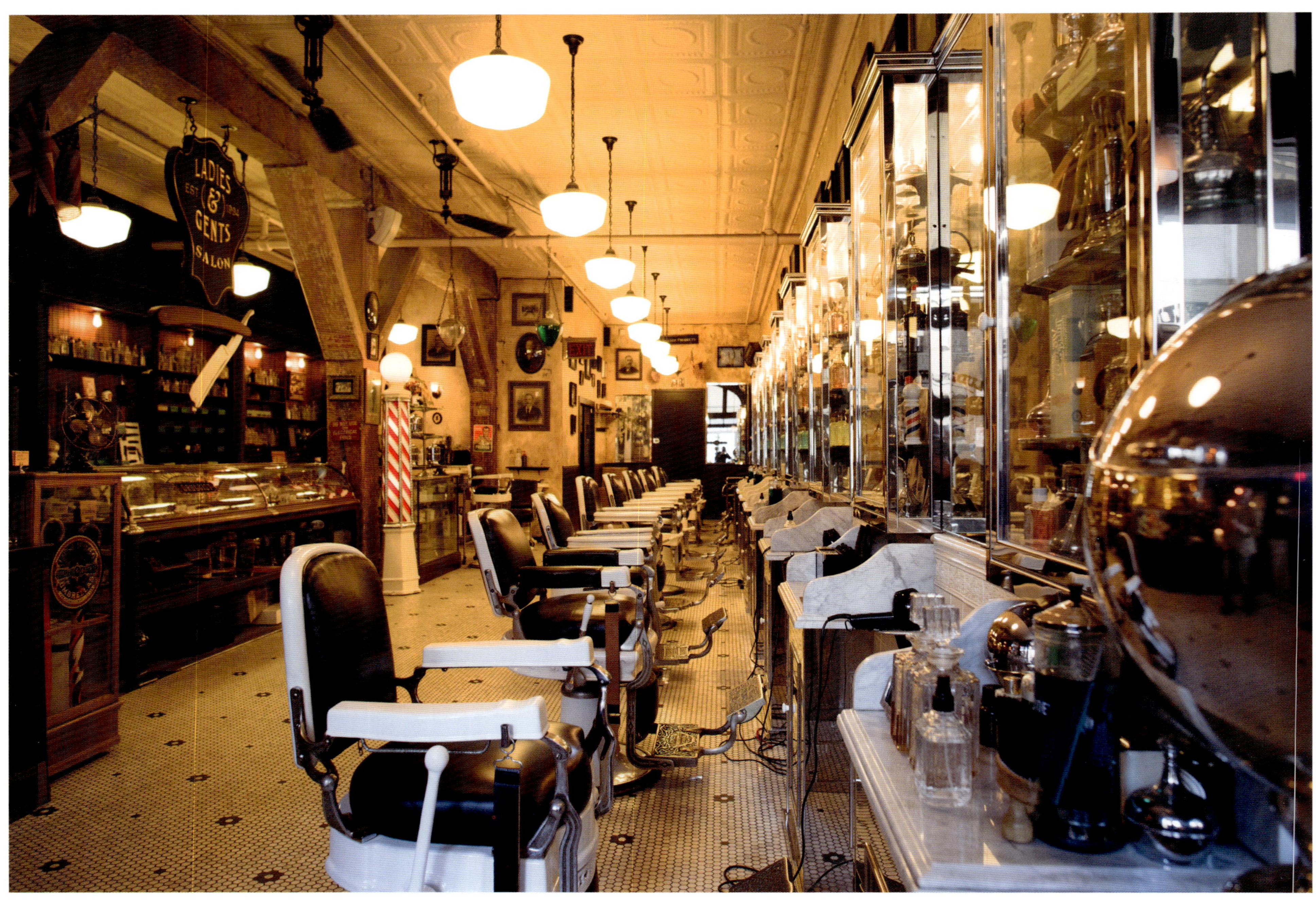

Ludlow Blunt, Brooklyn, New York

"For some of these guys, we go to the funeral parlor for their last haircut."

– Red, Red's Barbershop, Gulfport, Mississippi

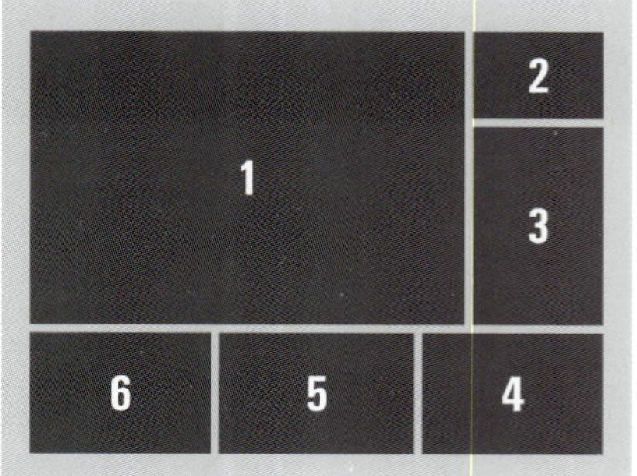

PAGE 15

1 Pat's Barbershop, San Diego, CA
2 City Barbershop, Ramona, CA
3 Johnny Lovato's Barbershop, San Diego, CA
4 Esquire Barbershop, Oceanside, CA
5 Unknown, KS
6 North 75 Barbershop, Topeka, KS

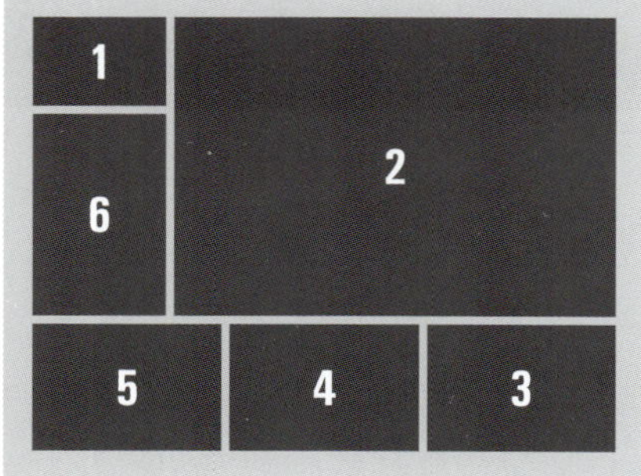

PAGE 23

1 North 75 Barbershop, Topeka, KS
2 Gene's Barbershop, Myrtle Creek, OR
3 Smith's Barbershop, Excelsior Springs, MO
4 Smith's Barbershop, Excelsior Springs, MO
5 Larry's Barbershop, Lawrence, KS
6 North 75 Barbershop, Topeka, KS

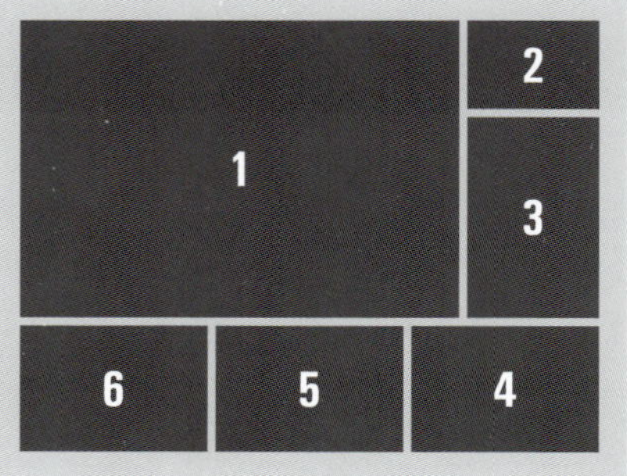

PAGE 24

1 Steimel's Barbershop, Vincennes, IN
2 Pip's Barbershop, Rutland, VT
3 Ken's Barbershop, Newport, KY
4 Ray's Barbershop, French Lick, IN
5 Unknown, IA
6 Jim's Barber and Style Shop, Winterset, IA

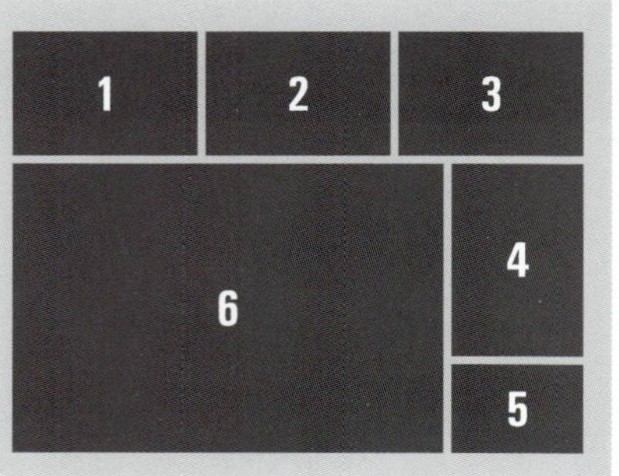

PAGE 27

1 Jones' Barbershop, Bennington, VT
2 Corey's Barbershop, Rock Springs, WY
3 Village Barber Styling, Dover, DE
4 Del's Barbershop, Escondido, CA
5 Don's Barbershop, Milford, DE
6 Unknown, Jefferson, SD

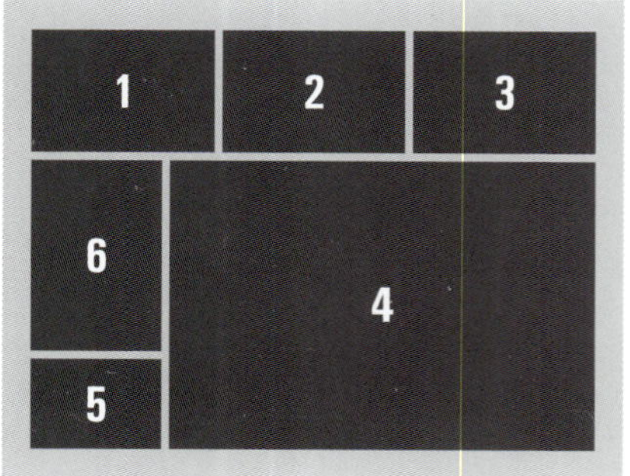

PAGE 28

1 Russell's Barbershop, Hurlock, MD
2 Tim's Barbershop, Portland, OR
3 The Park Slope Barber, Brooklyn, NY
4 Fausto Ferrari Barbershop, Cincinnati, OH
5 Russell's Barbershop, Hurlock, MD
6 Russell's Barbershop, Hurlock, MD

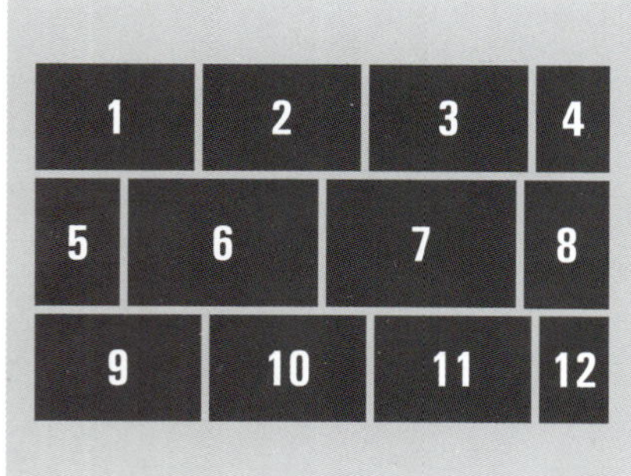

PAGE 31

1 Akemon's Barbershop, Paris, KY
2 Akemon's Barbershop, Paris, KY
3 Unknown, PA
4 Harold's Barber & Snack Shop, New Orleans, LA
5 Joe's Barbershop, Brooklyn, NY
6 Patrick's Barbershop, Winchester, KY
7 Don's Barbershop, Hudsonville, MI
8 Somewhere near Joshua Tree, CA
9 White's Barber College, Mobile, AL
10 White's Barber College, Mobile, AL
11 Rembert's Barbershop, Mobile, AL
12 Unknown, IA

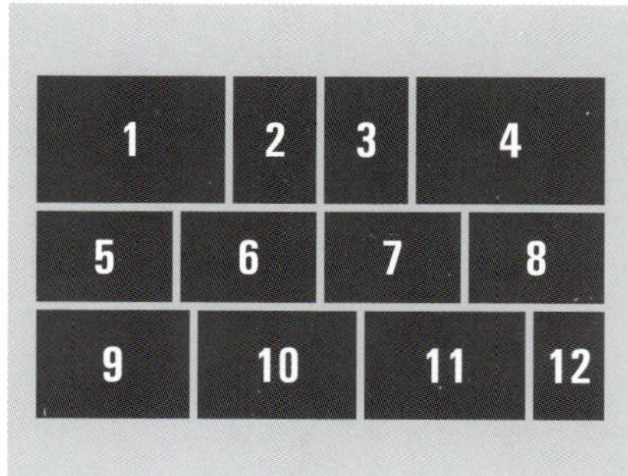

PAGE 32

1 The Barber Pole, Elkhart Lake, WI
2 Fausto Ferrari Barbershop, Cincinnati, OH
3 Vista Barbershop, Vista, CA
4 Duke's Barbershop, Hedgesville, WV
5 Vista Barbershop, Vista, CA
6 Canarsie Barbershop, Brooklyn, NY
7 Canarsie Barbershop, Brooklyn, NY
8 Canarsie Barbershop, Brooklyn, NY
9 Unknown, VA
10 Mark's Barbershop, Spearfish, SD
11 Stoneville Barbershop, Stoneville, NC
12 Mark's Barbershop, Spearfish, SD

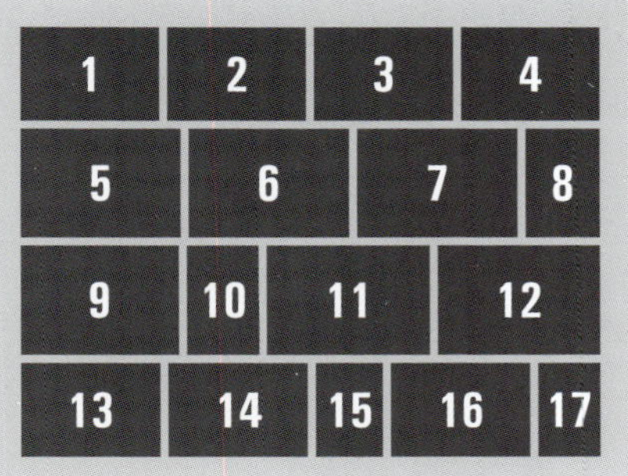

PAGE 35

1 Jim's Barbershop, Canon City, CO
2 Hunters Barbershop, Montrose, CO
3 Hunters Barbershop, Montrose, CO
4 Cortez Barbershop, Cortez, CO
5 Cortez Barbershop, Cortez, CO
6 Unknown, Rock Hill, SC
7 Jackson Barbershop, Chattahoochee, FL
8 Jackson Barbershop, Chattahoochee, FL
9 Senior Citizen Barber-shop, Portland, ME
10 McLean's Barbershop, Hyannis, MA
11 McLean's Barbershop, Hyannis, MA
12 Joe's Barbershop, Chicago, IL
13 Joe's Barbershop, Chicago, IL
14 Al's Barbershop, Webster City, IA
15 Bunn's Barber, Anchorage, AK
16 The Park Slope Barbers, Brooklyn, NY
17 La Legion Barbershop, Nashua, NH

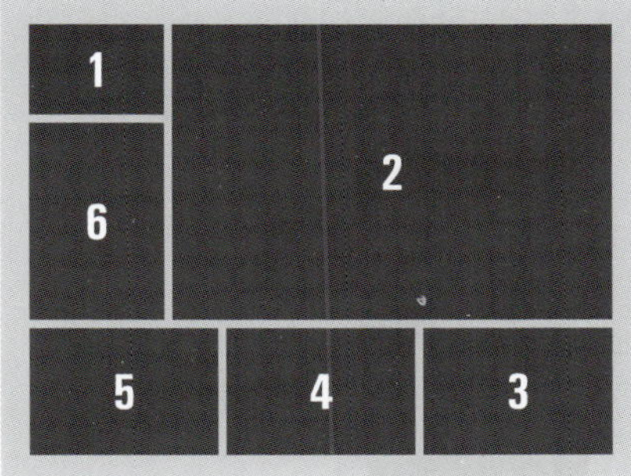

PAGE 39

1 Unknown, AZ
2 Los Muchachos Barbershop, New York City
3 A-Rod's Barbershop, Ellenville, NY
4 Loop Barbershop, Rock Falls, IL
5 Al's Barbershop, Webster City, IA
6 Unknown, AZ

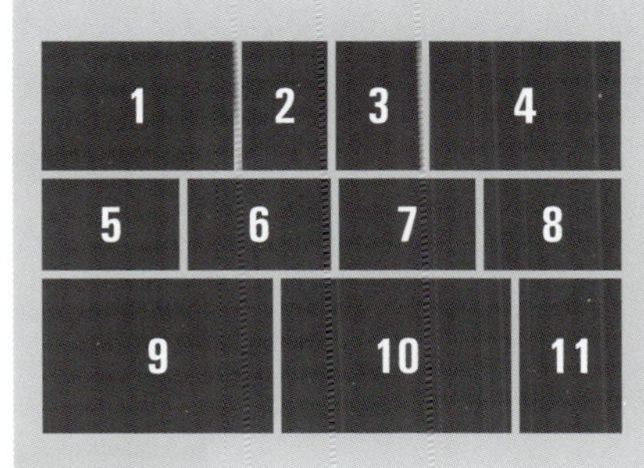

PAGE 49

1 La Legion Barbershop, Nashua, NH
2 Rome Style Barbershop, Brooklyn, NY
3 Sweeney Todd's Barbershop, Los Angeles, CA
4 Sweeney Todd's Barbershop, Los Angeles, CA
5 Elite Barbershop, Deming, NM
6 Holmes Barbershop, Cedar City, UT
7 Quality Cuts Barbershop, Amarillo, TX
8 Guico's Barbershop, Albany, NY
9 Craighead Barbershop, Nashville, TN
10 Tim's Barbershop, Portland, OR
11 Roseway Barbershop, Portland, OR

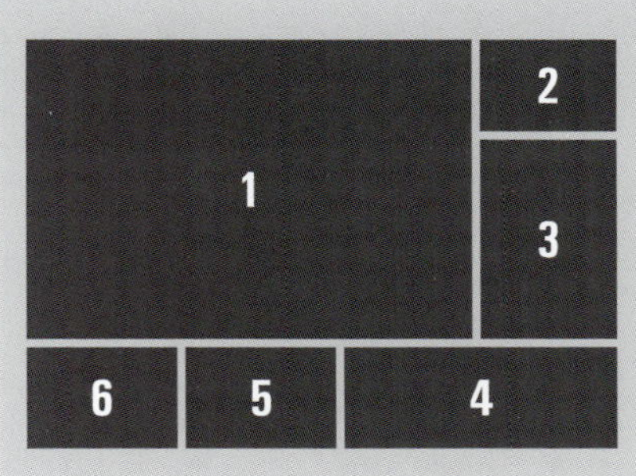

PAGE 50

1 Tony's Barbershop, Brooklyn, NY
2 Stancil's Barbershop, Albany, NY
3 A-Rod's Barbershop, Ellenville, NY
4 Ideal Barbershop, Taylor, TX
5 Rome Style Barbershop, Brooklyn, NY
6 Tony's Barbershop, Brooklyn, NY

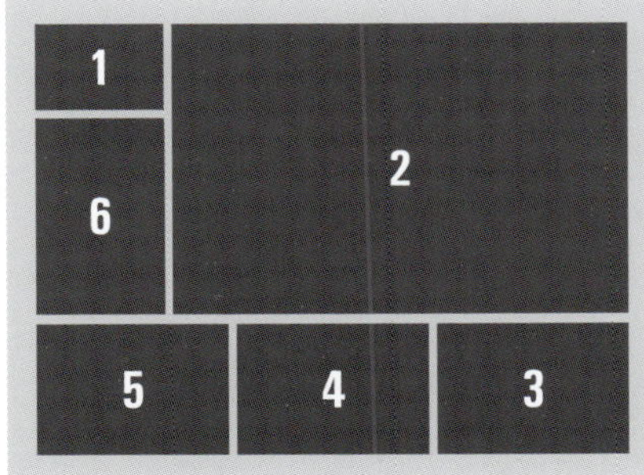

PAGE 53

1 Somewhere near Lake Tahoe, CA
2 Honest John's Barbershop, Burlington, KS
3 Len's Barbershop, Yakima, WA
4 Unique Barbershop, Cherry Hill, NJ
5 Allied Gardens Barbershop, San Diego, CA
6 OK Barbershop, Grants Pass, OR

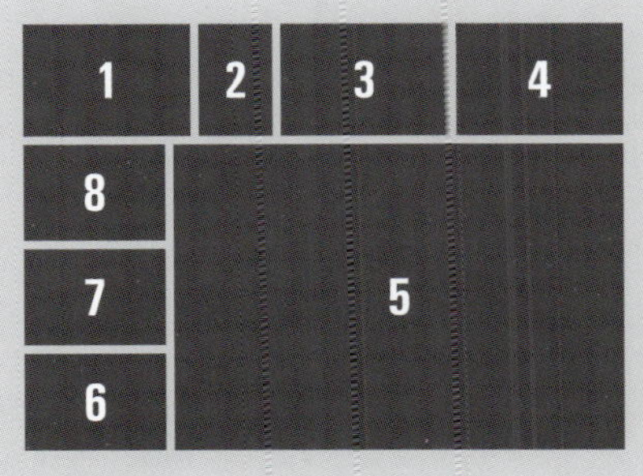

PAGE 54

1 Post Falls Barbershop, Post Falls, ID
2 Sweeney Todd's Barbershop, Los Angeles, CA
3 Commercial Barbershop, Elko, NV
4 Imperial Barbershop, Omaha, NE
5 Unknown
6 Joe's Barbershop, Chicago, IL
7 Deluxe Barbershop, Mandan, ND
8 Unknown, IL

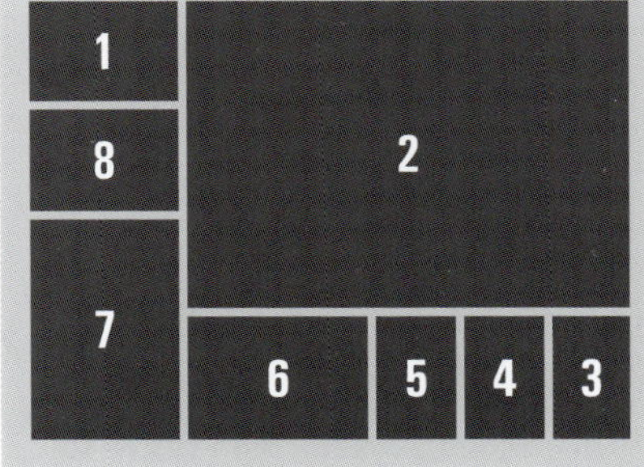

PAGE 57

1 Claudio's Barbershop, Harlem, NY
2 Duckett's Barbershop, Brooklyn, NY
3 OK Barbershop, Grants Pass, OR
4 Claudio's Barbershop, Harlem, NY
5 Unique Barbershop, Cherry Hills, NJ
6 Allied Gardens Barbershop, San Diego, CA
7 Bob the Barber, Fallbrook, CA
8 Murchinson Barbershop, Lancaster, SC

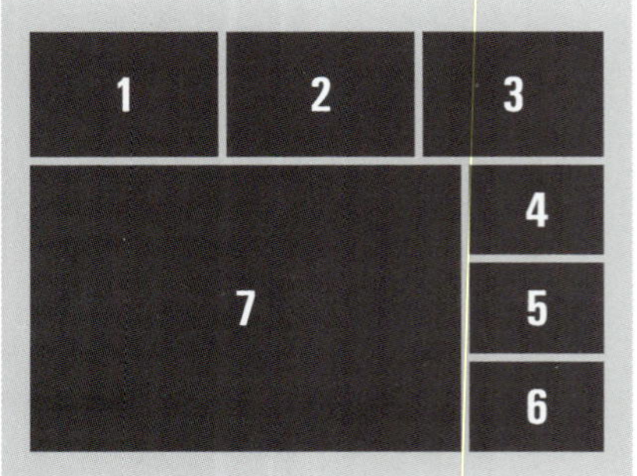

PAGE 63

1 City Barbershop, Ramona, CA
2 Pat's Barbershop, San Diego, CA
3 Johnny Lovato's Barbershop, San Diego, CA
4 Don and John's Barbershop, Springdale, AR
5 Back room (living quarters) at Post Falls Barbershop, Post Falls, ID
6 Penrod's Barbershop, Des Moines, IA
7 Woodard's Barbershop, Springdale, AR

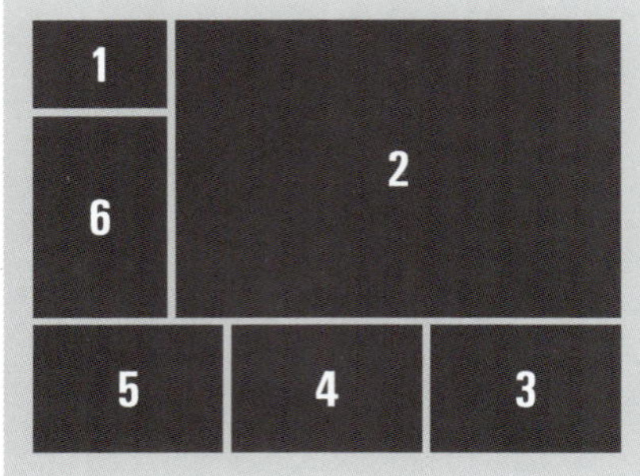

PAGE 64

1 Village Barbershop, Beaver, UT
2 Post Falls Barbershop, Post Falls, ID
3 Centennial Barbershop, Red Oak, IA
4 Jones' Barbershop, Bennington, VT
5 Capital Barbershop, Missoula, MT
6 Amherst Ave. Barbershop, Butte, MT

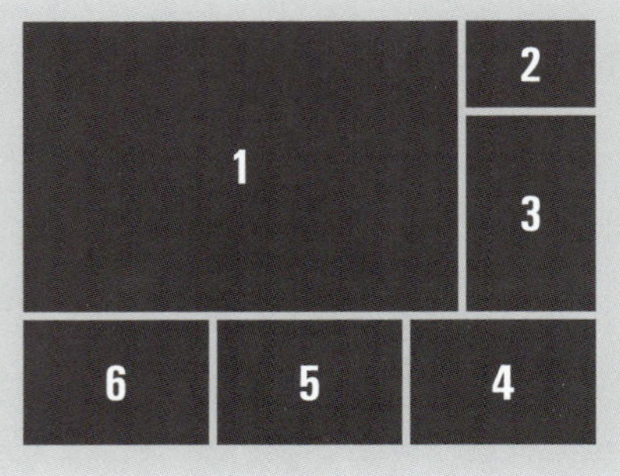

PAGE 73

1 Ed's Barber Salon, Oaklyn, NJ
2 Amherst Ave. Barbershop, Butte, MT
3 Jones' Barbershop, Bennington, VT
4 Jones' Barbershop, Bennington, VT
5 Amherst Ave. Barbershop, Butte, MT
6 Jones' Barbershop, Bennington, VT

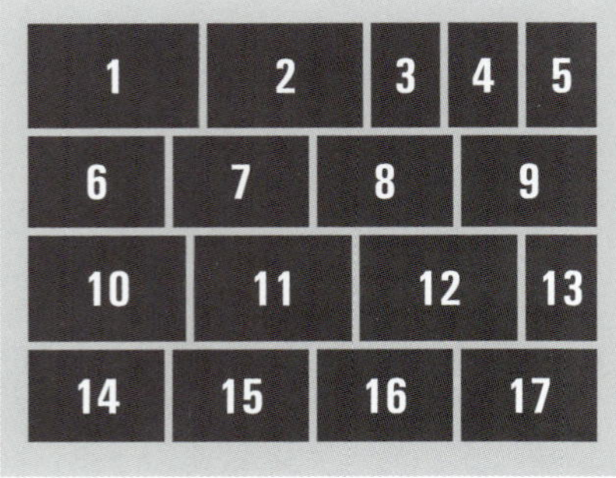

PAGE 76

1 Imperial Barbershop, Omaha, NE
2 The Haircut Co., Bozeman, MT
3 Unknown, UT
4 Scissor & Comb Barbershop, Oxnard, CA
5 Don's Barbershop, Milford, DE
6 Unknown, DE
7 Dick's Barbershop, Unknown
8 Craighead Barbershop, Nashville, TN
9 JB's Barbershop, Nashville, TN
10 JB's Barbershop, Nashville, TN
11 Damian Hair Styling, Brooklyn, NY
12 Akemon's Barbershop, Paris, KY
13 Joe's Barbershop, Brooklyn, NY
14 Harold's Barber & Snack Shop, New Orleans, LA
15 Don's Barbershop, Hudsonville, MI
16 Don's Barbershop, Hudsonville, MI
17 Harry's Barbershop, Biloxi, MS

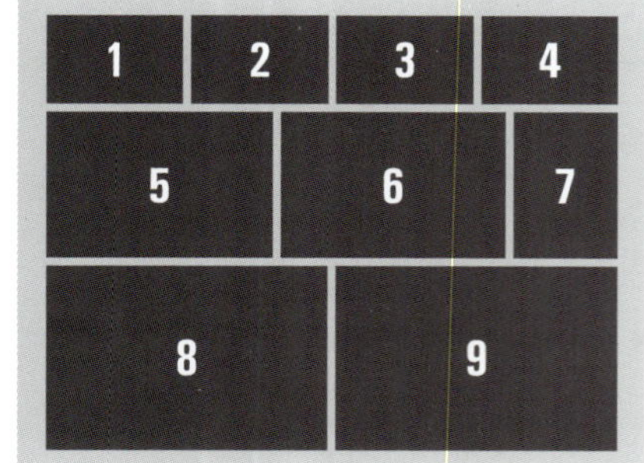

PAGE 81

1 Del's Barbershop, Escondido, CA
2 McLean's Barbershop, Hyannis, MA
3 Pat's Barbershop, San Diego, CA
4 Cortez Barbershop, Cortez, CO
5 Joe's Barbershop, Chicago, IL
6 Joe's Barbershop, Brooklyn, NY
7 Raymond's Barbershop, Lockhart, TX
8 Len's Barbershop, Yakima, WA
9 Craighead Barbershop, Nashville, TN

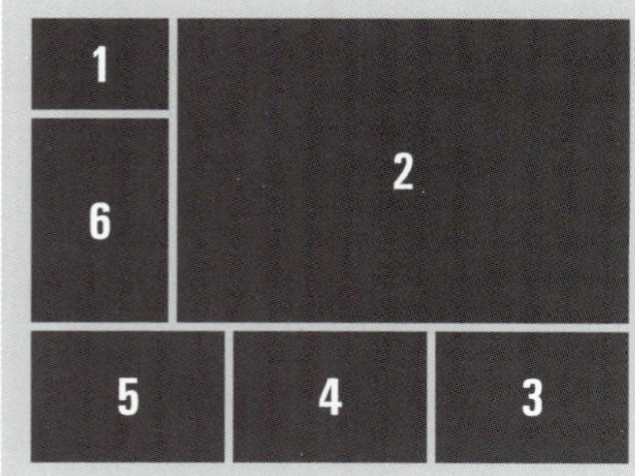

PAGE 82

1 Unknown, AL
2 Rembert's Barbershop, Mobile, AL
3 Tom's Barbershop, Winona, MN
4 Doug's Barbershop, Houston, TX
5 Doug's Barbershop, Houston, TX
6 White's Barbershop, Mobile, AL

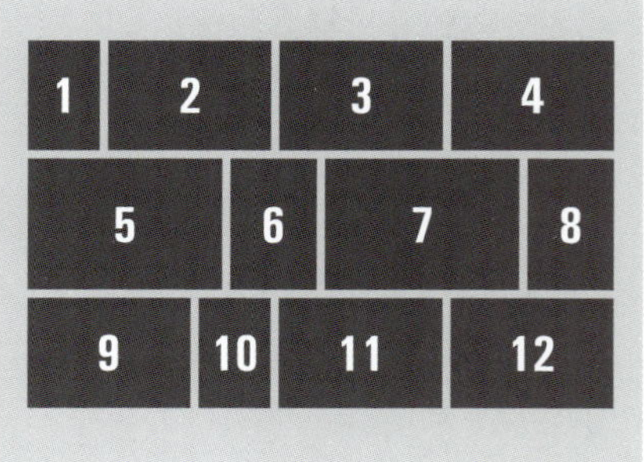

PAGE 85

1 Central Barbershop, Woodstock, VA
2 Central Barbershop, Woodstock, VA
3 Cowey Barbershop, Gonzalez, TX
4 Stoneville Barbershop, Stoneville, NC
5 Stoneville Barbershop, Stoneville, NC
6 Tommy's Style and Barbershop, Unknown
7 Woodall's Barbershop, Eden, NC
8 Mack Brooks Barbershop, Crestview, FL
9 Jackson Barbershop, Chattahoochee, FL
10 Blanche Barbershop, Lake City, FL
11 Smith's Barbershop, Excelsior Springs, MO
12 Central Barbershop, Woodstock, VA

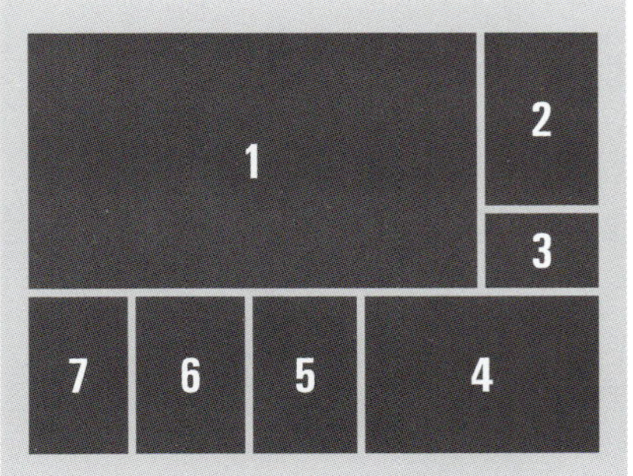

PAGE 86

1 Angel's Barbershop, Seligman, AZ
2 Unknown, AZ
3 Loop Barbershop, Rock Falls, IL
4 Unknown
5 Loop Barbershop, Rock Falls, IL
6 Del's Barbershop, Escondido, CA
7 Stancil's Barbershop, Albany, NY

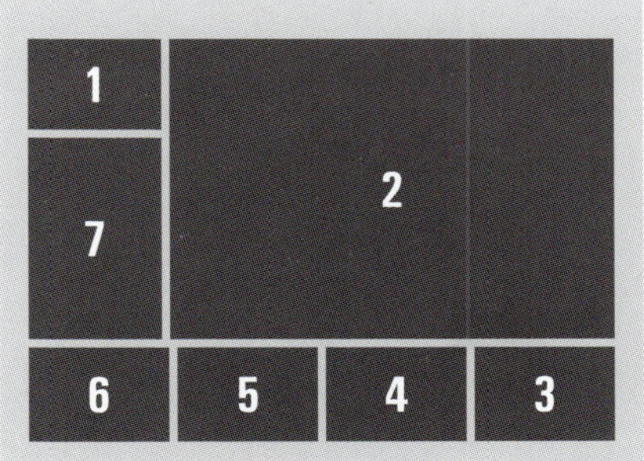

PAGE 89

1 Joe's Barbershop, Brooklyn, NY
2 Joe's Barbershop, Brooklyn, NY
3 Quintana's Barbershop, Marfa, TX
4 Quintana's Barbershop, Marfa, TX
5 Loop Barbershop, Rock Falls, IL
6 Penrod's Barbershop, Des Moines, IA
7 Duckett's Barbershop, Brooklyn, NY

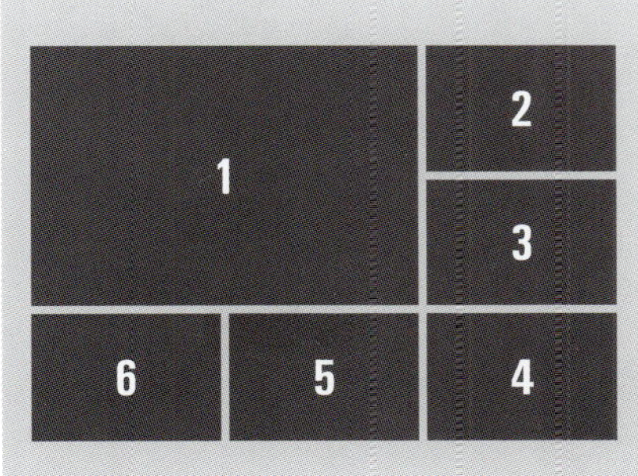

PAGE 90

1 Trophy Barbershop, Baytown, TX
2 Gene's Barbershop, Myrtle Creek, OR
3 Len's Barbershop, Yakima, WA
4 Continental Barbershop, Tulsa, OK
5 Los Gatos Barbershop, Los Gatos, CA
6 Unknown, Santa Maria, CA

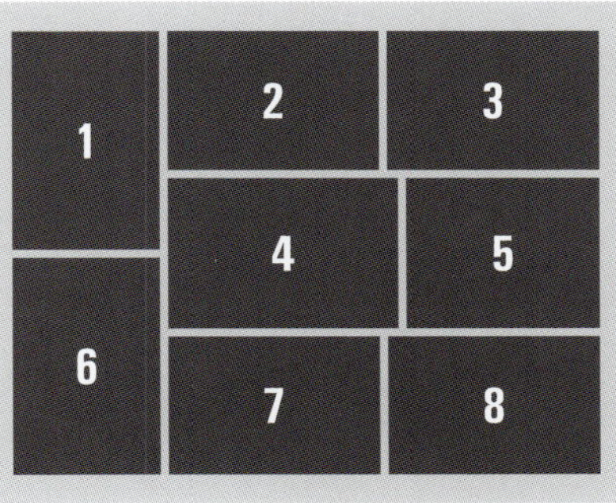

PAGE 109

1 Larchmont Barbershop, Los Angeles, CA
2 Duckett's Barbershop, Brooklyn, NY
3 Central Barbershop, Woodstock, VA
4 City Barbershop, Ramona, CA
5 The Park Slope Barbers, Brooklyn, NY
6 Tony's Barbershop, Greenwich, CT
7 Trophy Barbershop, Baytown, TX
8 Trophy Barbershop, Baytown, TX

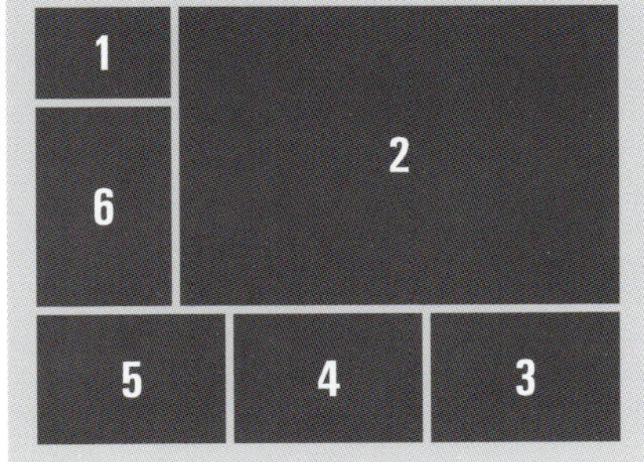

PAGE 121

1 Pappy's Barbershop, San Diego, CA
2 The Den Barbershop, Laguna, CA
3 Clifton Barbershop, Cincinnati, OH
4 Lyle's Barbershop, Portland, OR
5 Good Times Barbershop, Kearney, MO
6 Good Times Barbershop, Kearney, MO

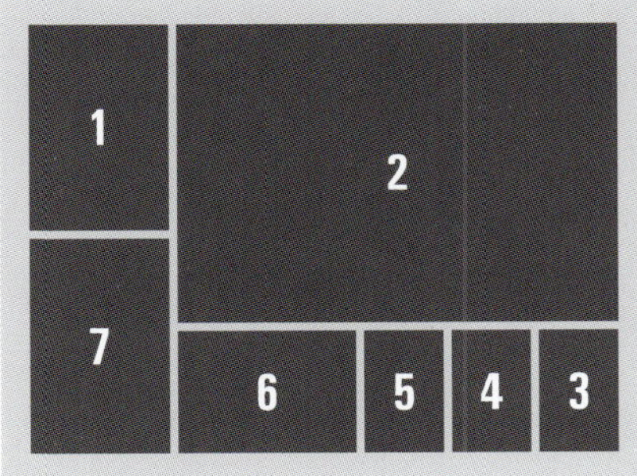

PAGE 122

1 The Den Barbershop, Laguna, CA
2 Kings Club Barbershop, Dana Point, CA
3 Kings Club Barbershop, Dana Point, CA
4 TipTop Barbershop, Whittier, CA
5 The Den Barbershop, Laguna, CA
6 Clifton Barbershop, Cincinnati, OH
7 Shane's Barbershop, San Mateo, CA

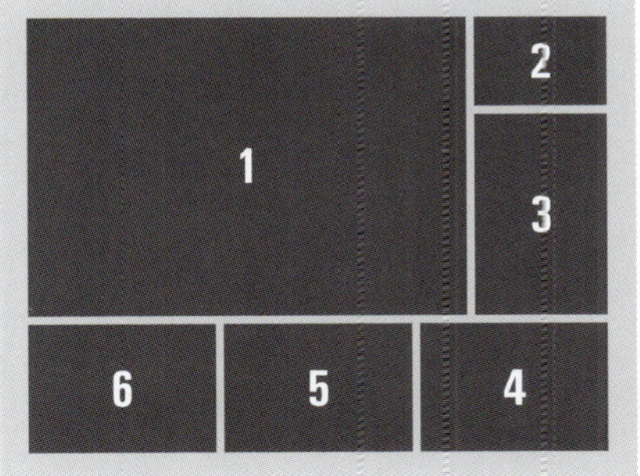

PAGE 127

1 Lyle's Barbershop, Portland, OR
2 Clifton Barbershop, Cincinnati, OH
3 Ferrari Barbershop, Cincinnati, OH
4 Lyle's Barbershop, Portland, OR
5 Golden Crown Barbershop, Laguna Niguel, CA
6 Mark-Jason Solofa Men's Grooming, Berkeley, CA

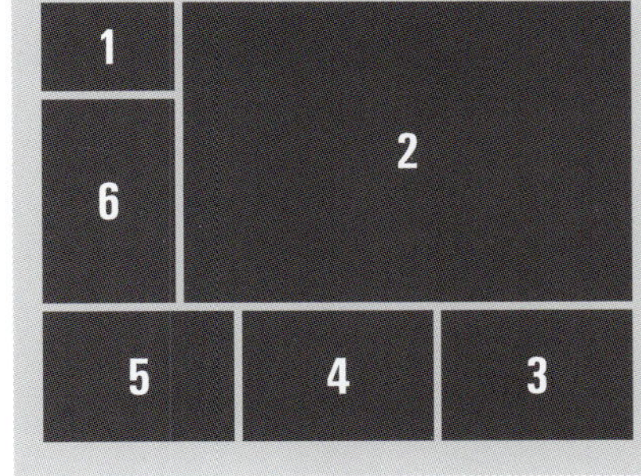

PAGE 133

1 Golden Crown Barbershop, Laguna Niguel, CA
2 Golden Crown Barbershop, Laguna Niguel, CA
3 Spanky's Barbershop, Newport, KY
4 Spanky's Barbershop, Newport, KY
5 Golden Crown Barbershop, Laguna Niguel, CA
6 Spanky's Barbershop, Newport, KY

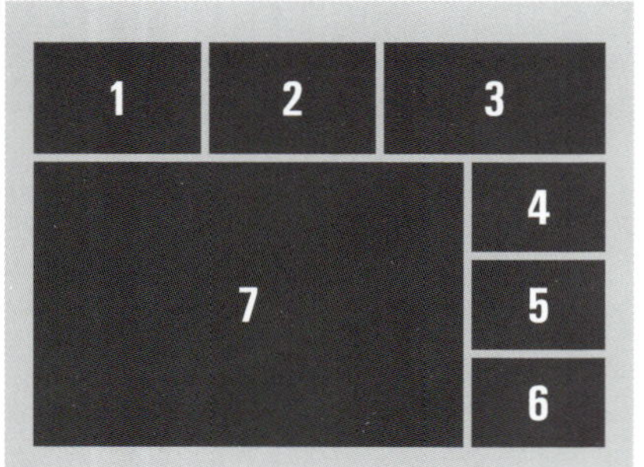

PAGE 134

1 Hawleywood's Barbershop, Long Beach, CA
2 Lefty's Barbershop, San Diego, CA
3 Painting on wall at 1927 Barbershop, Ventura, CA
4 The Blind Barber, Los Angeles, CA
5 Hawleywood's Barbershop, Long Beach, CA
6 Lefty's Barbershop, San Diego, CA
7 Spanky's Barbershop, Newport, KY

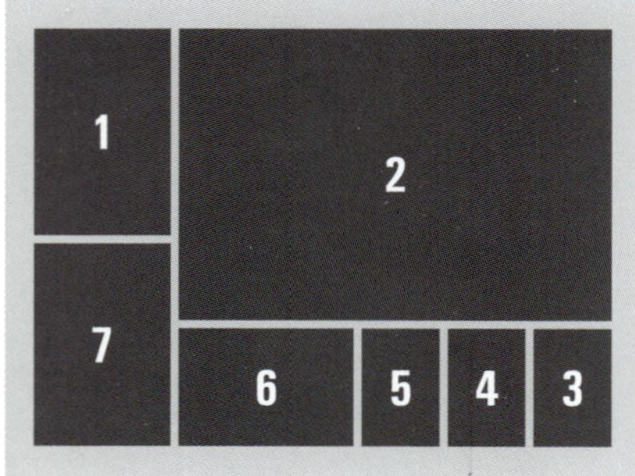

PAGE 139

1 Hawleywood's Barbershop, Long Beach, CA
2 Syndicate Barbershop, Long Beach, CA
3 Tip Top Barbershop, Whittier, CA
4 Unknown, Vista, CA
5 Deluxe Parlor and Shave Club, Long Beach, CA
6 Rooks Barbershop, Portland, OR
7 Deluxe Parlor and Shave Club, Long Beach, CA

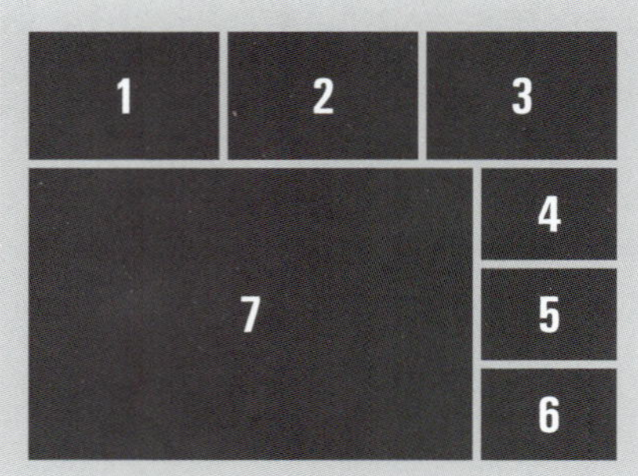

PAGE 140

1 Syndicate Barbershop, Long Beach, CA
2 Syndicate Barbershop, Long Beach, CA
3 Tip Top Barbershop, Whittier, CA
4 Syndicate Barbershop, Long Beach, CA
5 Vinnie's Barbershop, Los Angeles, CA
6 Syndicate Barbershop, Long Beach, CA
7 The Iron Society, Portland, OR

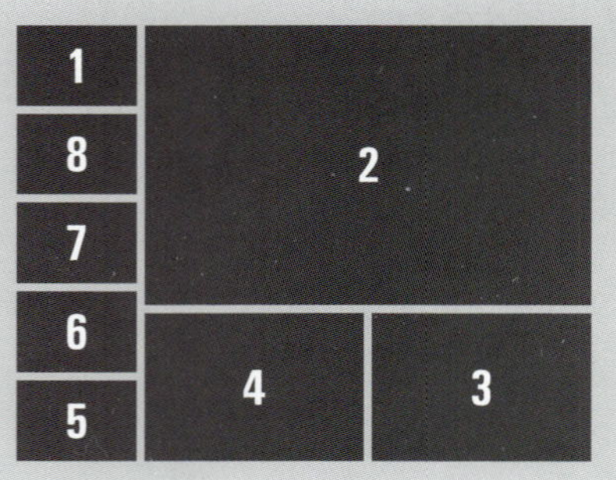

PAGE 145

1 Rooks Barbershop, Portland, OR
2 The Chop Shop, San Luis Obispo, CA
3 Shane's Barbershop, San Mateo, CA
4 Mark-Jason Solofa Men's Grooming, Danville, CA
5 Mark-Jason Solofa Men's Grooming, Danville, CA
6 Al's Barbershop, Alameda, CA
7 The Ritual, San Luis Obispo, CA
8 The Proper Barbershop, Los Angeles, CA

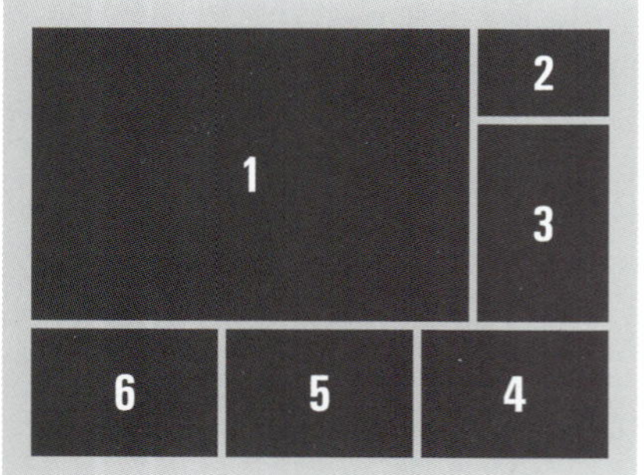

PAGE 146

1 Mark-Jason Solofa Men's Grooming, Berkeley, CA
2 Stepping Razor Barbershop, Brooklyn, NY
3 Stepping Razor Barbershop, Brooklyn, NY
4 Mark-Jason Solofa Men's Grooming, Berkeley, CA
5 Shane's Barbershop, San Mateo, CA
6 Unknown, Brooklyn, NY

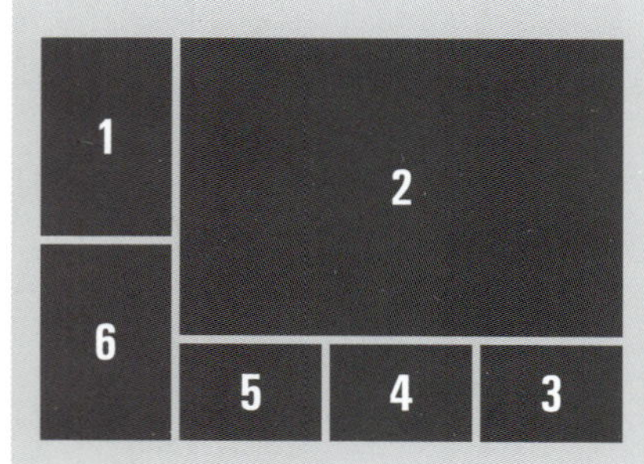

PAGE 155

1 Shane's Barbershop, San Mateo, CA
2 Rooks Barbershop, Portland, OR
3 The Iron Society, Portland, OR
4 Dover Honing Co., San Diego, CA
5 Oak Barbershop, Portland, OR
6 Poli's Barbershop, Sacramento, CA

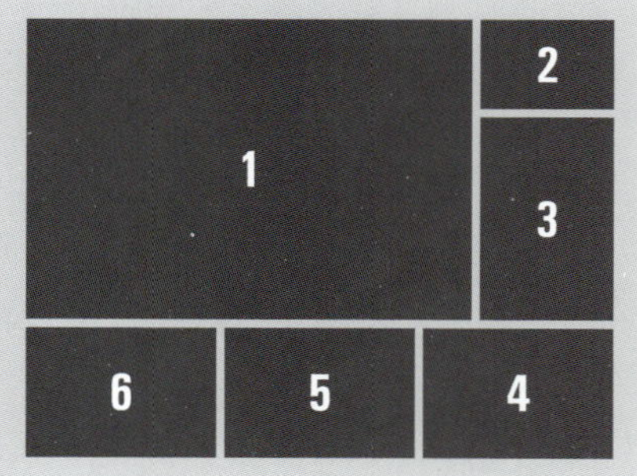

PAGE 156

1 Eagle & Pig Barbershop, Costa Mesa, CA
2 Eagle & Pig Barbershop, Costa Mesa, CA
3 Dover Honing Co., San Diego, CA
4 Rooks Barbershop, Portland, OR
5 Rooks Barbershop, Portland, OR
6 Rooks Barbershop, Portland, OR

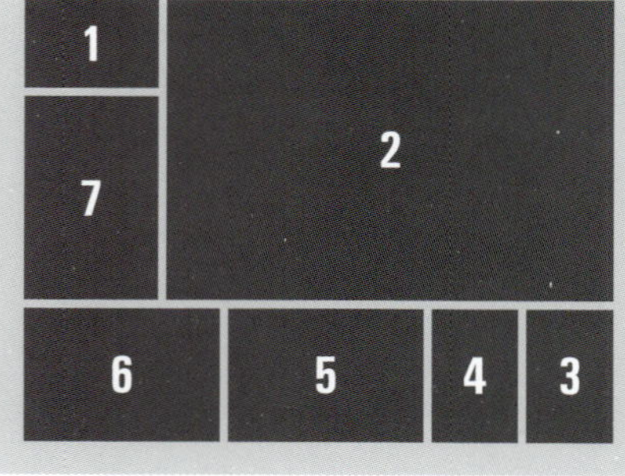

PAGE 161

1 Rooks Barbershop, Portland, OR
2 Squire Barbershop, Seattle, WA
3 The BlackBoard Barbershop, Bakersfield, CA
4 Squire Barbershop, Seattle, WA
5 Squire Barbershop, Seattle, WA
6 Squire Barbershop, Seattle, WA
7 Squire Barbershop, Seattle, WA

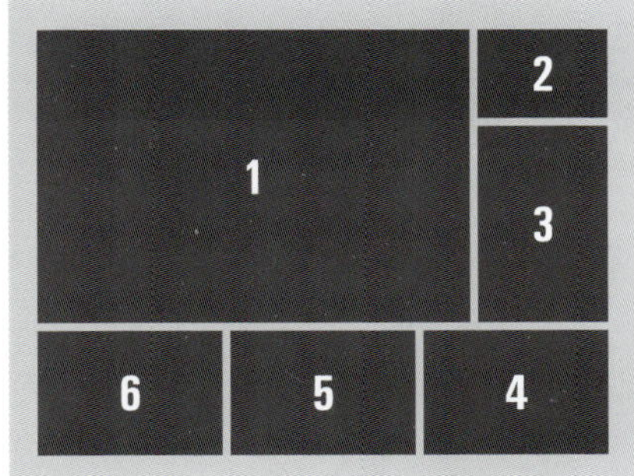

PAGE 162

1 The BlackBoard Barbershop, Bakersfield, CA
2 Stay Gold Barbershop, Fontana, CA
3 Good Times Barbershop, Imperial Beach, CA
4 Electric Barbershop, Riverside, CA
5 Lucky's Barbershop, Concord, NH
6 Lucky's Barbershop, Concord, NH

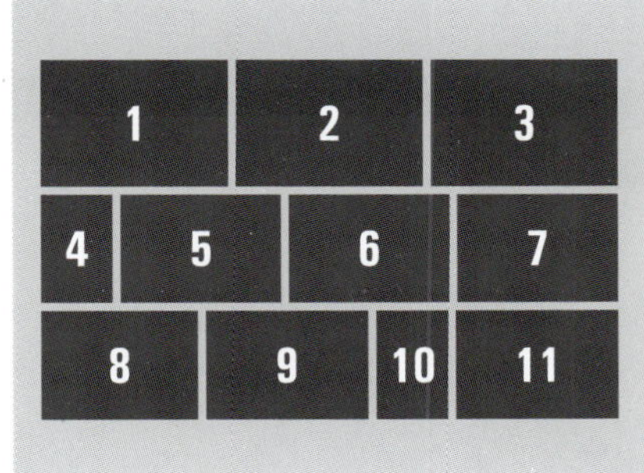

PAGE 167

1 Lucky's Barbershop, Concord, NH
2 Rooks Barbershop, Portland, OR
3 Pappy's Barbershop, San Diego, CA
4 The Den Barbershop, Laguna, CA
5 The Den Barbershop, Laguna, CA
6 Golden Crown Barbershop, Laguna Niguel, CA
7 Lyle's Barbershop, Portland, OR
8 Electric Barbershop, Riverside, CA
9 Lefty's Barbershop, San Diego, CA
10 Lefty's Barbershop, San Diego, CA
11 Electric Barbershop, San Diego, CA

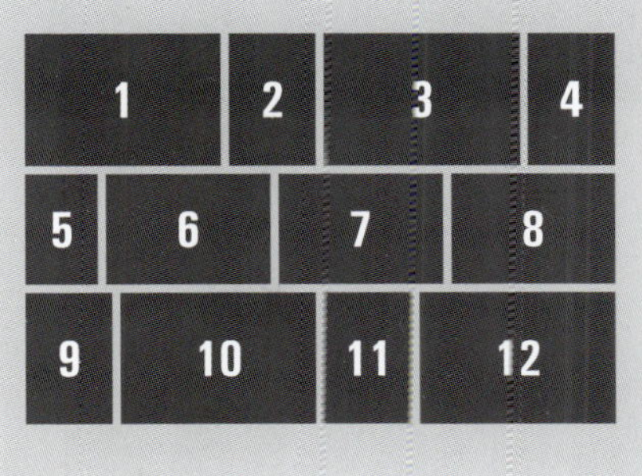

PAGE 168

1 1927 Barbershop, Ventura, CA
2 Lefty's Barbershop, San Diego, CA
3 1927 Barbershop, Ventura, CA
4 Lefty's Barbershop, San Diego, CA
5 Lefty's Barbershop, San Diego, CA
6 Circle City Barbers, Orange, CA
7 Dover Honing Co., San Diego, CA
8 Ludlow Blunt, Brooklyn, NY
9 Ludlow Blunt, Brooklyn, NY
10 Stepping Razor Barbershop, Brooklyn, NY
11 Stepping Razor Barbershop, Brooklyn, NY
12 Vinnie's Barbershop, Los Angeles, CA

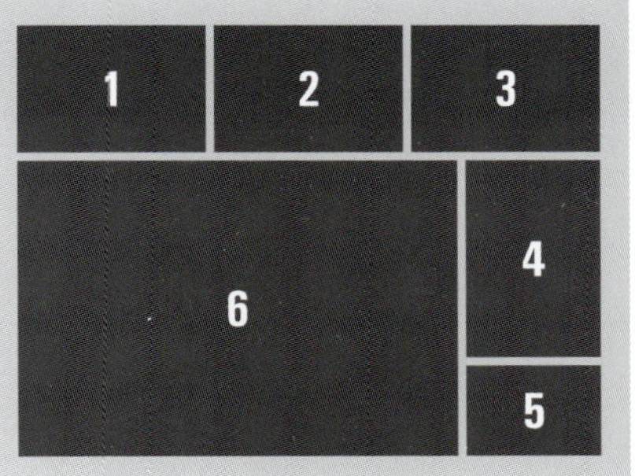

PAGE 171

1 Avenue Barbershop, Austin, TX
2 Rob's Chop Shop, Dallas, TX
3 Ford's Barbershop, Tulsa, OK
4 Rob's Chop Shop, Dallas, TX
5 Rob's Chop Shop, Dallas, TX
6 Yellow Rose Barbershop, Dallas, TX

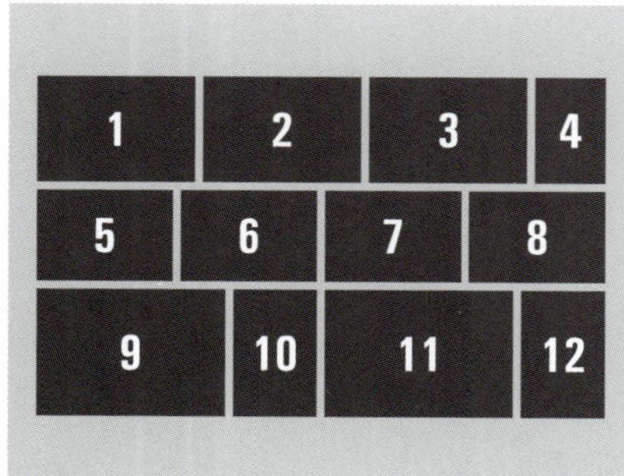

PAGE 172

1 Avenue Barbershop, Austin, TX
2 Vinnie's Barbershop, Los Angeles, CA
3 Vinnie's Barbershop, Los Angles, CA
4 Franklin's Barbershop, Philadelphia, PA
5 Avenue Barbershop, Austin, TX
6 Good Times Barbershop, Imperial Beach, CA
7 Pugsly's SideShow Barbershop, Kingston, NY
8 Franklin's Barbershop, Philadelphia, PA
9 Good Times Barbershop, Imperial Beach, CA
10 Pugsly's SideShow Barbershop, Kingston, NY
11 The Black Comb, Lancaster, PA
12 Unknown, Santa Maria, CA

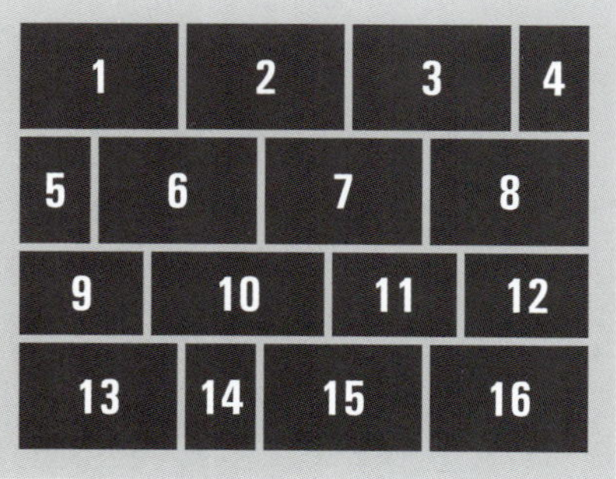

PAGE 174

1 Eagle & Pig Barbershop, Costa Mesa, CA
2 Eagle & Pig Barbershop, Costa Mesa, CA
3 Eagle & Pig Barbershop, Costa Mesa, CA
4 The Ritual, San Luis Obispo, CA
5 Lefty's Barbershop, Atascadero, CA
6 Eagle & Pig Barbershop, Costa Mesa, CA
7 Al's Barbershop, Alameda, CA
8 The Proper Barbershop, Los Angeles, CA
9 The Proper Barbershop, Los Angeles, CA
10 Al's Barbershop, Alameda, CA
11 Lyle's Barbershop, Portland, OR
12 Mark-Jason Solofa Men's Grooming, Berkeley, CA
13 Poli's Barbershop, Sacramento, CA
14 Syndicate Barbershop, Long Beach, CA
15 Syndicate Barbershop, Long Beach, CA
16 Eagle & Pig Barbershop, Costa Mesa, CA

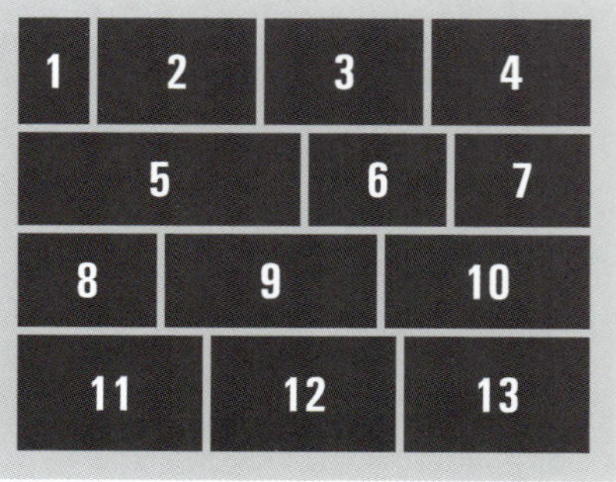

PAGE 175

1 Shane's Barbershop, San Mateo, CA
2 Kings Club Barbershop, Dana Point, CA
3 Stay Gold Barbershop, Fontana, CA
4 The BlackBoard Barbershop, Bakersfield, CA
5 The BlackBoard Barbershop, Bakersfield, CA
6 Lucky's Barbershop, Concord, NH
7 Good Times Barbershop, Imperial Beach, CA
8 Lefty's Barbershop, San Diego, CA
9 Circle City Barbers, Orange, CA
10 Ford's Barbershop, Tulsa, OK
11 Ford's Barbershop, Tulsa, OK
12 The Black Comb, Lancaster, PA
13 Pugsly's SideShow Barbershop, Kingston, NY